Marcel & Madeleine
Sabourin
342 Wisteria Crescent
Ottawa, ON K1V 0N5

RUSH TO DANGER

ALSO BY TED BARRIS

RUSH TO DANGER

MEDICS IN THE LINE OF FIRE

TED BARRIS

PATRICK CREAN EDITIONS
HarperCollins*Publishers*Ltd

Published by Patrick Crean Editions,
an imprint of HarperCollins Publishers Ltd

First edition

HarperCollins books may be purchased for educational, business,
or sales promotional use through our Special Markets Department.

HarperCollins Publishers Ltd
Bay Adelaide Centre, East Tower
22 Adelaide Street West, 41st Floor
Toronto, Ontario, Canada
M5H 4E3

www.harpercollins.ca

Library and Archives Canada Cataloguing in Publication
information is available upon request.

Maps and diagrams created by Lightfoot Art & Design Inc.
Photo inserts by Gordon Robertson.
Photo credits appear on pages 385–87.

ISBN 978-1-4434-4792-8

Printed and bound in the United States
LSC/H 9 8 7 6 5 4 3 2 1

*For my sister Kate Barris, who treasures the written word
as much as Dad and I, and who helped me reveal
our father's war.*

CONTENTS

FOREWORD

I'VE OFTEN SAID I became an emergency physician because the shift work gave me lots of time to develop my writing and broadcasting careers. In fact, I wanted to overcome my fear that I might rush into danger and not know what to do.

Experience and courses such as Advanced Cardiac Life Support and Advanced Trauma Life Support have made it possible for me to run toward the resuscitation room instead of away from it. Beyond the emergency room, I used that capacity to put aside doubts about my own abilities in shopping malls and at cruising altitude aboard passenger jets.

A few months back, I was returning home with my family from a vacation in Costa Rica. A Westjet flight attendant came on the intercom and asked if there was a physician on board. I raised my hand immediately and was escorted to the forward cabin, where I found a woman who was conscious but somewhat disoriented. I introduced myself and took a brief history while obtaining a blood pressure and pulse.

To the pilot's immense relief, I quickly ascertained that my patient did not require urgent medical attention. That meant he did not have to divert the aircraft to the nearest airport.

In the meantime, I put myself in the place of my patient and her startled husband.

"I know you're frightened about this," I told them. "But you're going to be okay."

I was exhibiting what psychologists call "cognitive empathy," the capacity to imagine things from the perspective of someone else, and to have that insight inform one's actions. It's a primary aspect of empathy. Another is affective or emotional empathy, which is the capacity to feel what another person feels. And a third aspect is the get-up-and-go that makes first responders rush to the aid of others.

In his book *Rush to Danger: Medics in the Line of Fire*, Ted Barris tells the gripping stories of men and women—recent and past—who have risked their own lives to tend to the bodies and psyches of the war wounded.

The book reminds us again and again of the quiet heroism of military physicians, nurses, and medics who have provided medical care to hundreds, sometimes thousands, of wounded and ill soldiers under enemy fire. Some of them enlisted. Many were drafted into the wars of their times. Others just rose to meet the challenge of a lifetime that they encountered by happenstance.

Augusta Chiwy was a twenty-three-year-old registered nurse originally from the Belgian Congo who just happened to be heading home to visit her parents in Bastogne, Belgium, in the days leading up to Christmas 1944. She arrived just as

Adolf Hitler had sent more than 400,000 German troops and 1,400 tanks into the Ardennes as part of Operation Watch on the Rhine, a desperate attempt to thwart the Allied advance toward Germany. Working beside US Army medic Jack Prior, Chiwy volunteered to lend her nursing skills to Allied troops. During a week-long siege of Bastogne, they treated hundreds of casualties while dodging enemy fire that destroyed the makeshift aid station where they worked.

Others performed medical miracles under conditions that can only be described as barbaric. Dr. Jacob Markowitz, a Canadian physician who enlisted in Britain's Royal Army Medical Corps, served as surgical officer during the fall of Singapore. He was eventually captured by the Japanese. Despite being given no medical equipment or supplies, Markowitz used his medical and surgical know-how to tend to thousands of fellow prisoners of war, often working up to eighteen hours a day for many days at a time. He even risked his own life by hiding meticulous accounts of their working and living conditions in amongst the many bodies of prisoners who died in captivity.

The medicine I practise every day owes a debt of gratitude to the medicine learned, practised, and improvised on the battlefield. Barris shows us that the modern ambulance was invented during the American Civil War, and the first blood bank was used by the British during the Great War. Sadly, modern asymmetrical and urban warfare have only increased the need for medical ingenuity and empathic human beings to step up.

And as Barris points out, the heroism and sacrifice shown by military medics comes at steep personal cost. Like combat soldiers, many of these battlefield healers developed post-traumatic stress disorder, or PTSD. That is yet another reason why we should not take their empathic work for granted.

—Brian Goldman, MD
Toronto, Ontario
May 2019

ACKNOWLEDGEMENTS

LIKE A COLUMN OF SOLDIERS, we walked in single file behind our guide. Then, as the narrow street of this small German town opened into a market square, the young man leading our historical tour painted a picture of this place in the winter of 1945. He pointed to the homes tucked neatly around the intersection. Because of the battle waged between German and US forces here during the Second World War, he told us, civilians had been evacuated.

"Well, that's not entirely true," said someone standing behind me—a man on the tour I hadn't met yet. He added, "Some of the civilians refused to leave."

I introduced myself to this fellow traveller, Al Theobald, from San Diego, California. We intentionally fell behind the rest of the walking tour to get acquainted. He told me that he'd been born in this part of Germany right after the war. His mother, Maria Fox, did eventually vacate her home in the nearby village of Borg on Christmas Day, 1944. Remarkably, when she returned to the family farmhouse after Borg was liberated, Al said, she found the home intact but full of medical supplies . . .

"Medical supplies?" I interrupted.

"Yes," he continued. "Bandages, medicines, utensils. Our home had been used by the Americans as a first-aid station."

I couldn't get the words out fast enough. "And where is this place, Borg?"

"About a mile from Campholz Woods."

I was nearly speechless. Campholz Woods, Germany, was one of the combat zones of the Battle of the Bulge, a horrific engagement in which upwards of 75,000 US soldiers were killed, captured, or wounded. It was from that woods that my father, a US Army medic, had rescued four men in his platoon in February of 1945. The action earned him a US meritorious citation. But until this trip to Germany in October 2017, I had never visited it. Until that moment, I had never come so close to knowing what he might have faced there. I read Al Theobald the citation the US Army had issued about my father's "total disregard for his personal safety."

"I've got goosebumps," Theobald said.

A few hours later, Maria Fox's son and I—my heart in my throat—walked through the bunkers, trenches, tank traps, and dense woods of Campholz. In some ways, Theobald told me, things there seemed just the same as in those final months of the war. The woods were just as dense, their look just as innocuous, the land just as pastoral. But when my father's medical battalion had rushed wounded from this battleground, it was during the coldest winter of the war; there was a foot of snow on the ground, and hidden there in Campholz lay some of the most lethal anti-personnel weapons of the war—*Schü* mines, tripwired booby traps, anti-tank ditches, and dragon's teeth (row-on-row concrete obstructions). Eventually, Al Theobald took me to the village of Borg and the location of his mother's former home, the farmhouse that my father's medical battalion had occupied that winter. It had been, in all probability, my father's first-aid station during his service as a medic on the front lines in the Battle of the Bulge.

"Now it's my turn for goosebumps," I told Al Theobald. And for the rest of our trip together I couldn't thank him enough for the chance to be where my father had served in the Second World War.

OTHERS HAVE GIVEN me unique access to my father's wartime trek. First and foremost, I am indebted to Tony Mellaci, at this writing, in his ninety-sixth year. In 2015, he and his wife, Sharon, and their family opened their home in Eatontown, New Jersey, as if I were their son; Tony, who'd served in the 319th Medical Battalion with my father, allowed me access to wartime photographs, mementos, battalion literature, and, most important to me, stories from times he shared with my father in training, at the front, and during the battalion's occupation service in Czechoslovakia. On that 2017 tour I mentioned, 94th Infantry Division vets Herb Ridyard Sr. and Jerome Fatora also helped me understand the conditions they and my father endured that winter in the Saar-Moselle Triangle. Like me, others on that trip were paying tribute to their fathers—Kurt Kinateder (remembering his father, Elmer H. Kinateder), Sharon and Brian Schell and Diane and Matt Creme (for Sharon's and Diane's father, Charles Remington), Matt and Rhonda Mulroy (his father, Paul Mulroy), Ellen and Mike McKinney (for her father, Bob Hibbs), Fran Bates Jr. (Fran Bates Sr.), and Bob Remsburg III (Robert Remsburg II).

The daily records of the 94th Infantry Division and my father's medical unit might never have been available to me for research if not for the efforts of David Yoakley Mitchell; his father Martin Hardin Mitchell's bequest to the Hargrett Rare Book and Manuscript Library at the University of Georgia, in Athens, gave the 94th's vast archives a permanent home, and its staff (under library co-director Chuck Barber) allowed me to plot my father's daily orders as a medic, his patient loads, and the reflections of fellow medical corpsmen throughout their service between 1943 and 1945. Others in the 94th Infantry Division Historical Society contributed via the archives, but veteran (and until recently the society's secretary) Harry Helms deserves my special thanks.

As well as the Mellaci family, other relatives of medical personnel allowed me vital first-hand access to letters, diaries, journals, and photo albums: Lisa Boyce (John Campbell Kennedy), Diana Filer (Grace MacPherson), Donna Henderson (Louise Spry and Frederick Lailey), Alison Pearce (Hubert Morris), Shirley McDonnell (Mildred S. Bates), Bo and Helen Fleischman (T. Arthur Henderson), Scott Elliott (Orvil A. Elliott), Kathy Varley (War Diary of No. 17 Canadian Light Field Ambulance), Carol Hodgkins-Smith (Arnold Hodgkins), Joe Reilly Jr. (Joe Reilly), Rob Alexander (Laurence Alexander); Scott Clare (Wes Clare), Clarice Wilsey (David Wilsey), Ray and Jim Duffield (Henry Duffield), and Ron Brittain (Jim Brittain).

As I have with past history manuscripts, while composing this one I turned to fellow writers who generously gave me access to their research and analysis (and permissions) on a variety of personal stories and valuable medical context, including: Mary F. Gaudet, author of *From a Stretcher Handle* (about her father Frank Walker); William A. Foley Jr., author of *Visions from a Foxhole* (memoir from the

Saar-Moselle Triangle battlefields); David O'Keefe, author of *One Day in August* (about Dieppe); Martin King, author of *Searching for Augusta* (regarding nurse Augusta Chiwy); Ellin Bessner, author of *Double Threat* (additional information on Jacob Markowitz); Malcolm Kelly, military historian (for his eleventh-hour editing notes); Lindy Oughtred, journalism professor (for her editorial eye); Robert H. Farquharson, author of *For Your Tomorrow* (about the Death Railway); George S. MacDonell, author of *One Soldier's Story* (about life in Japanese POW camps); Carl Christie, author of *Ocean Bridge* (for contacts at the Canadian War Museum); Hugh Halliday, co-author of *The Royal Canadian Air Force at War, 1939–1945* (for his data on Canadian military medical personnel who were decorated); Tim Cook, author of *No Place to Run* (about the Great War gas attacks); Adrienne Clarkson, author of *Norman Bethune* (about her biography); Harold Skaarup, author of *New Brunswick Hussar* (on mascot Princess Louise); Tom Taylor, author of *Brock's Agent* (for additional perspective on Grace MacPherson); Len Scher, CBC writer/producer of the film documentary *Emma's Battles: North America's First Female Soldier* (about Sarah Emma Edmonds); Paul Van Nest, Civil War historian (on Gettysburg); Cheryl A. Wells, author of *Civil War Time* (for data and images of Jonathan Letterman's first field ambulance); and Jody Mitic, author of *Unflinching: The Making of a Canadian Sniper* (regarding his experiences in the war in Afghanistan).

I am especially indebted to freelance journalist Marketa Schusterova, who took up the challenge of searching out the Krizek family, who billeted my father during the US Army occupation of Czechoslovakia after the war; not only did she find two surviving sons in Vodňany, Czech Republic, she interviewed them, translated those conversations, and retrieved other documentation about my father's role in the restoration of services to that Czech community in 1945. As well, I am blessed to have Marian Hebb as my contract lawyer in these literary works; always eager and exceedingly able, Marian rarely gets the credit for her long years of dedication to Canadian writers. I am also grateful to Kate Paddison, my interview transcriber, for her faithful and reliable attention to detail.

The eclectic nature of this manuscript sent me along traditional research paths—to museums, libraries, and archives I've long trusted—as well as to sources I've not explored before. In both cases I found professionals eager to help and deserving of praise for their assistance. At the Canadian War Museum in Ottawa, Jeff Noakes and Maggie Arbour assisted my search for photographs in both the CWM and at Library and Archives Canada. At Guelph Museums, in Ontario, curator Bev Dietrich provided me with vital biographical background on John McCrae and Alexis Helmer. At the National Personnel Records Center in St. Louis, Delphine Cage assisted me in tracking down my father's war records. My contacts at the (US) Army Medical Department (AMEDD) in San Antonio, Texas—Mary E. Hope and Carlos Alvarado—provided vital data on the composition of the 94th Infantry Division and its medical detachment, the 319th Medical Battalion, in which my father served.

When assembling the story of No. 3 Canadian General Hospital, I spent several days in the Osler Library of the History of Medicine, at McGill University, and in the capable hands of librarian Christopher Lyons (assisted by Gordon Burr and Bryna Cameron-Steinke). In search of Cluny Macpherson's invention of the first Allied gas mask during in the Great War, I gained access to his diaries and notebooks thanks to Melissa Glover, archival assistant with the Faculty of Medicine Founders' Archive at Memorial University in St. John's, Newfoundland. At the City of Toronto Archives, archivist Paul Gardiner expedited my acquisition of images of Frederick Lailey and Louise Spry. And over the years I've worked on this book, Jane Gibson and Barry Penhale, at Natural Heritage Books, regularly provided background, profiles, and leads for my research on the subject.

My pursuit of photographs beyond traditional sources led me to able volunteers working with historical organizations or on their own, among them: Angela Wallace at the Port Dover Harbour Museum of Norfolk County (Ontario), Glenn Kerr and Glenn Warner of the Central Ontario Branch of the Western Front Association, Tom McLaughlan with the 8th Canadian Hussars (Princess Louise's) Museum at Sussex (New Brunswick). For his care and expertise in scanning many of these aging and fragile images, I am indebted to photographer Stuart Blower. And to then create appropriate settings and arrangements for my photos, I turned to Gordon Robertson—he with a sharp eye and clever knack to make these photo sections come to life. Additionally, I asked artist and designer John Lightfoot to develop the maps I needed; his creations help readers visualize the part of Germany where my father's war proved the toughest—Campholz Woods in the Saar-Moselle Triangle.

As he has with six of my previous books on Canadian military history, publisher/editor Patrick Crean has urged me on with *Rush to Danger* from inception to completion. Partly because we are both the sons of fathers who served in the Second World War, partly because he too still wonders about their wartime service experience, but mostly because he believes these stories demand attention, Patrick is my editorial brother in this enterprise. Also, at HarperCollins Canada, I wish to thank production and editorial staff Natalie Meditsky, Noelle Zitzer, and Alan Jones, as well as publicist Melissa Nowakowski. I especially want to acknowledge the stellar work of copy editor Linda Pruessen, who has now guided me deftly through several military histories.

In 2008, as I assembled stories for a book about my journey with military veterans, I met and interviewed a medic with the Canadian Forces; at that time, Sgt. William Wilson had completed tours of duty in Somalia, Rwanda, Bosnia, and Afghanistan—including April 17, 2002, the night of the friendly fire incident at Tarnak Farm. Based on his coolness and competence in the resulting rescue operation, Bill received the Chief of the Defence Staff Commendation. I sensed Bill's experience and wisdom in military medicine gave him the expert eye my manuscript needed. He graciously agreed, and I am ever grateful for his assessment. Similarly, I want to thank Dr. Brian Goldman for his reading of the manuscript and the resulting foreword he has provided.

Because my father's story—that of a New Yorker drafted into the US army to serve as a medic in the Second World War—provides the thread for this book, I could not have brought his story to life without family members, including my father's older brother Angelo Barris, his daughter Christine Barris-Perigoe, Marion Andros, and my sister Kate Barris, who all provided insights into the times, our family, and especially my father, Alex. I thank my wife, Jayne MacAulay, who read and reread these pages to keep me on track and perhaps to learn more about her father-in-law.

ON THAT SAME TOUR of the Battle of the Bulge that I joined in 2017—when Al Theobald led me to my father's former aid station in Borg, Germany—I met a military historian named Giuseppe Castronovo. Of Italian parentage, he has lived in and around Saarburg, within the former Saar-Moselle Triangle battlefield, for most of his life. As a boy in the 1970s, he played in what was left of the trenches and foxholes. As an adult, he began collecting literature about the Battle of the Bulge and particularly about the 94th Infantry Division's engagement of German armies there that winter of 1945. The day we met in October 2017, Giuseppe told me that he'd taken time away from his work to join us and offer any assistance he could to our tour group; he gave me topographical maps that helped me understand the terrain that the American and German armies fought over. Then, I asked him why he cared so much about this story.

"The battle your father survived," Castronovo told me, "happened on ground that has been my home for forty-seven years. It's ground where my wife and I have raised our children. Your father and his comrades made this place worthwhile to live in again."

During rare moments when I stumbled writing this book, I was spurred on by such gratitude.

SAAR-MOSELLE TRIANGLE
(BATTLE LINE AS OF JANUARY 31, 1945)

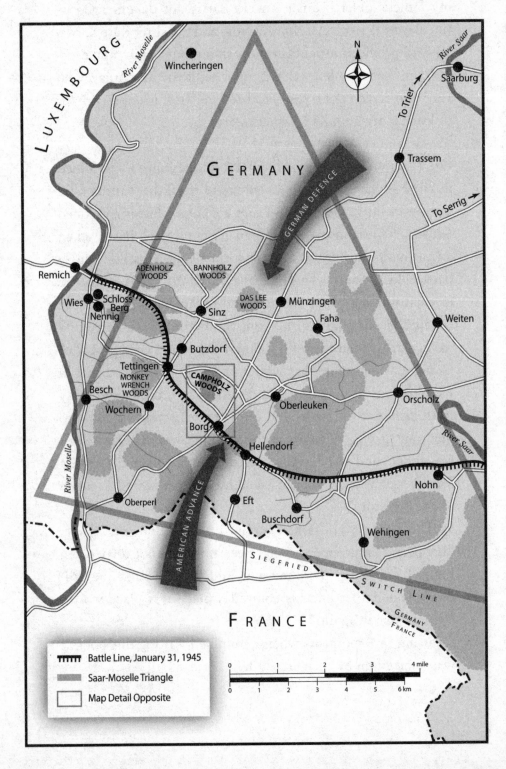

US Army Operations in Campholz Woods (February 1945)

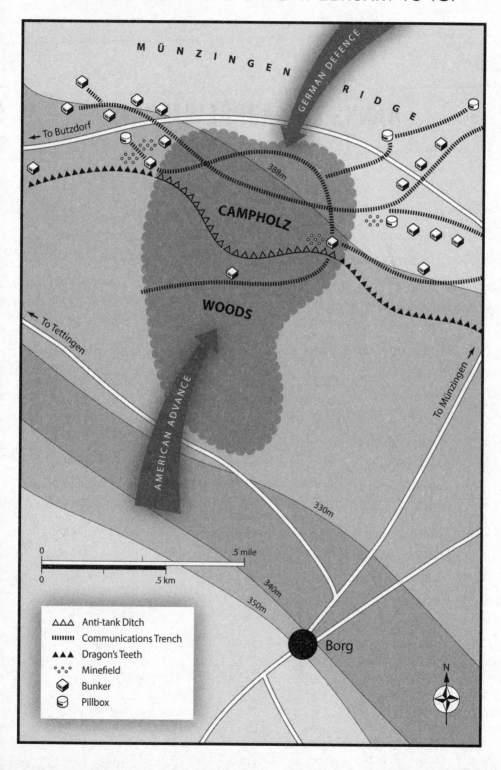

Legend:

- △△△ Anti-tank Ditch
- ||||||| Communications Trench
- ▲▲▲ Dragon's Teeth
- °o°o° Minefield
- ⬡ Bunker
- ⬭ Pillbox

RANKS AND ABBREVIATIONS

Canadian Forces

General	*Gen.*
Lieutenant-General	*Lt.-Gen.*
Major-General	*Maj.-Gen.*
Brigadier-General	*Brig.-Gen.*
Colonel	*Col.*
Lieutenant-Colonel	*Lt.-Col.*
Major	*Maj.*
Captain	*Capt.*
Lieutenant	*Lt.*
Warrant Officer	WO
Medical Officer	MO
Sergeant Major	*Sgt. Maj.*
Staff Sergeant	*S/Sgt.*
Sergeant	*Sgt.*
Lance Sergeant	*L/Sgt.*
Master Corporal	*M/Cpl.*
Corporal	*Cpl.*
Private	*Pte.*
Trooper	*Tpr.*

United States Army

Brigadier General	*Brig. Gen.*
Major General	*Maj. Gen.*
General	*Gen.*
Lieutenant General	*Lt. Gen.*
Colonel	*Col.*
Lieutenant Colonel	*Lt. Col.*
Major	*Maj.*
Captain	*Capt.*
Lieutenant	*Lt.*
Warrant Officer	WO
Medical Officer	MO
Sergeant Major	*Sgt. Maj.*
Technical Sergeant	*T/Sgt.*
Staff Sergeant	*S/Sgt.*
Sergeant	*Sgt.*
Corporal	*Cpl.*
Private First Class	*Pfc.*
Private	*Pte.*

CHAPTER ONE

"WHAT DID YOU DO IN THE WAR?"

I NEVER FOUGHT IN A WAR. I was born and raised in a time and a place that didn't require young men to sign up, take basic training in the country's armed forces, and leave its villages and cities to serve in a theatre of war overseas, the way my father did. And I certainly didn't have to witness the death and dying that he did. About as close as I ever came to serious injury in my youth, believe it or not, happened when I was participating in America's favourite pastime. It was during a competitive but relatively friendly game of baseball that I sustained my worst physical injury. On the final day of classes that year, my grade nine phys-ed instructor had no curriculum left to teach, so he gave us a bat and a ball and told us to go to the school diamond and play some work-up baseball. Not long into the game, I was playing at shortstop when the catcher and I chased the same infield fly and ran into each other head-on in the middle of the diamond. The collision broke my nose, knocked out my front teeth, and put me out cold for several minutes.

After the dentists and doctors sewed me back together, I spent several weeks recuperating at home in bed. My father happened to be working in his home office at the time, so he spent many hours trying to distract me from my pain and self-pity by telling me stories. It wasn't long before I popped the big question.

"What did you do in the war, Dad?" I asked former T/Sgt. Alex Barris.[1]

Never afraid to tell a good yarn, but in this case holding the power to choose what he would say and not say, my father used a ploy—a safety mechanism that many veterans of the Great War, the Second World War, the Korean War, and recent wars in Iraq and Afghanistan have used—to answer my question. Never tell the rough stories, the remembrances of destruction close by. Don't revisit the deaths of comrades on the battlefield. Under no circumstances let loved ones see you break down and cry. Instead, protect them from the truth. Always recall the antics, the quirky tales, and maybe the odd near miss. But never let them know the hell of your war.

That's what my father did. For several afternoons in a row, as I lay in bed recovering from my schoolyard wounds, Dad regaled me with just the war stories he knew would leave me laughing. I had a rough idea that he was a US Army medical corpsman during the Second World War. I knew from some of the stories he'd told at parties and occasionally around the family dinner table that he'd endured military training camps from Kansas to Mississippi. He rose to the rank of sergeant. During one stint in the winter of 1943, he recalled accidentally waking the battalion commander an hour too early for roll call outside in a freezing Kansas pre-dawn. My father told me about army food—K-rations, or "shit on a shingle," and coffee that tasted like mud. Everybody in the army hated the food, and the cooks hated everybody back. Nobody ever got any food he liked. So, from the moment he received his baloney sandwich ration each morning after breakfast until noon, when they stopped to each lunch, my father searched for anybody who hated the peanut butter sandwich ration as much as Dad hated his baloney sandwich ration. Only then could he eat lunch—two peanut butter sandwiches. Then there was the time at the end of the war, while part of the army of occupation in Czechoslovakia, that he and a buddy went AWOL and illegally snuck into the city of Prague, in the Russian sector, for the weekend.

What my father failed to mention, in all of his wartime descriptions, in all of the anecdotes he shared with me during those days when I was curious and convalescing, was an incident at Campholz Woods, Germany, during the Battle of the Bulge in February 1945. I didn't know about it, and as far as he was concerned, that's the way it would stay. Toward the end of my recuperation in that June of 1964, I asked my father one last question about his war.

"Were you awarded anything? A medal? Something?"

Presently my father retrieved a medal with five points on it, hanging from a short piece of striped ribbon. He made no fuss over it. He shrugged off any mention I made of his wartime bravery. He simply suggested that if I really cared about it I should put it away for safekeeping. So I tucked the medal into a dresser drawer and promptly forgot about it. While I'd managed to get an answer to the question "What did you do in the war, Dad?" it was, after all, the answer he'd chosen to give. He had gone only as far as he felt comfortable. Later, he wrote a memoir about growing up in New York City, and in it he offered some glimpses of his time overseas during the war. Then, in the 1990s, when he and I co-authored a book on the Second World War, Dad shared a few more of his wartime experiences and writings with me. But the rest would be left to my imagination or, as in the case of what happened at Campholz Woods, up to me to find out on my own.

FEBRUARY 12, 1945—CAMPHOLZ WOODS, GERMANY

IT WAS A TRAP. On the surface it looked like just another forest on just another hilltop. The trees were mature. But because it was the dead of winter, they had no foliage. The woods appeared dense, the outer trees—like dark sentries—hiding the inner ones. The only softening aspect of the woods' appearance was the blanket of fresh snow that dappled the tree limbs and covered the ground in the fields leading to the forest. But it was what lay beneath the snow, beyond the outer trees, and up the incline of the ridge on the other side of the woods that proved so deadly. On the battle maps this place had a name—Campholz Woods—and the American GIs approaching it that mid-winter morning would never forget it.

In the first week of February 1945, the fighting unit to which T/Sgt. Alex Barris was then attached—the 1st Battalion of the 302nd Infantry Regiment, supporting the 94th Infantry Division of the US Army—received orders to enter and clear Campholz Woods. My father served as a liaison sergeant on that mission. That meant, as a sergeant in the field with B Company of the 319th Medical Battalion, he maintained contact between aid men attending to the wounded of each fighting company and the doctors and technicians at aid stations behind the lines in the village of Borg. He ensured that casualties received treatment from front-line medics and that the wounded were then rapidly transported by stretcher-bearers to the regimental aid station—an evacuated farmhouse in the village—for further treatment. He regularly reported to a major at the aid station, informing him about the status of casualties—their numbers, their whereabouts, and the status of their evacuation to collecting companies, clearing companies, or field evacuation hospitals in rear echelons farther back from front-line fighting.

As a consequence of his duties—running between the battlefield and the regimental aid station in Borg, where motor transport might speed up an evacuation—and also because he'd never learned to drive (a born-and-bred New Yorker, he'd grown up travelling everywhere on transit), Barris faced an additional challenge. The army described his service, maintaining the chain of evacuation from battlefields to aid stations, as "being without organic transportation." In plain English, he carried out his duties on foot, "hitching rides with ambulances or other vehicles heading in the appropriate direction," he said. "But I managed."[2]

As American combat units advanced deeper into Germany that winter, this also meant that he was rarely in the same place twice—whether he was marshalling stretcher-bearers and medics to retrieve the wounded, managing the movement of those wounded to aid stations, or ensuring that wounded troops were quickly and efficiently loaded aboard ambulances. Conditions along the front line during both the German Bulge and the Allied counteroffensive meant that T/Sgt. Barris's whereabouts were nearly always in flux. He was something of a ghost—here one moment, gone the next. And in those infrequent times when he wasn't on the move, he might be found hunkered down in a foxhole, huddled in a parked ambulance, or resting on a vacant cot at the aid station in Borg.

Always a moving target, as it were, Barris felt on one hand that he'd formed a decent attachment to the medical unit he served, that he belonged to his outfit. There was a certain esprit de corps, he said, that was inescapable. The medical corpsmen were no longer New Yorkers or Southerners, no longer non-coms versus privates or even officers against enlisted men. In what he described as "this lonely little world of B Company, we knew each other as few citizens ever get to know their neighbours; and the cold shadow of death that hung over us all somehow made wherever the company was feel like home."[3] On the other hand, so peripatetic was his existence, dashing from front line to regimental aid station, that he also felt as if he were just a visitor, an outsider imposing on somebody else's small corner of the war.

But in February 1945, T/Sgt. Barris's feelings about whether he belonged or was an outsider didn't matter. The job at hand required his full attention and skill. By this stage in the Siegfried Switch Line campaign to undo damage inflicted by the Germans during the Battle of the Bulge, operations almost routinely began in the cold and darkness of the early morning. Just after dawn on a day in early February, advance troops of B and C Companies of the 302nd filed out of Borg and entered the southern edge of the woods in large numbers for the first time; they quickly captured a handful of prisoners who, it appeared, were a forward artillery observation group; that meant the Americans' exact position was known almost immediately by German gunners on the higher ground up Münzingen Ridge. It wasn't long before the enemy reacted. Rockets, artillery shells (also known as "screaming meemies"), and mortars were soon crashing into the advancing troops of the 302nd. Things went from bad to worse. Seeking shelter deeper into the woods, the American riflemen tripped into communication trenches, dragon's-teeth obstacles, and, worst of all, anti-personnel mines. The resulting chaos, reflected in the B Company sector, was typical.

As they moved from bunker to pillbox, inevitably the troops stumbled into more *Schü* mines—wooden boxes with a spring-loaded lid, a detonator, and 200 grams of explosives. Working with G Company, a group of 319th Combat Engineers tripped one of the mines, wounding three of them. A corporal leading a rescue party moved in to carry out the wounded, but he triggered a second mine; the corporal was temporarily blinded and two corpsmen wounded. A second aid party assisting another wounded rifleman set off a third mine; this explosion killed the medic and wounded a lieutenant and an infantryman who'd both volunteered to assist. And each new *Schü* mine explosion brought down more German artillery and mortar fire on the advancing troops. This domino-like process continued every costly step of the way into Campholz Woods. One staff sergeant witnessed the carnage at close range.

"Suddenly a mine went off killing the scout, and the platoon leader set two men to probing," he wrote. "No sooner had they started than they were blown up. The explosions alerted the Krauts in a bunker not fifty yards away and the machine gun opened up. . . . Men hit the ground setting off more mines as they landed. Legs and feet were blown away. Men began screaming. Others cried, 'Medic! Medic!' The enemy was throwing mortars and 88s and a machine gun was adding to the hell."[4]

At the first sign of trouble, the medical corpsmen of the 319th Medical Battalion began dashing from their positions at the starting line of the operation near Borg, forward into Campholz Woods to retrieve the wounded, and then back again. An indication of the frenzy T/Sgt. Barris's unit faced during this one engagement alone is reflected in the patient case lists of previous days. On February 10, between 9:15 a.m. and 9:36 p.m., for example, the 319th Regimental Aid Station processed 119 wounded (including seven medics and two prisoners of war.)[5] In other words, litter-bearers, medics, surgeons, and orderlies attended on average six wounded every minute, all day long. It's perhaps no surprise then, that somewhere in the haste and confusion of the next forty-eight hours, a squad of litter-bearers had failed to return to its rendezvous point. As many as four men dispatched to bring back wounded from the killing zone concealed in the woods had disappeared.

Waiting, watching, listening, and attempting to hasten the evacuation of casualties that day—February 12, 1945—T/Sgt. Barris was first to realize that the four corpsmen and the men on their stretchers were long overdue. With no other way to learn where the squad was located or what had caused the delay, and, as usual, with no "organic transportation" to get him there, he felt he had no choice but to set out on foot to find them.

"Tech 4 Sgt. Barris personally entered these woods, which

were heavily sown with mines and booby traps," an official report later described, "and located the members of this squad. Two of the members of the squad were wounded and the remaining two were disoriented. He managed to extricate [all four of them] and further their evacuation through medical channels."[6]

Perhaps it is a result of the chaos that day at Campholz Woods, up Münzingen Ridge, where 119 wounded needed full attention, and of the wartime medical system that always had difficulty labelling, treating, and cataloguing such injuries as disorientation and shell shock, that neither T/Sgt. Barris's written accounts nor the battalion's case lists show which litter-bearers were extricated from that battlefield. Apparently they survived their initial wounds and either returned to active service nearly immediately or disappeared quietly beyond the evacuation hospitals, on their way home to the States. In either case, it appears that T/Sgt. Alex Barris never gave his actions another thought. He had to be reminded, a month later, of his meritorious service. Meanwhile, the battle of the Saar-Moselle Triangle dragged on for several more bloody weeks before the 94th Infantry Division established a bridgehead over the River Saar and commenced the final stage of the war, on its way to VE-Day in Düsseldorf, Germany.

IT'S THAT ATTITUDE—not giving his actions another thought—that has haunted me, not just about my father but among other veterans whose stories I've listened to for half my life. In fact, my library of recorded conversations, stacks of stenography pads full of notation, unpublished letters and diaries, and walls of books I've collected all harbour passages revealing such thinking. Those moments in interviews, references in documents, or images in film or video all have that unique selflessness, dedication to service, and disregard for one's safety to save others.

From my earliest awareness of warfare and the history of battles, I knew of Florence Nightingale, who transformed a British base hospital in Constantinople—where patients were often abandoned amid contaminated water and vermin to face certain death—into a functioning facility with attendants, soap, bandages, and hope; in the process she and her staff of thirty-four nurses reduced horrific mortality rates in Crimea by two-thirds. During tours I've led to historic spots of the Great War, I've stood many times in the entrance to John McCrae's advanced dressing station at Essex Farm, near Ypres, Belgium, and wondered how he could steady his hand for first aid as well as for writing those evocative lines of "In Flanders Fields" with the German artillery firing relentlessly so close by.

Since the Second World War was my father's war, and since I was born right after it, I had access to more veterans from Dad's war than any other; consequently, my travels and research have led me to hundreds of first-person accounts of medics in the front lines between 1939 and 1945. Among my father's books, in the Time-Life series, I was always struck by the story of Pfc. Desmond Doss, a conscientious objector who served his faith and his country not by bearing arms but by saving lives. According to both the *Time Capsule* story and the 2016 big-screen movie *Hacksaw Ridge*, during the Battle of Okinawa, medical corpsman Doss climbed a four-hundred-foot escarpment and under relentless Japanese infantry fire managed to lower seventy-five wounded men down the rock face to safety. A photograph accompanying the *Time Capsule* story shows President Harry Truman placing the Medal of Honor around his neck, with the caption: "Medal for a pacifist."[7]

As compelling, the six hours of Frederick Topham's battle-field heroism have always resonated. The former northern Ontario miner, who enlisted in the 1st Canadian Parachute Battalion, jumped first into Normandy on D-Day, and then across the River Rhine on March 24, 1945. On the ground that morning near the end of the war, the battalion came under heavy fire; orderlies from a field ambulance attempted to attend a wounded paratrooper but were killed as they knelt next to the casualty.

"Without hesitation and on his own initiative," a citation read, "Cpl. Topham went forward through intense fire to replace the orderlies. As he worked on the wounded man, he was himself shot in the face. He never faltered and carried the wounded man to shelter."[8]

But Topham didn't stop there. When he finally consented to evacuation to be treated for his head wound, he came across a carrier vehicle struck by enemy fire; despite warnings not to, Topham rescued all three of the carrier's wounded occupants. His selfless acts under fire remain among the most extraordinary in Canadian military medical history. He received the Victoria Cross at the war's end.

Awards came to many deserving survivors (and others posthumously) who exhibited what the citations routinely called uncommon acts of bravery. But when those courageous feats also involved trying to save the lives of others—as with Sarah Emma Edmonds at Bull Run, Francis Scrimger at Ypres, Grace

MacPherson at Etaples, Jacob Markowitz along the "Death Railway," Dane Harden in Iraq, and Alannah Gilmore in Afghanistan—somehow the citations fell short of explanation. Sure, one could argue that saving lives came with the job description. Signing up to be a field surgeon, a nursing sister, a military dentist, an operation room orderly, a battlefield ambulance driver, a stretcher-bearer, or a medical corpsman brought with it an "in the fine print" acknowledgement of perceived peril. And I dare say that none of those taking on such official wartime medical roles ever considered themselves immune from attack in a war zone. Even if the articles of the Geneva Convention clearly stated that shooting a medic on the battlefield was considered a war crime, too much history of atrocity in warfare proved such articles weren't worth the paper they were printed on. In short, being a medic was not a bombproof job.

And yet, for so many of these individuals, even when conditions appeared to be at their worst, where the risk seemed its greatest, or in what seemed a suicidal action, the perceived peril didn't seem to matter. I have always found myself in search of answers to very basic questions about such people: Why would these military medical personnel go so far beyond job function and duty? Were these people so hotheaded, or cold-blooded, that nothing could stop them? Did something intangible inside—a faith, an obligation to do better, a call for what seemed right—drive these men and women to defy the law of averages and override their instincts for survival?

As I have devoted more and more of my life to studying war, researching its context, interviewing its warriors, and writing and publishing the stories of its participants, I have come to realize that I never really asked my father the most important question about his time as a medic in the Battle of the Bulge. In 2017, when I returned to Campholz Woods in Germany to walk the same mile my father did to save those four corpsmen in 1945, I kept asking—right into my cellphone recorder—how he could have accomplished such a mission and survived. Maybe the more relevant question—and, in fact, the motivation for this book—is why? Why, against his better judgment to stay within the safety of friendly lines, would my father instead choose to pick his way through a snow-covered mine-field and into a forest infested with booby traps, find those wounded and dazed young litter-bearers, and bring them safely back? Why, when all the world was dashing the other way, would he choose to rush to danger?

CHAPTER TWO

"MEDICAL DICTATOR"

S ECURITY MEASURES have made the facility virtually impregnable. Nobody without authorization can gain access, even digitally. It's kind of the Fort Knox of veterans' vitals in the United States. That's how impenetrable the National Personnel Records Center (NPRC) is today. In fact, even though I'm a member of my father's nuclear family, the centre required full documentation of our blood connection. I had to provide cross-reference material on his working life, his military serial number, and his death certificate before officials would even consider my request for data on his service record. And they would provide me with nothing until each application form was complete, every document checked, and all my identity files verified. The NPRC is so particular about protecting its clients, living or dead, that each page of the centre's outgoing correspondence includes its primary mission: "We value our veterans' privacy," it says, and, "Let us know if we have failed to protect it."[1]

Only once did the National Personnel Records Center in Overland, a suburb of St. Louis, Missouri, fail its clients in that promise to protect. On July 12, 1973, the fail-safe system at what was then known as the National Archives and Records Administration could not prevent a fire from racing through its sixth floor—destroying the records of 80 percent of the US Army personnel discharged between November 1, 1912, and January 1, 1960. My father's honourable discharge occurred in December 1945. I waited patiently for six months, not expecting that the NPRC would have salvaged much of my father's records. When I finally received the return package in the mail, the contents showed just how close his records had come to incineration. The photocopies clearly reproduced the singe marks around the edges of his military records. Remarkably, though, some of my father's wartime data survived.

I learned from them, for example, where my father had served in the US Army on Christmas Day 1942 and New Year's Day 1943—in a military hospital at Camp Phillips, a base just outside Salina, Kansas. The singed NPRC records showed that as a member of the 319th Medical Battalion, 94th Infantry Division, he had been admitted to the base hospital just before noon on December 25, 1942, with a diagnosis of "pharyngitis catarrhal acute" and a temperature of 102 degrees.[2] Not just a severe cold and fever, this bacterial invasion of his chest, throat, and sinuses was more like pneumonia or influenza.* It was so debilitating that he was admitted to the base hospital

---

* Canadian Army medic William Wilson (deployed to Afghanistan in 2002) explained that pharyngitis catarrhalis, sometimes referred to as moraxella catarrhalis, is like strep pneumonia and hemophilus influenza, which in some cases has led to bacteremia with a 21 percent mortality rate if left untreated.

and confined to bed for most of the next ten days.[3] No Christmas or New Year's pass to Salina for him. The New York–born draftee in his first days as a medical corpsman—just a buck private in training—was himself in need of close medical attention.

Among the other fire-damaged documents enclosed, the record centre also sent details of my father's service overseas—in particular, some of the actions of his medical unit, the 319th Medical Battalion, between January 15 and March 1, 1945. Previously "restricted," the dossier was released to me as I pieced together the day-to-day experiences of my father as a wartime medic.

DECEMBER 1943—CAMP PHILLIPS, KANSAS

WHEN THE UNITED STATES entered the Second World War, my father was nineteen. Alex said a lot of his contemporaries volunteered, partly out of eagerness to serve and partly because those who enlisted had a better chance of getting into the branch of the service they preferred, rather than being drafted and told where to serve. He admitted, too, that many joined up seeking some sort of adventure. Nobody in his family was so bloodthirsty as to want to rush overseas to kill Germans, Italians, or Japanese right away. Nor did any of them consider shirking the service. They knew their country's armed forces would eventually come calling. The husband of my father's older sister, Jim Chilaris, was drafted and served in the Aleutian Islands. Alex's older brother, Angelo Barris, answered his draft notice on his twentieth birthday, February 7, 1941, and eventually served with the US Army's 67th Antiaircraft Artillery in North Africa, Italy, France, and Germany.

"From the time I was drafted in October of 1942," Angelo said, "besides the odd letter that said, 'I'm okay. Are you okay?' I didn't see my brother again for almost three years."[4]

Alex followed suit. As required, on his twentieth birthday—September 16, 1942—Alex registered for the draft. The fall went by and the army didn't call. He'd heard through the grapevine that if he weighed less than 130 pounds he wouldn't be accepted. He weighed 125. So he tried a so-called weight-gaining diet of bananas and water. It didn't help at all. By November he still hadn't been called up, so he paid the draft office a visit. An exhaustive search for his file ensued, until it was found stuck to the underside of a filing cabinet drawer. For years afterward, his sister Irene chastised him for fussing enough to get his file unearthed at the enlistment office, else he might never have had to go to war.

If the army's draft system seemed a mystery, my father was equally flummoxed in his attempts to discover the yardstick used for deciding which branch draftees were assigned to. It was pretty clear that a prerequisite—having a medical background, say, or at least an interest in medicine—had little or nothing to do with his being assigned to the medical corps. In his B Company of trainees at Camp Phillips in early 1943, Alex remembered only one or two pre-med students and another who'd worked as a hospital orderly. He came to the conclusion, therefore, that the yardstick was *need*. In other words, draftees were assigned to units that the army decided were below their prescribed strength, without regard for the trainees' educational background, civilian experience, or specific aptitudes. Upon Alex's arrival at Camp Phillips, those assigned to "the medics" reported to one or another of the units comprising the medical battalion—the 319th Medical Battalion—eventually attached to a combat unit, the 94th Infantry Division.

Within a day or two of his arrival, orientation lectures began. These were designed to explain the functions of a medical battalion and, more loftily, the spirit of the medical corps. Another lecture dealt with the meaning of the medical corps, stressing the good fortune he and his comrades enjoyed being in the branch of the army devoted to saving lives. My father wrote later that he took some comfort in the thought that as a medic he wouldn't be expected to take lives. Not that he was either an outspoken pacifist or a conscientious objector, per se. He claimed he had never given the matter much thought before he landed in the medical corps and was forced to think about the basic function of a soldier, which was to kill. Alex sensed he did not have the "killer instinct" and wondered how many others were of the same frame of mind but who—unlike medics— would have to acquire it.

Tony Mellaci had no better understanding of his posting to Camp Phillips than my father did. Born into an Italian working family in Rumson, New Jersey, Tony recalled living above a garage with his parents and older brother, Lou. The owner of the garage, a New York lawyer, had employed Tony's father, Frank Mellaci, in the 1930s to tend the surrounding grounds and gardens. With his dad tending the estate vegetable garden and raising chickens and quail, and his mother, Barbara, jarring the produce, Tony said, "my family didn't really know what the Depression was."⁵ Still, the Mellaci elders instilled in both sons the need to be respectful, save their pennies, and study hard. Lou proved to be an A student and graduated second in the University of Pittsburgh's dental class of 1941. Tony preferred sports to studies, and when the University of Miami invited him for a football tryout, he jumped at it. But in the meantime, the Japanese bombed Pearl Harbor, bringing America into the war, and the New Jersey draft board ordered Tony to report to the US Army at Fort Dix, ending his dream of starring on a college football team.

"What branch of the service do you want to be in?" the receiving officer asked at the New Jersey army base. "Signal corps? Machine guns?"

"I don't give a damn where you put me," snapped Mellaci, still smarting from losing out on the football scholarship.

"Okay, wise guy, it's infantry for you."⁶

That fall, instead of heading to Miami, Mellaci was posted to Fort Bragg, North Carolina, for six weeks of basic training, and then sent west. He didn't know where he was heading until the train stopped in the middle of the country, where he read the station sign for Salina, Kansas. Off the train and into troop trucks, the draftees were transported to Camp Phillips—past the barracks for the rifle companies, Signal Corps, quartermaster's, reconnaissance, and engineers to the tarpaper huts housing the medical corps. Mellaci figured that his mentioning an interest in teaching physical education in his draft papers had caught their attention, so they streamed him into the medical corps. There, in the winter of 1942–43, he met my father, who hadn't figured out how they'd chosen him for medics either. But unlike so many of the others streamed into the 319th Medical Battalion at Phillips, Mellaci and Barris at least had a couple of things in common. They had grown up within a few miles of each other in New Jersey and New York; they both loved their Yankees come World Series time; and, at least initially, they had a common enemy.

"Ah, you Rebs," Mellaci and Barris would taunt the Southerners in camp.

"You Yanks!" they'd shout back.

"What do you guys from the backwoods know anyhow?"[7]

My father's wariness around some of his Southern comrades was amplified during a class on blood transfusion. The interaction between the rookie medics and the instructor somehow arrived at a discussion about whether blood could be pure or not. My father wrote that a young man from Alabama wanted assurance that no blood from a black man would ever be mixed with "white blood"; he was concerned lest he ever got wounded or had to administer blood plasma to an American in the battlefield. My father was astonished to learn that, at the time, the US Army did indeed give assurance that no blood from African-American troops would be transfused into whites, or vice versa. That seemed to satisfy the Alabaman's concern,[8] although it surely mystified Alex's personal code of ethics.

To start with, at least, except for some of the real physicians who'd come from civilian medical practice, few of the draftees had much sense of their new roles in the medical corps. B Company of the 319th Medical Battalion, as my father remembered it, had five officers and some ninety-eight enlisted men. There were three medical corps officers—qualified doctors, who in army parlance would command medical units—and two medical administrative corps officers, non-doctors who were thus relegated to running the ambulance and litter-bearer platoons of the company. The medical battalion consisted of three "collecting" companies, a "clearing" company, and a headquarters detachment, some five hundred officers and men in all. But the finer aspects of becoming medical corpsmen lay ahead. For the newcomers, it was down to the basics in every respect.

"First it was a five-mile hike," Mellaci remembered. "Then up to ten miles. Then fifteen. And the big test—the twenty-five-mile hike—with full pack, in the heat or the cold in the middle of the country, where there wasn't a tree to be seen."[9]

If the bald prairie wasn't conducive to hiking, neither were the tarpaper shacks particularly stimulating as classrooms for the novice medical corpsman. And it didn't seem to matter whether the new draftee was going to end up in the motor pool, as Tony Mellaci did, or orchestrating litter teams, as my father did. Everybody had to know something about first aid and anatomy. And the medical officer in charge of training B Company apparently made no distinction between those in the battalion who were training to administer drugs, dress wounds, and apply splints, and those keeping records, driving ambulances, or cooking meals. Alex recalled an instance when a major entered the classroom in the middle of a map-reading session. No matter, the major was on a mission. He walked up the centre aisle between the desks and chairs and handed out three human bones to three different soldiers.

"Who has the tibia?" grinned the major.

Each of the student medics looked at his piece of bone uncertainly. Then the medics looked at each other and back at the major; none of the three was able to identify if he had the tibia or not.

"Then let's see who has the fibula," the major continued.

More silence as the three men gazed at the bones they held with even more ill-disguised incomprehension.

"Speak up now," said the major, losing his jolly demeanour. "Who has the femur?" But again, no answer came back. Finally, in frustration, the major ordered the three men to identify what they held.

"Tibia?" said one.

"No," the major barked.

"Tibia?" said the second, holding his bone in the air.

"No."

"Tibia!" blurted out the third man, holding his up with delight.

"A little late, soldier," the major admonished. And he lurched at the three men, grabbed the bone samples from their hands, and stomped out of the classroom.[10]

Another of the vital foundation skills required in preparing medics for war, according to the Camp Phillips trainers, was guard duty. The routine called for the medical corpsman to march along the boundaries of his outdoor post for two hours, have four hours off, and then repeat the process. On an overnight posting that winter, my father recalled, he had the additional responsibility of waking up the officer of the day at six o'clock in the morning to take reveille; that is, to listen to the shouted-out responses of the first sergeants of each company, who would be assembled before the commanding officer (CO) out on the parade ground. That required the sentry on guard duty to wake the officer of the day—a Lt. Swigert—at 5:45 a.m. so that he could arrive on the parade ground in time to take the verbal reports. With that additional responsibility top of mind all night, Pte. Barris conscientiously went to the headquarters building while it was still dark and woke Lt. Swigert. He recalled the officer rising, putting on his boots and heavy coat, and striding out of the building into the still-dark Kansas morning.

"Battaaalion . . . reeeport!" he heard Swigert roar.

There was no answer from the opposite side of the parade ground, where the company sergeants were supposed to be shouting back their status. Nothing.

Swigert repeated the call even more loudly. Even with the wooden door of the headquarters building shut tight, my father could hear Swigert calling again and again, his voice growing increasingly hoarse. Both the officer outside and the private inside were baffled by the lack of response. After five minutes of this painful experience my father realized in horror that it was now 4:55 a.m. In his anxiety to get the lieutenant up in time, he'd misread his own wristwatch and woken the poor man a full hour too early. The officer must have realized the same thing; a few moments later, he appeared in the doorway looking for an explanation.

"Private Barris," he said, looking at my father in disgust, "the United States Army assumes, perhaps unwisely, that the minimum requirement for a soldier to perform guard duty is that he be able to tell time."

"Yes, sir. Sorry, sir."

"Dismissed!"

Perhaps the motto on the crest of the 319th Medical Battalion—*Prodesse quam conspici*, or "Accomplish without being conspicuous"—was more a rationalization of limited skill than a recognition of selfless service. At least in basic training, Privates Barris and Mellaci and their comrades had left a lot to be desired that winter at Camp Phillips, Kansas. Nevertheless, in just months, their instructors had imparted sufficient knowledge and skill for the draftees to graduate. And later that year the battalion moved to manoeuvres in Mississippi and Tennessee. In name, at least, the army now considered them medics.

JANUARY 11, 2007—MASUM GHAR, AFGHANISTAN

As a green private in basic training in the infantry— fifty years later—Jody Mitic had an attitude toward medics that was pretty common among newcomers to the Canadian Armed Forces, in which he served. He and the others looked at medical personnel, at least during their basic training, as a necessary inconvenience. Medics regularly inspected the recruits' uniforms and their barracks for bugs. Often they went even further, checking the soldiers' feet, underarms, and crotches, looking for rashes or fungus or worse. Mitic recognized that the medics' hearts were in the right place. When they got a chance to talk to the recruits, the medics asked how they were feeling. Were they getting enough sleep, sufficient food? Still, at that stage of his young military career, Jody Mitic generally dismissed medics who seemed purely interested in the troops' well-being. They were "kind of like your mommy," he wrote, even if they happened to be men.[11]

Cpl. Mitic's view hadn't changed a great deal through his time in the militia, or even after he joined the regular army in 1997, when he was twenty. As a combat soldier, he considered it his job to be tough, to dismiss any discomfort, even if he actually had blisters running the entire length of his foot, churning guts, or a rash on his backside. It was a matter of turning the other cheek, so to speak. After his first full deployment overseas, when he came home to take specialized training as a basic reconnaissance patrolman and then a basic sniper, that sense of mind over matter took on even greater significance. During sniper training, for example, Mitic learned that the job wasn't just about marksmanship. Being a capable sniper meant more than proficiency on the shooting range, making an accurate shot at 6,500 feet. It demanded that a marksman on a mission, almost as an involuntary reflex, could deny his own needs and put the mission first. As Mitic put it, if occupying a two-man snipers' position required him to "sit in a hole, get rained on, not eat, piss on each other, and still make an accurate shot four days later," so be it.[12] The objective of the mission trumped just about everything. And coincidentally, if it meant hiding an injury or malady from medical personnel along the way, well, suck it up.

Mitic gained a grudging respect for the medical side of soldiering during his first operational tour of duty in Afghanistan, as part of Task Force Kabul at Camp Julien. In the fall of 2003, an Iltis Jeep containing three fellow Royal Canadian Regiment (RCR) troops ran over a land mine. Two of the occupants—Cpl. Robbie Beerenfenger and Sgt. Robert Short—died immediately in the explosion; they were the first Canadian soldiers killed by enemy fire in the post-9/11 Afghanistan mission. Meanwhile, the driver, Cpl. Thomas J. Stirling, was rushed into surgery. Afterward, Mitic and other members of the mission visited him to offer moral support. Not only was Stirling the first comrade-in-arms Mitic had ever seen injured by a land mine, he was also the first casualty Mitic had ever seen. As Mitic explained in a memoir several years later, with his buddy conscious, there was time for small talk among fellow Royals and even a chance to give Stirling a few puffs on an (illegal) cigarette.* Oddly, it wasn't the smell of the cigarette smoke that remained in Mitic's nostrils.

"I took in every detail," Mitic said, "what it smells like when someone's been wounded as badly as he was and the look in his eye. And the swelling in his face; his teeth had been all smashed by the concussion of the explosion. . . . You need to see that. The first time shouldn't be when you're putting your buddy in a body bag."[13]

That "wounded" smell would indeed come back to Mitic, on his next deployment three and a half years later. After the improvised explosive device (IED) incident in October 2003, there would be numerous similar attacks against Canadian troops by the Taliban—one in 2004, six in 2006. With another sniper course behind him and a promotion to master corporal on his record, Jody Mitic returned to Afghanistan in August 2006 for a second tour of duty. This time, however, M/Cpl. Mitic arrived at the Canadian base at Kandahar Airfield as part of an elite sniper team. The group participated in several different missions—Operation Rocket Man to track down Taliban targeting the airport with rockets, and Operation Medusa attempting to push the Taliban out of Panjwaii

---

* Born and raised in Calgary, Alberta, and a veteran of four years in the military, Cpl. Thomas Jared Stirling was serving in his second tour of duty in Afghanistan on October 2, 2003, when wounded in the land mine explosion. Married and a father of two, he would die by suicide on August 19, 2009. He was twenty-nine.

district—partnering with Joint Task Force troops. His sniper team included Barry, whom Mitic called "a real soldier's soldier," Kash, "a laid-back Jamaican killing machine,"[14] and Gord, who joined Mitic later on the tour in a stakeout during which all they tangled with was a mouse that ran up Gord's leg. Any levity on that tour ended in the middle of the night on January 11, 2007.

That night, about 3:30 a.m., the sniper team left a friendly position called the "Ant Hill" near Masum Ghar to set up sniping positions in a village before daybreak. En route, the foursome came to a doorway that would give them easier access to the village. At intervals about thirty feet apart, the snipers moved through the darkness up to and through the opening, each assuring the next in line that the way was clear. Mitic was the last of the four to reach the doorway, stop, let the man ahead advance, and then step ahead himself. As his next step touched the ground a fireball erupted in front of him—a land mine.[15] Mitic remembered being airborne and weightless for a moment, and then hitting the ground and blurting out "oh my God" several times. His foot had triggered a mine "about the size of a hockey puck"[16] that accomplished only half of what was intended. The explosion blew off Mitic's right foot. It also triggered a second explosion—a mortar shell beneath the mine. Had any of the three men ahead of him stepped on the initial mine, the additional mortar shell would likely have severely injured or killed those following. But since he was bringing up the rear, the mortar shrapnel cost Mitic his other foot too.

As soon as the rest of the patrol realized the explosion wasn't the start of a Taliban ambush, they launched into rescue mode.

One began first aid, applying a tourniquet to Mitic's leg and wrapping his wounds, while another pulled the radio from Mitic's pack and called for a medical evacuation.

Mitic remembered the next hour as "the longest of my life," trying to stay conscious and calm so as not to go into shock.[17] Not surprisingly, he worried aloud about the extent of his injuries and how far up his body the explosion had inflicted damage. The thought crossed his mind that no one on the sniper team had bothered to take a tactical combat casualty care course in first aid. He even flashed back to the 1970s TV show *M*A*S*H*, in which the Alan Alda character, Hawkeye, would tell his wounded patients not to gulp down water. But the realities of the situation—it was the middle of the night, some distance from actual medical assistance, and an even greater distance to where a chopper could land and then fly him out—began to play on his thoughts even more. A recce platoon arrived with a medic, who applied more tourniquets— he now had three on each leg—to reduce the amount of blood Mitic was losing. In response to the pain Mitic was feeling, the medic administered a shot of morphine. Minutes later, because he couldn't feel any difference, Mitic demanded another. The medic hesitated but then, unsure of Mitic's chances, gave him the second dose. Then Mitic became aware of a new player on the scene. He recognized a voice from the base.

"What's going on here?" the female voice asked. "Give me an update."

The leader of the recce platoon responded: "It's all good. Our medic has it under control."

"That's great," said the female voice, "but I'm taking over from here, so I need an update."

This wasn't about pulling rank and it wasn't about machismo. This was about situation awareness. M/Cpl. Alannah Gilmore needed to know details of the injury, that tourniquets had been applied, and what medication Mitic had received: tactical combat casualty care—what every infantry soldier in theatre is supposed to know, but certainly medics. Gilmore discovered that the medics at the scene did have things under control; they'd stopped the bleeding on both of Mitic's legs, packed the wounds, and done their best to prevent the patient from slipping into shock.

"I heard the patient talking," Gilmore said. "My focus, as soon as I hear someone talking, is breathing. Good, he's conscious. But my brain has moved on. I'm thinking, 'What more does he need? How do I get him out of here? Where do I have to go?' My job is extrication, getting him to a safe landing zone for evacuation. That's my priority."[18]

It was going to be complicated. Just getting to the Ant Hill had been a challenge. An armoured bulldozer, called a Badger, had literally plowed a roadway into the site—with a light armoured vehicle (LAV) and Gilmore's Bison ambulance following—in total darkness. Next, the medical response team would have to retrace that drive to a landing zone. By the time the Bison reached the chopper, Gilmore had put an IV into Mitic's arm and prepared him for air evacuation to Kandahar Airfield.

"I felt awful," Gilmore said, because she knew what the loss of both legs below the knee would mean to Jody Mitic's soldiering career. "But I wasn't fearful. You're running on such a level of adrenaline. It's constant. The whole time you're in react mode."

Despite this natural adrenaline, in Alannah Gilmore's

case there was much more at work. First, she'd acquired a healthy sense of self-confidence; she said that operating in a male-dominated environment suited her perfectly. She'd grown up with two older brothers, while her father, Maj. Ben Gilmore, had served thirty-four years in the Canadian Forces with the Royal Canadian Regiment. She'd trained as a gymnast, excelled at dance, and at age seventeen had visited an army recruiting centre to inquire about service in the reserve; at the E.J.G. Holland VC Armoury in Ottawa they had a medical platoon, so on weekends and one other night of the week she trained as a medic. And she learned to deal with the unspoken suggestions that as a woman she'd be slower, weaker, or a liability to the platoon.

"I had to work a heck of a lot harder to prove my ability," she said, "but I always loved the challenge."

By 1999 she'd completed post-secondary education, gone to Japan to teach ESL, and come home to enter Canada's regular armed service. But she never stopped upgrading her medical skill set; as a medical technician in the army, she took courses and instructed others, all the while acquiring what she called "muscle memory" on the job. In 2003 the army deployed her "as the mini doc" to Alert, Nunavut, about 460 miles south of the North Pole. Naturally she dealt with seasonal affective disorder and frostbite, but on the base they also trained for the possibility of a fire or a plane crash.

Gilmore treated every aspect of her work as a way to sharpen her ability to react without having to think. The less she felt she had to rely on what her head told her hands—the greater her muscle memory—the more effective her ability to react to anything new. By the time the army deployed her to

Afghanistan in 2006, M/Cpl. Gilmore was bringing all her innate and acquired skills—her competitiveness, her thirst for knowledge, her leadership, her muscle memory—to the job of saving lives in a war zone.

During the first weeks of September that year, the 1st Battalion of the RCR battle group led an offensive against the Taliban in Panjwaii to establish government control over that area of Kandahar Province. Operation Medusa tested the mettle of both the front-line troops and the support units, including M/Cpl. Gilmore's Bison ambulance crew. Stationed at a command post known as Patrol Base Wilson, Gilmore was now crew commander in the Bison, assisted by junior medic Dave Pridham and driver Kurt Nelson.

Right after they joined the operation, her crew received a LAV full of patients who'd sustained shrapnel wounds from a rocket attack. Working with an officer, Gilmore triaged the five wounded, their mantra being *identify, recognize, treat.* At the same time, Nelson, her script, made note of casualty names and medical information, while Pridham and the rest of the medical team checked vital signs, cleaned wounds, set up IVs, and administered painkillers. It was the first time they'd faced a "mass cals" situation, but whether it was individuals or "mass casualties," the principle was the same.

"I didn't have to think about it; it just happened," she said. "I just calmed right down and did what I had to do. I was doing muscle memory."

Gilmore and her crew took a three-week leave during their tour, but when they returned to duty, their enemy had introduced a new array of weapons and methods of attack. The Taliban were now packing civilian vehicles with explosives and detonating them where people gathered, or using children as suicide bombers and secondaries; in other words, one suicide bomber would set off a device and a second would wait for a crowd to gather and set off another one in the same place. As well, setting IEDs and laying land mines had become the Taliban's tactics of choice. Sniper Jody Mitic had triggered one such land mine at the Ant Hill that night in January 2007 —dispatching medic Alannah Gilmore to treat and extricate him to the landing zone for safe evacuation.

Despite his semi-conscious state, M/Cpl. Mitic remembered hearing the unmistakable sound of a Black Hawk medevac helicopter and being lifted aboard.

"These American medevac guys are highly trained," Mitic said later. "They're called air rescue. If they have to, when they land, they will go into a gunfight to extract you. That's how hard-core these guys are. Then you're into a helicopter and it's basically like a flying surgical room."

With another IV line in him as the medevac helicopter flew toward Kandahar Airfield, about twenty minutes away, Mitic felt revived enough to carry on a conversation with the flight surgeon. And he obliged, keeping Mitic engaged and talking about Afghanistan, the war, anything to distract him until the chopper arrived at the base, where he was rushed into surgery. As they wheeled Mitic into the operating room, the medical team passed him a phone to call his parents back in Canada, to let them know what was happening and that he'd be okay. It was only on the other side of the anesthesia and surgery, hours later, that he learned the OR surgeon had had to remove both feet. Mitic recognized that the decision had not been easy, but that, in the surgeon's view, amputating both limbs below the knee would give Mitic a fighting chance to function one day on two roughly similar prosthetics.

It didn't take M/Cpl. Mitic long to begin thinking ahead—perhaps more optimistically than most—about getting home, doing some rehabilitation, acquiring a set of prosthetic legs, and, after some rehabilitation, getting redeployed to Afghanistan for another tour of duty. "After all," he said, "most prosthetics for legs, besides what they're made of, they're almost the same design as they were during the Civil War. Now they're carbon fibre and stainless steel . . . Back then it was wood and plaster."

He was right. Prosthetics had not changed much in their functionality since the war between the northern and southern states. But everything else had. In 2007, M/Cpl. Mitic had the evolution of nearly 150 years of military medicine to help save his life in the field, get him to an operating theatre to repair catastrophic damage to his lower body, and then facilitate his physical and mental recovery to relative normalcy. In the 1860s, wounded soldiers might never make it off the battlefield.

DECEMBER 13, 1862—FREDERICKSBURG, VIRGINIA

IN A SPACE barely large enough to erect a small block of downtown buildings, about 8,000 soldiers of the US Federal Army were killed outright, maimed, or died of wounds in the hours after just one battle. In that space—about six hundred yards west of the mid-nineteenth-century city of Fredericksburg, Virginia—the open ground features a gentle incline rising to about forty or fifty feet above the town, known as Marye's Heights. As fog lifted from the area on the morning of December 13, 1862, Union Maj. Gen. Ambrose Burnside launched what he considered a diversionary attack toward a four-foot-high stone wall with an impromptu trench and sunken road behind it. From relative safety behind that wall, about 2,000 Confederate troops, under Gen. Thomas Reade Rootes Cobb, stood four ranks deep. They poured down continuous rifle fire, while from higher ground 3,000 more men in reserve and artillery rained shells on the advancing Federals. Attempting to make his way over about a half-mile of open field to his enemy's lines, a Union soldier recorded that he and his comrades ran forward "as though breasting a storm of rain and sleet, our faces and bodies being only half-turned to the storm, our shoulders shrugged."[19] Confederate artillerist Edward Alexander told his superiors before the battle, "We cover that ground now so well . . . a chicken could not live on that field when we open on it."[20]

He was right. In one hour, the Union Army of the Potomac lost nearly 3,000 men. Still the madness of the Union assault continued. Through the afternoon, no fewer than fifteen Union brigades attempted charges against Marye's Heights. Not a single Northern unit reached the stone wall. That day the Southerners recorded fewer than 1,200 casualties,* but that included the death of Gen. Cobb. That December evening, as the sun set, the temperature dropped, and some light snow fell on the battlefield, thousands of Union wounded lay out in the

---

* Civil War scholar Cheryl A. Wells, editor of Jonathan Letterman's accounts in *A Surgeon in the Army of the Potomac,* pegs Fredericksburg's total losses at 12,653 on the Union side and 5,000 on the Confederate side.

open within range of Confederate guns. American poet and journalist Walt Whitman later met a survivor at a hospital in Washington, DC.

"He got badly hit in his leg and side," wrote Whitman, then a Civil War hospital volunteer. "He lay the succeeding two days and nights helpless on the field between the city and those grim terraces of batteries; his company and his [Pennsylvania] regiment had been compell'd to leave him to his fate." Unable to move because of his wounds, the rifleman was forced to spend nearly fifty hours lying with his head facing downhill. Just when the scenario seemed at its worst, the Pennsylvanian awoke in this no man's land to find a man leaning over him. "Moving around the field among the dead and wounded," Whitman continued, "[he] treated our soldier kindly, bound up his wounds, gave him a couple of biscuits, and a drink of water." Remarkably, the Confederate soldier knew enough about first aid not to move the Union soldier, else blood that had clotted might burst from his wounds. In his journal, Whitman referred to the benevolent soul as "this good Secesh,"[21] or Secessionist. He was, in all likelihood, Sgt. Richard Kirkland.

The day after the Union attack on Marye's Heights, Confederate Gen. J.B. Kershaw sat in a makeshift headquarters in an upstairs room of a farmhouse about 150 yards behind the sunken road and stone wall. From his vantage point he could see most of the half-mile of fields over which nearly 8,000 Union troops had dashed in vain to reach the sunken road where Kershaw's brigade had stood its ground. In a memoir about the aftermath, Gen. Kershaw recalled that a soldier had suddenly arrived in his office with "an expression of indignant remonstrance." The nineteen-year-old wore the insignia of the 2nd South Carolina Volunteers.

"What is the matter, Sergeant?" the general asked.

"General, I can't stand this," Kirkland blurted out. "All night and all day, I have heard those poor people crying for water. . . . I come to ask permission to go and give them water."

"Don't you know that you would get a bullet through your head the moment you stepped over the wall?"

"I know that," Kirkland said; he was a veteran of battles at Manassas, Savage Station, Maryland Heights, and Antietam.[22] "But if you will let me, I am willing to try it."

The general paused a moment and said, "I ought not to allow you to run a risk, but the sentiment which actuates you is so noble that I will not refuse your request."

According to Kershaw's account of the dialogue, the sergeant stopped on the stairs outside his office. Kershaw listened in case Kirkland might have changed his mind. Instead, the young sergeant called out a final request.

"General, can I show a white handkerchief?"

"No, Sergeant, you can't do that," Kershaw said definitively.

"All right," Kirkland said. "I'll take my chances."[23]

In the next few minutes, Kershaw and some of his South Carolinian comrades watched "with profound anxiety" as the sergeant filled as many canteens as he could carry. Then, shortly after noon on December 14, Kirkland stepped over the stone wall that had been witness to the worst one-day carnage of the Civil War to that point and moved to the first wounded Federal soldier. Some reports said that when troops on the Union side saw the Confederate sergeant out in the open, several took shots at him, but they were too distant to be effective. And once they saw Kirkland cradling the first of the wounded and offering water, they ceased firing. Sgt. Kirkland's mission of mercy went on for ninety minutes. He tried to deliver blankets to as many as he could and made certain every wounded man's cry for water was answered. Kirkland later died at the Battle of Chickamauga and was buried at his family's White Oak plantation in South Carolina.*

In 1965, a sculpture by Felix de Weldon was unveiled in front of the stone wall at Fredericksburg where Kirkland had performed his humanitarian act.[24] "At the risk of his life, this American soldier of sublime compassion brought water to his wounded foes at Fredericksburg," the inscription beneath the sculpture reads. "The fighting men on both sides of the line called him the Angel of Marye's Heights."

Despite the compassion shown by Sgt. Kirkland in front of that infamous stone wall, the odds did not favour survival for a soldier wounded in the American Civil War. In spite of the availability of qualified battlefield medical officers and limited anesthetics, some of the most inhumane conditions awaited troops injured in combat as they were transported from the battlefield and attended by surgeons behind the lines. Ambulances consisted of little more than crude wagons, and they were generally overflowing with wounded men being tossed about like rag dolls; the civilian drivers had no battlefield

---

* After Fredericksburg, Richard Kirkland served in the Battles of Chancellorsville and Gettysburg, where—at age twenty—he received a field promotion to lieutenant; on September 20, 1863, he and two others took command of a charge at Snodgrass Hill during the Battle of Chickamauga, where Kirkland was mortally wounded. Civil War historian Paul Van Nest points out that long after Kirkland's body was moved from the family farm to the Quaker Cemetery in Camden, visitors to the site left water canteens behind in tribute.

experience and often bolted from the scene without bringing out the wounded.

And if transport to field hospitals wasn't detrimental enough, the treatment, considered the realm of military surgeons, proved little better. Even though the opposing armed forces claimed extraordinary numbers of surgeons in their ranks, most of them had little experience treating gunshot wounds, nor had they conducted battlefield surgery. Of some 11,000 physicians in the service of the Union, only five hundred had actually performed in-theatre operations; of the 3,000 doctors serving the Confederacy, only twenty-seven had operated on wounded soldiers. The medical men signed up for army service were often political appointments or "quacks" admitted by ill-informed medical boards.[25] Too often, that meant a surgeon, sometimes with less than two years' experience, learned how to operate on the job. The patients paid the price.

The Civil War infantry used the cylindrical soft lead, slow-moving Minie bullet in their muskets. At 1,000 yards, such projectiles had the capacity to kill, due to the gaping holes, shattered bones, shredded muscles, and torn arteries they inflicted on a victim. If a soldier took a Minie ball to the head or torso, doctors would not expect him to live. When the roughly .58-calibre bullet hit a man in the gut, it tore intestines or other internal organs irreparably; when it struck a limb, it expanded, crushing or smashing a man's bones, leaving doctors little alternative but to amputate. When army statisticians got around to tallying battlefield injuries, they concluded that nearly three-quarters of all wounds occurred to soldiers' extremities, their arms and legs. Amputation became the most common procedure performed by Civil War surgeons.

TED BARRIS

Among the Union commanders serving in the Army of the Potomac in 1862 was a former journalist and future senator of Missouri, Gen. Carl Schurz. Amid his eloquent accounts of courage and prowess on the battlefield, he found space in his memoirs to include scenes behind the front lines, where the wounded fought for their lives on the operating tables of military surgeons—hell on earth.

Schurz admitted to becoming conscious of a strong sympathetic emotion to the scenes of death and dying before him. Suddenly he heard the moans and exclamations of the men going under the knife. He noted "the stretchers coming in dreadful procession" to operating tables placed out in the open, where the light was best, or occasionally protected from the elements by blankets stretched over poles. There beside their medicine chests and piles of bandages, Schurz depicted the surgeons, "their sleeves rolled up to their elbows, their bare arms as well as their linen aprons smeared with blood, their knives not seldom held between their teeth, while they helped a patient on or off the table." His gaze caught the heaps of cut-off legs and arms and "the beseeching eyes of the dying boy who, recognizing me, says with his broken voice: 'Oh, General! Can you not do something for me?' And I can do nothing but stroke his hands and utter some words of courage and hope, which I do not believe myself. I feel a lump in my throat which almost chokes me."[26]

Despite the horrific conditions Gen. Schurz described, there was actually more to offer those beseeching eyes and dying pleas than ever before. Remarkably, a revolution in military medicine was about to begin on the very battlefield where Union wounded languished that cold December night

40

in 1862. In May of that same year—for the first time since he'd been posted to serve as a full surgeon and major in the Army of the Potomac—Jonathan Letterman had successfully gained the attention of the US War Department and the military brass leading the Army of the Potomac. His painstaking work gathering data on casualties and crafting the logistics of a medical response, as well as his resulting recommendations, were about to get a chance to prove themselves—and perhaps save lives.

Later described as "the father of battlefield medicine," Letterman had followed in his father's footsteps as a civilian surgeon, gaining his medical certificate in 1849. But Letterman had also passed his exams at the Army Medical Board, which promoted him to officer in the field and assistant surgeon behind the lines. Between 1853 and 1860, Maj. Letterman received his baptism of fire as a surgeon during US military campaigns against the Navajo, Gila Apache, and Pah-Ute bands in the western and southern US territories. However, from the moment of his installation as a full surgeon and major in the Union Army, his attention shifted to the woeful conditions of field medical care, inadequate supplies of medicine, jury-rigged hospital facilities, and insufficient numbers of qualified medical officers. During the Peninsula campaign in the spring and early summer of 1862, the Union's Army of the Potomac had sustained unprecedented casualties—as many as 27,000 killed, wounded, or missing—attempting to capture the Confederate capital, Richmond, Virginia. In the wake of such carnage, as the newly installed medical director of the Army of the Potomac, Maj. Letterman had to find a better way to deal with the wounded. "To accomplish [this]," he said in his report, "the entire system then in vogue must be abolished."[27]

In August 1862, based on his analysis of the campaign and his template for change, Maj. Letterman introduced a new and far more qualified medical player to the Civil War battlefield, the field ambulance. His Special Orders No. 147 document offered a template for saving lives: an ambulance corps and the management of ambulance trains. In the revised system, all ambulances came under the control of the medical director (in this case Letterman). His principal initiative was to introduce non-physician officers—captains, lieutenants, and sergeants— to command ambulance units, to relieve physicians from duties that distracted them from the primary mission of patient care and to give higher priority to attending to the needs of the wounded. In addition, the Letterman plan assigned vehicles to the direct control of the medical director, three for each infantry regiment, two for each cavalry regiment, and one for each artillery battery. Only medical personnel were permitted to accompany the sick and wounded to the rear, and only patients were allowed to ride in the ambulances.

A Union Army chaplain, recognizing the seismic shift in control over the wounded, described Letterman as "virtually a medical dictator."[28]

Following the implementation of Letterman's field ambulance concept, the Army of the Potomac accepted and implemented his subsequent recommendations for field hospitals too. In October 1862, Letterman's directives assigned a field hospital to each division, each housing a surgeon to provide food and shelter and an assistant to keep records. Each facility would include three medical officers to perform operations and another nine medical officers to assist the three. In addition, an administrative staff was responsible for pitching the hospital tents; providing straw, fuel, water, and blankets; and organizing kitchen facilities with staffs of hospital stewards, nurses, and cooks assigned to each. Staff would also triage to determine the expediency and character of serious operations and record interment of the dead (complete with a headboard showing name, rank, and company "legibly inscribed upon it"). Letterman accounted for discipline, guard duty, inspection, regular reporting, and medical service to enemy wounded. "These institutions," Letterman commented in his memoirs, "were the first of the kind attempted in this country."[29]

The efficiency and efficacy of Letterman's concepts were borne out in the major Civil War battles that followed in the fall of 1862 and into 1863. Even though the Battle of Antietam, on September 17, 1862, resulted in 23,000 casualties—the bloodiest single engagement of the war to that point—the field ambulance and field hospital system managed to remove and attend to all of the wounded within twenty-four hours. At Fredericksburg, even as the Union troops fell by the hundreds attempting to overrun the stone wall, Maj. Letterman supervised as his medical officers set up field hospitals in sheltered areas along both banks of the Rappahanock River, easily within cannon shot of the Confederate artillery. Nevertheless, he ensured that each field location had three operating tables, as well as surgeons, attendants, instruments, and dressings "all arranged with order, precision, and convenience rarely excelled in regular hospitals."[30]

Letterman recognized the futility of the assault but marvelled at the enthusiasm of his field ambulance medics as they recovered and carried the wounded to the riverside field hospitals as quickly as stretcher-bearers could move them. He noted the difficulty his corpsmen faced after dark on December 13, since "they could not use their lanterns, as the glimmer of a candle invariably called forth a shot from a sharpshooting picket; they were obliged to grope their way and search for their wounded comrades, who lay on the field covered by the fire of the enemy's musketry. . . . The officers and men of this corps persevered so well, that before dawn all the wounded were taken to the hospitals prepared for them in the rear."[31] Maj. Letterman's novice ambulance corps managed to process almost 10,000 wounded during three intense days of close combat at Marye's Heights.

Among the lessons Letterman delivered between the lines of his Special Orders recommendations was the paramount need for sanitation among procedures of the field ambulance corps, and even more so at the field hospitals. For every Civil War soldier who died in battle there were two who died of disease; on the Union side 620,000 troops died in total, and 250,000 of them died from disease.[32] The unsanitary conditions of the campsites, sleeping quarters, kitchens, and overcrowded hospitals bred all manner of disease, including malaria, typhoid, scurvy, pneumonia, smallpox, measles, skin infections from mosquitoes and lice, and intestinal infections; dysentery and diarrhea on their own killed more men during the Civil War than did battle injuries. In his reports to the chief army surgeons that same autumn of 1862, Letterman noted that the sick soldiers in the Army of the Potomac numbered 200,000 men, or 8 percent of the force. Early in 1863 Letterman called for a hospital in Washington, DC, dedicated to attending the Army's sick soldier population.

Volunteer hospital worker Walt Whitman witnessed this carnage during his regular stops along "hospital row" in Washington, DC. On the afternoon of July 22, 1863, Whitman visited with Oscar Wilber, who'd served with the 154th New York Volunteers at the Battle of Chancellorsville. Along with a fractured femur, chronic diarrhea had left the young soldier bedridden. During one of several visits, Wilbur asked Whitman to read from the New Testament. Whitman wondered which passage.

"Make your own choice," the patient said.

Whitman chose to read chapters describing the final hours of Christ's life and the scenes of the Crucifixion.

The New Yorker asked Whitman to go on to the following chapter, when Christ rose again. Tears welled in his eyes as Whitman finished the passage. Wilber and the young volunteer spoke about death.

"Why, Oscar, don't you think you will get well?" Whitman asked.

"I may, but it is not probable," he said. He talked about his wound, but more so about the diarrhea that had prostrated him. Then Wilber gave Whitman the address of his mother in Cattaraugus County, New York.

Whitman gently embraced and kissed the man, who returned the affection. But it was the last time they saw each other. Wilber died a few days later of the diarrhea and infection from his wound.[33]

If the blow of the wound didn't kill a soldier, then in many cases spreading infection would. Since doctors often took over barns to function as hospitals, and since the battles took place in farmers' fields enriched by animal manure, the majority of battlefield wounds became infected. Often the field surgeons did have anesthesia, in the form of ether or chloroform administered via a soaked cloth placed over the patient's nose and mouth. But at best the surgeons probed battle wounds with their fingers, used knives repeatedly as scalpels, and performed operations in coats smeared with what doctors called "laudable pus,"[34] whose appearance they calculated was a good sign. However, pus in a patient's blood—or blood poisoning—usually triggered fevers and gas gangrene. Without oxygen present, bacillus microbes from manure or other toxic sources quickly multiplied and mixed with severed blood vessels, shattered bone, and ripped muscle tissue to form a septic swill bubbling up like gas in a wound, turning green in the process. Gas gangrene proved as much a killer as any Minie bullet or piece of cannon shrapnel. If patients survived the operating table under these conditions, they still might face deadly surgical fevers and agonizing pain until they died. A full three-quarters of those whose limbs were amputated in the Civil War died of complications from infection.

Despite the experience that nearly a year under his new field ambulance/hospital system gave him, what may have been Maj. Letterman's greatest test came in the summer of 1863, as the Confederate and Union armies clashed at Gettysburg, Pennsylvania. With the battle looming, Letterman faced problems he thought he'd solved in previous campaigns. Maj. Gen. Joseph Hooker, Burnside's replacement as commander of the Army of the Potomac, appeared to commandeer Letterman's ambulance corps wagons for his own supplies, tents, and manpower. The ambulance corps also lost access to rail transport and had most of its supplies sent to the rear of the battle formation, in lieu of ammunition and artillery transport. In Letterman's view, "this order would deprive the department almost wholly of the means for taking care of the wounded until the result of the engagement was fully known." What wasn't fully known, until the Ambulance Corps arrived on July 3, was that the battle had caused 22,000 casualties. And when "Camp Letterman" finally opened its medical-aid campsite about a mile from Gettysburg, the doctor who had so thoroughly reconfigured ambulance and hospital services in his army faced what he called "a field of blood, on which the demon of Destruction revelled."[35]

Nevertheless, in the middle of it all, Letterman's reorganized and rejuvenated medical corps soldiered on. Letterman's legion of ambulance corpsmen—some 650 of them—rushed to their field positions right behind the front-line fighting and led their ambulance crews through the next three days and nights, some of them fainting from exhaustion and overexertion.

"The ambulance corps throughout the army acted in the most commendable manner during those days of severe labor. Notwithstanding the great number of wounded, amounting to 14,193 . . . from my own observation . . . not one wounded man of all that number was left on the field within our lines early on the morning of July 4," Letterman reported. "The corps did not escape unhurt; one officer and four privates were killed and 17 wounded while in the discharge of their duties. I know of no battlefield from which wounded men have been so speedily and so carefully removed."[36]

Camp Letterman had attended not only to all of the Union wounded, but also to the Confederate, numbering 6,802; the total attended to was 20,995 wounded.

In January 1864, at his own request, Jonathan Letterman was relieved of his position as medical director of the Army of the Potomac, and his connection with the army ceased. He offered a summary of his feelings about the work completed in his *Medical Recollections of the Army of the Potomac*. He wrote that his time with the army had proven to be arduous and eventful, yielding friendships with the best and the bravest comrades on the road to restoring peace and the Union. "But whether the grass grows over them, or they are wanderers, far from the scene of their perils and victories," he concluded, "those who labored together with but one heart, in their country's hour of agony, will live among [my] many memories."[37]

In March 1864, Brig. Gen. William Hammond, the War Department surgeon general who had appointed Letterman to come up with logistical solutions for evacuating the wounded, shared the limelight with the "medical dictator." Petitions and lobbying efforts had finally moved Congress to establish a permanent ambulance corps in the US Army. The law authorized corps commanders to direct officers and enlisted soldiers to form ambulance organizations and ensured that boards of medical officers would search long and hard to find ambulance corps candidates to "at least equal the best of the fighting men in gallantry."[38] The War Department also issued a directive giving commanders the authority to create a distinctive ambulance corps uniform.

...

THROUGH THE NINETEENTH CENTURY and into the twenty-first, Jonathan Letterman's protocols have persisted. They dictated the way Second World War medical corpsmen evacuated a war zone in the Rhineland and they provided for the rapid high-tech removal of IED victims in the war in Afghanistan—with the equivalent of a surgical theatre at the flight surgeon's disposal.

It's safe to say that, innovative as he was, Jonathan Letterman could never have imagined Jody Mitic's evacuation from Masum Ghar; that scenario would have been beyond my father's comprehension as well. But it's just as unlikely that my father or Mitic were aware of how much they owed to Maj. Letterman's innovations.

CHAPTER THREE

"OUR PLOTS FILL UP RAPIDLY"

ONCE THE AXIS POWERS had unconditionally surrendered in Northwest Europe on May 8, 1945, and in the Pacific on August 15, most military outfits that weren't assigned to occupation duty packed up their veterans, invited some to join the regular force, and sent the rest back to civvy street to pick up where they had left off. Since most Allied nations were war weary, veterans didn't seem particularly interested in keeping up correspondence and staying in touch, much less preserving their combat experiences. My father's 94th Infantry Division of the US Army proved an exception; a surprising number of them decided to hang on to the outfit's wartime past. In 1950, survivors formed an association; they wrote up a charter, elected an executive, and staged memorials and reunions, the first in Boston (the division's birthplace was actually the Boston Army Base, in 1921), to keep the spirit of the 94th alive. They revived their wartime newsletter, *The Attack,* and made a conscious effort to gather artifacts, photographs, diaries, and correspondence as a living archive of the division's wartime record.

Along the way, the next generation got involved. Long-time association secretary Harry Helms noted that the original constitution of the 94th Infantry Division Association allowed only veterans as members. "You could only join if you were a 94ther," he said. "But with numbers dwindling, we created an alliance. We changed the name to the 94th Historical Society and allowed 94th family members to join."[1]

David Mitchell's second cousin, Raiden Winfield Dellinger, had served as a medical officer with the 94th. Eventually Dellinger began to share stories and the names of his comrades-in-arms with his young relative. Mitchell attended the reunions to listen to the veterans' recollections and, having won their confidence, to save some of their memorabilia. Mitchell, who calls himself a "hunter-gatherer,"[2] felt comfortable, if not driven, trying to keep the division's history growing and active. Then, following the premature death of his father, Martin Hardin "Buddy" Mitchell, David founded M.H. Mitchell, Inc., a non-profit organization to raise awareness of the state of Georgia's unique history. Among the projects the organization supported was a donation of the 94th Infantry Division Association archives to the Hargrett Rare Book and Manuscript Library at the University of Georgia in Athens (UGA).

"When my [son] was born in 2006, I realized these men weren't going to be around forever," he said in the association newsletter. "I needed to [ensure that] their legacy and their sacrifice is remembered."[3]

Connected to the 94th Infantry Division Association through my father's story, I accepted David Mitchell's invitation to explore the division's archival collection at UGA, seventy years after the first veterans began assembling it. Inside the atmospherically controlled reading room at UGA, I found data to give my father's medical corpsman experience some context—a third dimension, if you will. In roughly the same length of time as my father's medical battalion would have handled a thousand casualties during the Battle of the Bulge—about a week—I went through a thousand documents. I felt as if I were opening a family album featuring my father's brothers-in-arms, as well as the patients they treated during the toughest ordeal of the family's history.

During those days at the reading room, I pieced together the daily routine of the division's wartime trek from America to Germany and back. In the dozens of archival boxes I found memoirs by trainees who complained about the same food my father did. I read reminiscences by non-commissioned officers (NCOs) who'd shared cabins with him aboard the troopship *Queen Elizabeth*, bound for England in August of 1944, recalling the cramped conditions and lineups for meals. And from alphabetically arranged sleeves I carefully pulled letters written and mailed home, recounting the bitter cold, platoon mates killed in action, and the quick actions of the medics who treated their frostbite, trench foot, and battle wounds during those last pivotal months of the war.

SEPTEMBER 8, 1944—NORMANDY, FRANCE

T/Sgt. Alex Barris joined the liberation of France at Utah Beach on September 8, 1944, three months and two days after American GIs had begun the historic Allied invasion of

Normandy there. He saw plenty of evidence of the D-Day struggle of June 6: masts, funnels, and the bows and sterns of the wrecks of landing craft and Liberty ships sticking grotesquely out of the shallow water—what the official divisional war diary described as "spewed bits of military equipage." Beyond Utah Beach, my father's unit passed the obliterated or abandoned remains of the pillboxes, gun emplacements, firing pits, communications trenches, dugouts, and shelters that had once formed the defensive Atlantic Wall of Hitler's Fortress Europe. With Allied reinforcements and fresh machinery swarming everywhere, the beachhead seemed "a place of utter confusion."[4]

Nevertheless, my father's 319th Medical Battalion, attached to the 94th Infantry Division, landed in France with relative ease. For the next three months, their commanders assigned them to a holding action on the western coastline of France, preventing a pocket of some 50,000 German troops, cut off in the Brittany ports of Lorient and St. Nazaire, from escaping by land. The job of the 94th was simply to contain these two German garrisons. Restrained by orders against offensive action, the division's work was more like an occupation than a battle. American infantry and armoured groups limited their actions to combat patrols and artillery exchanges. Foot soldiers coordinated actions with tank units, and prisoner-of-war (POW) interrogation teams worked with military intelligence and photo reconnaissance to keep tabs on the Germans in the pockets. Occasionally the two sides agreed to an armistice to allow French civilians to evacuate or to exchange prisoners of war. For my father and his medical battalion, the war became comparatively routine. They even had time and materials to fashion more comfortable quarters they called "Brittany bungalows."[5]

"Some of us built huts out of scrap lumber to live in more comfortably as the winter drew closer," he wrote. "In our leisure time, we learned to drink Calvados, sometimes mixed with grapefruit juice. Some days we would get passes to Nantes, where most of us soon discovered the attractions of some of the numerous bordellos in the area. All of them were, of course, 'Off Limits' to Allied soldiers, a fact of which we were occasionally reminded by the MPs, when we ran into them in those same establishments. They, like we, were off duty."[6]

Three months into their "front-line" service "fighting" in Brittany, the corpsmen of my father's medical battalion had earned an additional leave; the respite marked a first in his life. He and a number of his NCO buddies received three-day passes to Paris. In the city of lights the GIs played tourists. They visited Napoleon's tomb at Les Invalides, took in the famous *Folies Bergère*, attended a production of Bizet's "Children's Games" at the Paris Opera, and took photographs of each other posing in front of the Eiffel Tower, but none of the snaps turned out because the film jammed in the camera. On the final night of his leave, my father returned to the hotel commandeered to house US Army troops in Paris in the lead-up to Christmas. To my father's surprise, the lobby was buzzing.

"You mean you haven't heard, Sergeant?" one nervous-looking private queried Barris. "The Germans have broken through in the Ardennes."

On December 16, Hitler had launched his breakout plan, *Unternehmen Wacht am Rhein* ("Operation Watch on the Rhine"), sending hundreds of thousands of German troops, backed by artillery and tanks, across the River Our and into the Ardennes. Their objective? To recapture Antwerp, Belgium. The sudden bulge in the Western Front line sent American commanders into a panic as they scrambled to find reinforcements to slow the German advance; the 94th would join the Allied response to the Bulge. Lt. Gen. Omar Bradley, commander of the US 12th Army Group, was eager to get the 94th away from Brittany and "into the big picture."[7] So was the commander of the US Third Army. Through the fall of 1944, Gen. George S. Patton had chased the Germans across former First World War battlefields all the way to the fortress city of Metz, France, on the western edge of the Rhineland, where the *Wacht am Rhein* offensive had begun. However, by early January 1945, Field Marshal Gerd von Rundstedt's Ardennes offensive was spent. It had ripped a forty-five-mile gap into the American and British front lines and penetrated formerly Allied-controlled territory to within four miles of the River Meuse, near Celles, Belgium. It stalled there just as my father's 94th Infantry Division was racing from Brittany to Reims, France.

Plans called for the 94th's four-hundred-mile trek northeast to take three days.[8] Those on foot boarded the boxcars marked *Hommes 40, Chevaux 8*, railcars that dated back to nineteenth-century warfare and could carry "comfortably" forty men or eight horses. Meanwhile, those in motor transport, including medical corps ambulances, rumbled through the ancient city of Chartres, on the outskirts of Paris, en route to an assembly area near Reims to join the rest of XX Corps, which the Germans had nicknamed Patton's "Ghost Corps."

"I was mostly conscious of discomfort," my father wrote of that cross-country dash. "No matter how stoically I tried to endure the chill wind and the cold K-rations and endless nights of blackout where no cheery fire was permitted, I was sure the whole business was insane and I wondered what the hell we were all doing there."[9]

On January 3, 1945, the US First Army counterattacked against the Germans from the northwest while Patton's Third Army advanced from the south, like a great pincer into the flanks of von Rundstedt's breakout. The Allied counteroffensive against the Bulge had begun. At the far eastern end of Patton's push from the south lay the so-called Saar-Moselle Triangle. Just beyond the apex of the triangle stood Trier, Prussia's first city. Between the eastern leg of the triangle (the River Saar) and the western leg (the River Moselle), the Germans had created a fortified defence zone, and along the base of the triangle a "switch position" extending from the original Siegfried Line (built on the east bank of the Saar during the First World War, and then strengthened in 1938 to stretch from the Netherlands to the Swiss border). This defensive triangle encompassed about thirty square miles of rolling, often densely wooded terrain that the Americans eventually named the "Siegfried Switch Line." Any aggressive action into this zone brought an immediate and violent enemy reaction. It was here—in the thawing and freezing, the advancing and retreating, and the living and dying within that Saar-Moselle Triangle—where the 94th spent its strength of 15,000 troops and sustained the majority of its 10,000 casualties.*

On January 6, trucks transporting my father's medical unit

---

* Consistent with other US Army infantry units deployed in the Second World War, the 94th Infantry Division was organized to create a relatively small but independent battle group. The division comprised three rifle regiments (301st, 302nd, and 376th), each made up of three battalions with rifle companies and heavy weapons companies. Attached to the division were one medium and three light field artillery battalions (390th, 301st, 356th, and 919th, respectively), the 94th Ordnance Light Maintenance Company, the 94th Signal Company, the 94th Quartermaster Company, the 94th Reconnaissance Troop, the 319th Engineer Combat Battalion, and the 319th Medical Battalion. Total strength: 14,253. When needed, the division could add anti-aircraft, tank, tank-destroyer, and chemical warfare battalions, and military police, growing its overall strength to 15,000.

and the men of the 301st Infantry Regiment, the leading contingent of the 94th Infantry Division, crossed a pontoon bridge over the River Moselle into the southwestern corner of the Siegfried Switch Line. Those troops and medics were the first of their division to step into Germany, but the only memory my father had of that New Year's was the cold. En route to the battle lines in front of the fortified town of Tettingen, transport drivers lost control on icy roads, sometimes skidding into ditches, while the steel floors and flimsy canvas truck coverings "sucked the warmth out of a man's feet, and woolen gloves proved inadequate."[10] Some of the first assistance T/Sgt. Barris and his medical squad administered was treating frostbite; in fact, they had neither the training nor the means to relieve such a malady.

Through the early weeks of the year, to the frustration of its commanders, the 94th's missions into the Saar-Moselle Triangle were restricted to holding and consolidating and testing the enemy's fixed defences, in some respects what the 94th had done in Brittany throughout the fall. Eventually their field orders were elevated to "limited-objective attacks . . . not to exceed one reinforced battalion"[11] in order to draw German reserve units into the battle and to inflict heavy casualties, wearing out the enemy to exhaustion. Call it what they liked, for the ground-level GIs and those units going forward with them—anti-tank specialists, mortar batterymen, engineers, and medical corpsmen—it proved to be their first taste of winter combat. Initially the Americans clashed with troops of Germany's 416th Infantry Division, which Allied intelligence claimed was at about 60 percent effective strength and had limited combat experience. That quickly changed, however, when the Germans moved their 11th Panzer Division (a.k.a. the "Ghost Division") into the Triangle. Suddenly Patton's Ghost Corps found itself facing the Germans' Ghost Division, with its proven strength in artillery, tanks, and shock troops. That left the 94th at a sudden and severe disadvantage, attempting to hold any gains in the Triangle with only men and anti-tank weaponry. In other words, unlike the 11th Panzers, the 94th had no offensive tank support and no air support.

And the challenge intensified. As foot soldiers of the US 376th attempted to take the villages of Nennig, Schloss Berg, and Wies in the western sector of the Triangle, and their sister regiment, the 301st, moved forward in the eastern sector toward Orscholz, the GIs in the advance quickly learned what defensive obstacles the Germans had laid in their way. Dragon's teeth (unending lines of concrete obstructions) and anti-tank ditches criss-crossed the terrain, making any attack with vehicles treacherous. Meanwhile, most open fields or clearings had been sown with anti-personnel *Schü* mines. Beyond those obstructions, the defenders relied on a network of pillboxes, bunkers, communications trenches, and field entrenchments for protection. And ultimately, from the high ground of the woods, German batteries equipped with mortars, anti-aircraft/anti-tank guns, and howitzers held a commanding view of the landscape should an enemy move against them. Some of these fortified areas had names on existing maps, such as Bannholz Woods and Campholz Woods, while another, because it looked like the head of a plumber's wrench, was nicknamed Monkey Wrench Woods. For my father and the medical corpsmen of his battalion, these fortified areas became notorious for other reasons.

In the morning hours of January 16, when Capt. George Whitman's F Company of the 376th advanced into Monkey Wrench Woods, his troops faced knee-high snow and then the challenge of crossing anti-tank ditches that were ten feet wide and equally deep. With the trench traversed, the company had to walk single file through woods where each tree appeared to be strung with a tripwire barely above the surface of the snow. Beneath the snow, waiting for any unsuspecting invader, lay booby-trapped explosives and anti-personnel mines. Whitman's group had entered a German position fortified by a dozen machine-gun nests and a below-ground hospital bunker three storeys deep. The surprise attack netted the Americans sixty-two prisoners at a cost of four lives, among them a company medic.

According to Whitman, during the advance, eighteen-year-old medical corpsman Bill Cleary came forward to attend to a wounded rifleman. Despite wearing a helmet clearly marked with a red cross, the corpsman was shot dead by enemy fire. In his first action in the Saar-Moselle Triangle, Whitman insisted Cleary's body be left where it fell so that all members of F Company moving past it would understand what American troops were facing. But combatants in the Battle of the Bulge soon learned that killing begets killing. Upon seeing Cleary's body, a squad leader in the company was so incensed that when he spotted two Germans with their hands in the air in surrender, he shot them dead.[12] A Browning automatic gunner in G Company, Guy Fisher, referred to the incident as his introduction to war. "This, God help us, is what is termed 'being blooded,'" he wrote. "We were coming of age."[13]

An equally grim scenario played out several days later at the eastern end of the Saar-Moselle Triangle, as the 1st Battalion of the 301st Infantry Regiment began its assault on the village of Orscholz. Already naturally defended by the topography—Orscholz sat atop a four-hundred-foot-high hill and was flanked by the steep, heavily wooded banks of the River Saar on one side—the village was further protected just below the hilltop by an arc of pillboxes a quarter-mile long. Infantryman Richard Bertz, of D Company, remembered officers sketching the objective in the snow the day before the attack. So as not to stand out against the snow-covered terrain in their "olive drab" uniforms, troops were ordered to camouflage themselves. Some used appropriated white lace curtains to do the job. Bertz tore up some bedsheets to cover his helmet and field jacket. He also packed an extra pair of socks, should his feet get wet. As the men formed up in the dawn, Bertz wrote, he could see crystals of snow glinting in the night air, and the snow, then about twelve inches deep, crunched loudly underfoot. The temperature was well below freezing, just above zero Fahrenheit.

D Company had barely moved a few steps down a grade leading to German trenches when rifle shots and machine-gun fire began kicking up the snow. As the men around him began to scatter, Bertz realized they were triggering anti-personnel *Schü* mines under the snow. Most of those spooked by the sudden chaos were the recently arrived Army Specialized Training Program (ASTP) replacement troops, including one who was carrying 81 mm mortar rounds in a backpack, just yards ahead of where Bertz had stopped.

"Turn around slowly," Bertz called out firmly but calmly to the ASTP soldier ahead of him.

With bullets still whizzing around them and wounded

members of D Company screaming for medics, the youngster surprisingly responded to Bertz's directions and calmed down.

"Turn around slowly in your own tracks," Bertz repeated. "Stay calm and we'll get out of this."[14]

The ASTP began stepping smartly into the already imprinted snow where he had stepped safely moments before; presently, both Bertz and the reinforcement reached cover safely. They were among the few fortunate ones. Later reports from the medical corpsmen showed that one of the advancing companies had sustained sixty casualties from anti-personnel mines in a matter of minutes. The remaining companies had scattered in the confusion and were fruitlessly seeking cover at the base of the hillside in front of Orscholz. All that day and into the night German artillery fired down on them, inflicting further casualties and killing one of the company commanders.

Medical corpsmen had a disaster on their hands. The incoming shells exploded in the treetops, sending piercing shell shrapnel and wood splinters down on unprotected troops below. Each time the platoon and squad leaders did a casualty count, more shelling made their totals obsolete. Even a captured pillbox gave little protection; several wounded GIs had frozen to death overnight, and eight others lay shivering on the concrete floor. After two days cut off, without ammunition and near death from the cold, the survivors of B Company, with others from Companies A and D—some 240 American officers and enlisted men of the 301st—surrendered.

If further proof of the deadly cold on that night of January 20, 1945, was needed, infantryman Richard Bertz saw it firsthand. Now in some safety back behind his own lines, Bertz sought some shelter from the elements. He spotted a sergeant brushing away snow between the treads of a disabled tank, where he curled up for the night. "With the first light of dawn the next morning," Bertz wrote, "the sergeant was found dead, frozen in the same bent-over position I'd last seen him in. A man pried him out with an iron bar."[15]

The frozen sergeant who'd been unable to find refuge from the cold or the combat symbolized—at least to some—the plight of the 94th in this horrendous winter campaign. Units of the division had been ordered to fight a limited engagement: in other words, to avoid a reinforced divisional assault. It had artillery support but was forced to advance without tank or air support. It now faced a formidable well-armed and well-entrenched enemy out there in the Triangle that had caused the surrender of a couple of hundred men of the 301st Regiment. And if the enemy didn't throw the Americans back, the bitter winter chased whoever was left into waterlogged and freezing foxholes. In this section of the Saar-Moselle Triangle, the water table lay only four inches below the surface of the ground; within a matter of three or four hours, an unbailed foxhole would fill with water to within inches of the rim. As a consequence, it was impossible for the men of the 94th to stay dry.[16]

The job of finding a solution fell, in part, to medics such as T/Sgt. Barris and his battalion. Somehow members of the 319th found empty buildings or farmhouses just behind the front lines. Away from the snow and cold, they established first-aid facilities where the wounded could be treated, but also heated spaces where GIs could find dry boots and shoes, sometimes hot food and coffee, and, if there were a cellar, mattresses to sleep on. These so-called hash houses provided medical assistance and at least momentary refuge from the fighting and the winter.[17] The watchwords for military medics in the Battle of the Bulge had become *move* and *adapt*.

AUGUST 1914—MONTREAL, QUEBEC

THE CONCEPT OF MILITARY MEDICAL adaptability, while not born in 1914, took on a unique shape as Canada joined Britain in the Great War. The dean of medicine at McGill University had seen his summer holidays interrupted that August of 1914. With past experience as an officer in the non-permanent Canadian Army Medical Corps (CAMC), Dr. Herbert S. Birkett realized that Canada would quickly become directly involved in the war in Europe. During the Boer War, he had witnessed the work of the Royal Army Medical Corps (RAMC) at Aldershot, England, and he foresaw the need for hospital accommodation in support of the British armies in France and Flanders.

Birkett sensed that Canadian expertise could deliver such support. He consulted his medical colleagues at McGill University, and together they forwarded an idea to the Canadian minister of militia and defence. They would assemble "a completely equipped general hospital, of 520 beds, officered by men from the staff of the Faculty of Medicine of the University, with the ranks including a high percentage of medical and other students, and with the nursing personnel selected from graduates of the Training Schools of the Royal Victoria and Montreal General Hospitals."[18]

In December, the War Office in London, England, finally reviewed the offer and acknowledged that Birkett's plan for a field hospital in France had merit. London informed Birkett that McGill would have the winter to prepare and would then embark overseas in the spring. Birkett began selecting his senior and junior officers—a who's who of military and medical experience in the country at that time. Lt.-Col. H.B. Yates, second in command to Birkett, had served as medical officer of the 3rd Regiment, Victoria Rifles of Canada, for seventeen years. Lt.-Col. J.M. Elder, who became the officer in charge of surgery, had served in the militia against Louis Riel, and for an additional thirteen years with the 2nd (Montreal) Brigade, Heavy Artillery. Lt.-Col. John McCrae, soon to become the field hospital's senior officer in charge of medicine, had earned the Queen's Medal in South Africa and was already serving on the Western Front in France as medical officer for the Canadian Field Artillery. Meanwhile, over the winter, the War Office wired Birkett to say all future general hospitals had to support 1,040 beds, a doubling of his original offer. With little time to consider the implications, he agreed.

Of course, the new requirement immediately put greater demands on equipping and supplying the planned Canadian field hospital—from scalpels to syringes, bandages to kit bags, and tents to surgery tables. But it also meant that those placed on the reserve list when the commitment was announced in the fall of 1914 could now expect an immediate call-up. If the size of the hospital had to double, so did its staff of doctors, nurses, and other ranks. Despite the pressure, McGill's medical school appeared ready and able, with men and women who had not only medical skills but also military experience.

There were, for example, twenty-six captains whose military medical credentials included service with the RAMC, the CAMC, the Royal Highlanders of Canada, the 17th Hussars, the Duke of York's Royal Canadian Hussars, and the Victoria Rifles of Canada, as well as seventy-two nursing assistants from the Montreal General and Royal Victoria Hospitals. Also stepping up were highly respected members of McGill's surgical and medical staff, including Majors W.H.P. Hill, A.C.P. Howard, J.C. Meakins, and E.W. Archibald.

"We have a very congenial crowd," Archibald wrote to his parents in the days before arriving at the front. "We are so well organized that we could start work at any time."[19] In contrast with others at McGill, Edward Archibald had little or no military experience. However, then in his forties, the seasoned surgeon had risen to prominence in a variety of medical fields well before his country called on him to serve at an army hospital in the Great War. Born in Montreal in 1872, Archibald initially appeared more interested in the arts than the sciences; he studied Latin and German and was fluent in French, graduating in arts from McGill with a gold medal in modern languages in 1892. But he immediately enrolled in the medical school, and graduated four years later. Along the way, at the University of Montpellier in France and in Edinburgh, he received traditional instruction in bedside manner. He completed his residency at Montreal's Royal Victoria Hospital and served as house surgeon there from 1896 to 1899.

One of Archibald's earliest bedside challenges actually involved one of his fellow housemen in the Royal Vic hockey club. The night before a key game, teammate Tom Graydon complained of a severe toothache. Following a shot of brandy and several attempts to remove the tooth while Graydon was seated in a chair, an impromptu dentist brought in some help.

"He called in two attendants, took me out of the chair, seated me on the floor, [and] placed one attendant on each leg. He stood up behind me and pulled," Graydon explained. "The tooth would not move. Finally, with the two pushing upwards and him pulling, he got the tooth extracted."

Trouble was, the stand-in dentist had yanked out the wrong tooth. So the process started all over again, with more brandy and a second extraction, this time removing the actual offending tooth. "I promised the young intern I would not say anything about the tooth extraction stunt," Graydon concluded, "as I was as much to blame as he was, and I kept my word."[20] The intern, of course, had been house surgeon Edward Archibald.

Though his skill set may not have included dental surgery, Archibald excelled in much else that would make him an ideal battlefield surgeon. He studied clinical surgery abroad, resolving that he should explore and research unknown territory while maintaining direct contact with patients' everyday needs. In 1901 he contracted tuberculosis; while recovering in a sanatorium, he began research on the debilitating lung disease that would continue for twenty-five years. As assistant surgeon at the Royal Victoria Hospital in 1904, Archibald learned from chief surgeon Sir Thomas Roddick about Joseph Lister's method of antiseptic surgery while attending to public patients two days a week.

Since surgical hospital staff received no salary, Archibald sustained himself by opening a private practice. Operating on ailments as varied as gunshot wounds, fractures, and vital organ diseases, he employed new surgical procedures and restorative medicine (analeptics) and even performed autopsies to widen his knowledge and better serve his patients. He became a workaholic, expanding the hospital's emergency service, leading tutorials with his medical students, and attending to patients in his office, all while he assembled his accumulated knowledge into presentations to medical societies and articles for journals of medicine; in the decade before the Great War, Archibald compiled twenty-five different papers, single-handedly developing "the whole of surgery."[21]

But the war forced him to apply his knowledge and skill to military medicine. At forty-three, citizen Edward Archibald joined 1,700 other volunteers enlisted in this mission by completing an attestation form, pledging allegiance to His Majesty King George V. So too did he receive his inoculation against typhoid, with the others at the Royal Vic and Montreal General. And overnight, assistant surgeon Archibald became Major Archibald with No. 3 Canadian General Hospital (CGH), as it was officially named on March 2, 1915. Meanwhile, any question that Canada's first field hospital for the war effort might not have community support was quelled as friends of McGill in Canada and the United States pledged to a fund totalling $25,598.10.[22] Within days of its official designation, No. 3 CGH received correspondence from Sir William Osler, a McGill alumnus and Regius Professor of Medicine at Oxford University in England. In the letter Osler quoted Alfred Keogh, director general of British Army Medical Services. "I hope that the McGill unit will not delay," Keogh wrote. "Everything points to our wanting them as soon as possible."[23]

On May 6, 1915, No. 3 CGH began its march to fulfill that

commitment. Following reveille at four o'clock that morning, the entire complement paraded outside its Montreal barracks, received inspection from Lt.-Col. Yates, and marched to the docks for embarkation. Well-wishers lined the parade route, the same one used by the 33,000 members of the First Canadian Contingent of the Canadian Expeditionary Force (a.k.a. First Canadian Division) when it had departed for overseas service the summer before. As they stepped in time through the streets, many of the field hospital volunteers sang the McGill fight song:

> Hail, Alma Mater, we sing to thy praise.
> Loud in thy Honour, our voices we raise.
> Full to thy Fortune, our glasses we fill.
> Life and Prosperity, dear Old McGill.

At the wharf, little time was lost as the Canadian Pacific Steamship *Metagama* welcomed all aboard. At 11 a.m. lines were cast off and a sea of handkerchiefs waved goodbyes as the sounds of the ship's engines and cheers from ashore and on deck mixed with the on-board band's playing of "O Canada" and "The Girl I Left Behind Me." In all, there were 1,700 Canadians aboard, including the 21st Battalion of the Canadian Expeditionary Force (CEF); Nos. 4 and 5 Stationary Hospitals, from Laval University and Queen's University, respectively; and No. 3 CGH, with an overall strength of thirty-three officers, 205 other ranks, and seventy-three nursing sisters, among them Sister Harriet Tuttle Drake. "I saw you until the very last, at the end of the wharf," she wrote to her sister Daisy later that afternoon. "I think that the people that went home this morning had the hardest time. Be sure not to pity us just yet."[24]

Harriet Drake was born in 1872, the third daughter of gold prospector William Wilson and his wife, Elizabeth Cronyn, in Salt Lake City, Utah. The family had travelled to the US western plains aboard the First Transcontinental Railroad. Harriet's mother taught school in the community, but she suddenly fell ill and was packed off with all three daughters for home in Simcoe, Ontario. En route east, at the home of relative John Drake in Michigan, Elizabeth died. The Drakes adopted the two youngest daughters, who remained in Michigan until Harriet was thirty-two, in 1904. That's when she emigrated to her mother's original home and took up nursing, graduating from the Royal Victoria Hospital in 1907.

Sister Harriet considered her acceptance into No. 3 CGH a most serious one. Barely settled aboard CPS *Metagama* that morning, she told her sister in that first letter that she had already begun attending to the soldiers. "I have been talking to two of the husbands I was asked by family to look after," she wrote. "[I] think I will look up two a day."[25]

Medical demands of a more serious nature tested the field hospital personnel en route to England. A day out of Quebec City, Lt.-Col. Elder operated on the gangrenous appendix of a young private with the 21st Battalion. Five days later, Lt.-Col. W.G. Anglin of No. 5 Stationary Hospital operated on a sergeant major, also with the 21st, who'd come down with appendicitis. There was one case of pneumonia and another of measles on board *Metagama* for No. 3 CGH to address as well. But the greatest life-and-death story during their crossing occurred just miles away, off the south coast of Ireland, where a

German U-boat torpedoed and sank the *Lusitania*, killing 1,198 of the ship's 1,962 passengers and crew. Early on the morning of May 15, when *Metagama*'s crew and company docked at Devonport on Plymouth Sound, Sister Harriet learned an axiom about the place and time she was entering—that truth was the first casualty of war. "[Please] save the clippings about the McGill Hospital," she asked her sister Daisy. "Will you mail me what the papers had to say about us being sunk? . . . It had been rumoured that the 'Metagama' had been lost."[26]

As No. 3 Canadian General Hospital dispelled rumours of its demise at sea, its medical personnel regained their land legs by assembling at the training camp at Shorncliffe, in southern England, and prepared for the Channel crossing in June. As some of its members enjoyed short leaves in London or a badger hunt on the property of Sir Arthur Markham, Lt.-Col. Birkett fought off a War Office suggestion to break up No. 3 and send its personnel to reinforce existing units in France. Meanwhile, Lt.-Col Elder visited the Royal Victoria Military Hospital and the British and Welsh Red Cross Hospital in Southampton, and Lt.-Col. John McCrae was officially installed as the officer in charge of medicine for No. 3.

Joining the hospital's staff as it prepared to embark at Southampton for France, McCrae had a chance to decompress and reunite with medical colleagues from Montreal—Bill Francis, Bill Turner, Edward Archibald, and Revere Osler, son of Sir William Osler. Now forty-one and therefore among the older volunteers in the CEF, McCrae had already served through the winter as brigade surgeon with the 1st Canadian Field Artillery. He instantly brought awareness of trench warfare, artillery barrages, and battlefield medicine from the front lines to share with his new officer subordinates at No. 3 CGH. McCrae had participated in the First Canadian Division's baptism of fire in Flanders. During the British advance against Neuve Chapelle, McCrae was attached to the Royal Artillery, guiding the evacuation of the wounded in a sector of the front plagued by flooding trenches, meagre sandbag protection, and murderous sniper fire from nearby woods. Despite the support of three hundred artillery pieces, the Allies had suffered 13,000 casualties.

"The wounded and sick stay where they are till dark, when the field ambulances go over certain ground and collect," McCrae wrote to his brother Tom. "A good deal of suffering is perhaps entailed by the delays till night, but it is dangerous for wheeled vehicles to go on the roads within 1,500 yards of the trenches . . . ."[27]

McCrae described coming upon a pool of blood around a wounded man and speculating as to the kind of impact the soldier had sustained from a bullet or an artillery shell, as well as the length of time he might have had to wait to be evacuated. In other correspondence, after describing his efforts to administer first aid or lifesaving surgery, McCrae wrote about his own clothes, boots, and kit being covered in the blood of his patients. He would look up for a moment and focus on the sight of the dead, the wounded, and the maimed all around him.[28] "Our Canadian plots fill up rapidly," he concluded to his brother.[29]

McCrae would watch things get worse. In April the Canadian units in Belgium joined the Second British Army, relieving French troops in what military strategists called "the salient," a semicircular protrusion eastward from the Western Front around the moated town of Ypres. The salient cut into the area opposed by the Fourth German Army. On three sides of the salient—to the north, east, and south—high ground on Passchendaele ridge gave the occupying German artillery the opportunity to bring enfilade fire down on Allied positions and the medieval town itself. German guns had open sightlines to prominent features in downtown Ypres, including its cathedral, its busy markets, and its Cloth Hall.

Elsewhere around Ypres, the countryside was flat, the ground composed of heavy clay, and the water table high, as evidenced by the network of irrigation ditches that criss-crossed the land in every direction. The farmland posed a number of logistical and, as it turned out, medical problems for the Allied armies attempting to defend it. Elevated roadways proved practical for transit in peacetime but presented hazardous exposure to enemy fire in time of war. As well, farmers in the region regularly fertilized their soil with manure of every type. And since most combat between the opposing armies occurred across those open farm fields, medics and doctors on both sides recognized that any open wound could quickly, and often fatally, become infected.

On penetration, a bullet or a piece of shrapnel likely carried with it dirt enriched for centuries by animal and human manure, tiny shreds of uniform made filthy by the same earth staining its fibres, and the outer layers of the victim's skin, made septic by bacteria-filled perspiration or louse infection from the trenches or barracks behind the lines. A witch's brew of infection awaited even the slightest cut or scrape. And field medics and surgeons were helpless to prevent it from becoming a death sentence.[30]

Pte. Bert Goose, a member of the No. 3 Canadian Field Ambulance, diarized about the helplessness he felt at his post. "[There were] 1,800 . . . put through inside 24 hours," he wrote. "Many of my chums have been through. The wounded came at such a great pace, it was a great job to attend them all. . . . Some awful wounds were attended to, gashes large enough to put your fist in, many came with bullet wounds, many poor boys will have to have their arms or legs taken off. Other poor fellows will never live to tell the tale."[31]

For five days in mid-April, the Canadian 2nd Brigade entered the former French trenches north and east of Ypres and began excavating. They dug, sandbagged, built up, cleaned up, and reinforced what had been little more than depressions in the soil and shell holes the French had used as latrines, refuse pits, and graveyards to bury their dead. As Allied troops all along that portion of the salient were about to discover, the Germans had been preparing too. In violation of the Hague Conventions of 1899, the Fourth German Army had brought forward canisters of chlorine gas to spearhead a planned advance against the north front of the salient. All that remained for German planners to unleash their deadly weapon was winds blowing in the same direction of the projected infantry advance. They arrived on April 21, and the historic German attack would occur the next day.

At the time, McCrae and his 1st Brigade of the Canadian Field Artillery were located at Poperinge, conducting exercises behind the lines, but they heard the increased frequency and intensity of German artillery on the afternoon of April 22. Coincidentally, one of McCrae's former students, Francis Scrimger, now a medical officer with the 14th Battalion of the Royal Montreal Regiment, was walking with George Nasmith, a chemist from Toronto and lieutenant-colonel now attached to No. 5 Canadian Mobile Laboratory. Looking northwest from their vantage point near St. Julien at about 5 p.m., Scrimger and Nasmith could see the vanguard of the German advance—a yellowish green cloud along a three-mile front rising a hundred feet into the air.

"[It's] the poison gas that we have heard vague rumours about," Nasmith noted. "It looks like chlorine and I bet it is."

"Probably is," Scrimger agreed.

"With perhaps an admixture of bromine," Nasmith added.[32] He had previously advised Allied commanders about the potential appearance of poisonous gas in the Germans' arsenal on the Western Front and had recommended the introduction of hyposulphite of soda and gas masks to protect Allied front-line troops. His warnings and his suggested antidotes had gone unheeded. The thickest concentration of the chlorine cloud crossed no man's land into the 45th Algerian (Colonial) Division and the 87th French Territorial Division, to the left of the Canadians. Some thought what they were seeing was simply a new form of gunpowder or a smokescreen to veil the advancing German infantry. To their left, the Canadians heard the guns of the French troops fading away; moments later, choking Algerian troops, gasping "Asphyxiate," staggered through the Canadian lines. The gas was settling into the French trenches and smothering the defenders. The chlorine would be on top of the Canadians momentarily.

Capt. Scrimger was one of the first medical men among Allied officers to concoct an impromptu way for front-line troops to survive the effects of noxious gases. He told the men of the Royal Montreal Regiment to "urinate on your handkerchief [and] tie it over your mouth,"[33] since the ammonia in the urine would crystallize and partly neutralize the chlorine.[34]

If they had time amid the confusion to witness it, the Canadians saw their French and Algerian comrades writhing on the ground, their complexions turning green as they gasped for oxygen. When mixed with the tears in their eyes, the chlorine gas formed hydrochloric acid, burning or blinding the men.[35] The poison in their bronchial tubes triggered the membranes to swell and increased blood flow into their lungs, causing the men to suffocate, drowning in their own fluids. Canadian artillery officer Andrew McNaughton watched in horror as the Algerians fled past him, "their eyeballs showing white, and coughing their lungs out."[36]

On the battlefield, the French army sector had been decimated, and although they didn't immediately recognize the extent of the annihilation in front of them, the Germans had opened up a mile-wide gap along the north edge of the salient. As many as 50,000 British and Canadian troops, along the south side of the salient, were in danger of being cut off. The gas technicians who unleashed the chlorine from the German front lines had been issued cotton pads soaked in a solution of potassium bicarbonate and sodium thiosulphate as an antidote to the poison gas. However, the advancing German infantry had no respiratory protection, no gas masks; their officers—prodding their troops with pistols and swords—assured them they'd be unaffected as long as they remained a safe distance behind the southwesterly flow of the gas. Consequently, their advance was more tentative than it needed to be. Still, the Germans moved onto Pilckem Ridge, an objective that had exceeded their grasp for months.

Meanwhile, the inexperienced Canadian troops shifted their defences to keep the Germans from flanking them from the left. The 1st Canadian Brigade, in reserve, joined the counter-offensive. While some of the German troops sensed the advantage and moved deeper into the salient, others, uncertain of the numbers of Canadians they were suddenly facing, entrenched themselves in French positions, unable to take full advantage of the breakthrough before Allied reinforcements arrived to halt the German advance.

The next day, the Germans launched a second gas attack against the positions that remained in their way, principally the Canadian ones. Again the waves of German assault troops advanced cautiously behind the wall of gas. Word had spread along the Canadian lines to use the urine-and-cloth method of defence against the chlorine; consequently, the advancing Germans—despite the effectiveness of the gas the day before—encountered Canadians still standing, partially blinded, gasping for air, some vomiting, but desperately firing their weapons against the oncoming German infantry. If nothing else, the Canadians' stubborn resistance at the Second Battle of Ypres temporarily neutralized the Germans' most hideous weapon of the war thus far. The same could not be said of the frantic rush to save lives at the aid posts and clearing stations behind the lines.

Two days earlier, stretcher-bearers and surgeons had faced an overwhelming tide of wounded. Hundreds needed gashes from bullets and shrapnel cleaned, dressed, and bound. The backlog of limb amputations was reminiscent of Civil War–era field surgeries. Suddenly field ambulances, regimental aid posts, and stationary hospitals faced a horror no one had imagined. James Walker, a member of No. 2 Canadian Stationary Hospital, at Le Touquet, France, described his frustration as the first all-Canadian medical staff faced a seemingly endless parade of gassed soldiers.

"Staggering, dumbfounded and stupefied, they were brought in, after having been conveyed from the ambulance train," he noted. "The effect of these gas fumes which wrought such deadly havoc is a noticeably watery running of the eyes. Later, the features become discoloured by a sort of green and yellow-ish hue. Many took the precautions to stuff handkerchiefs in their mouths. However, once too much gas had been inhaled its action has the same effect upon the lungs as a slow process of drowning."[37]

Attending to men in such condition had not been part of the Boer War, in which some experienced medical officers, including John McCrae, had served. And even the most contemporary medical manuals did not include poisonous gas inhalation. And so, to cope with men who flailed around on hospital cots or who gagged, choked, and vomited, some medical personnel simply resorted to placing damp cloths over their mouths. One patient who survived reported that the doctor had examined his throat and stuck needles up his nostrils.

At a casualty clearing station (CCS) manned by the Royal Army Medical Corps, a medical officer treated a Canadian soldier with the 15th Battalion, but the man died after two agonizing days. A post-mortem showed that "the body showed definite discolouration of the face and neck and hands. On opening the chest the two lungs bulged forwards. On removing the lungs there exuded a considerable amount of frothy light-yellow fluid. . . . The veins on the surface of the brain were found greatly congested, all the small vessels standing out prominently."[38]

John McCrae was an accomplished pathologist, but even he admitted that no medical school practicum had ever prepared him to treat such a malady, let alone cure it. Nevertheless, the experience at Second Ypres hardened his resolve. "We would be terrible traitors to the world and the future, if we stopped any time before the snake is scotched," McCrae wrote to his mother, Janet McCrae. "Germany has got to get a lot of lessons yet."[39]

Second Ypres had not only proven McCrae's worth as a field surgeon, it had also inspired him to write what he'd witnessed in letters, diaries, and poems. From his vantage point on the west side of the Yser Canal, he recorded the landscape in his journal (without revealing military secrets): "The Censor will allow me to say that on the high bank between [the road and canal] we had our headquarters. . . . Where the guns were I shall not say, but . . . all along behind us at varying distances, French and British guns: the flashes at night lit up the sky."

In the lee of that high bank, in a dugout he called a "square hole," McCrae fashioned a dressing station eight feet square, roofed to keep out the rain and sandbagged at the entrance to absorb artillery shrapnel. During the gas attacks, some of the fumes descended into trenches and depressions near enough to cause his eyes to burn and his breathing to be laboured. Sometimes his own troops, shot atop the bank above him, would tumble down in front of his dressing station, and he commented that even Montreal hospitals didn't possess that efficient a delivery service.[40]

But whimsy proved a rare commodity in front of Ypres, even

for an officer as hardened as McCrae had become. From his dressing station he had a clear view of the road parallel to the canal. The Canadians coined it "Devil's Corner"—with reason. Wounded infantry, supply trains, army mules, ambulances, and bicycle messengers took advantage of its relatively smooth surface, but they had to dodge German shelling, which too often for McCrae's liking "killed or wounded . . . straggling soldiers . . . horses, ditto, until it got to be a nightmare." Indeed, McCrae and his fellow medical officers worked day and night, weeks on end, processing 5,200 cases through the last weeks of April 1915,[41] Canadian batteries returning fire nearly shell for shell against their German battery foes. When it seemed things couldn't get any worse, at the beginning of May, Allied commanders consolidated their positions, realigning Allied troops cheek by jowl within the Ypres salient, consequently giving their enemy even more to shoot at.

On May 2, 1915, heavy shelling in the sector took the life of a young lieutenant with whom McCrae had served in the Canadian Officers' Training Corps in artillery in Montreal. Alexis Helmer was a McGill graduate, and his death cut emotionally deep wounds among his battery mates. When the shelling ceased, a couple of gunners excavated a grave as others gathered sandbags containing Helmer's remains, placed them in a blanket and pinned the ends and sides to approximate a body length for the burial.*

---

* When John McCrae completed his eulogy, incorporating extracts from the Church of England "Order of Burial of the Dead," a plain wooden cross was planted at the gravesite. Given the burial ground's proximity to the front line, many of the graves and their contents were lost during the remainder of the war. Lt. Alexis Hannum Helmer is commemorated on Panel 10 of the Menin Gate Memorial to the Missing, unveiled in 1927. He is one of 54,896 soldiers who have no known graves in the battlefields of the Ypres salient.

No chaplains were near enough to lead the funeral, so McCrae, reciting the Anglican service from memory, bid his friend farewell. Others attending the ceremony observed the pain in McCrae's delivery. It proved a seminal moment for a doctor seemingly numbed by the death around him. The morning after Helmer's funeral, Capt. Lawrence Cosgrave, who had studied with Helmer at both the Royal Military College and McGill, and who shared the Ypres salient dugout with McCrae, watched the colonel apparently lost in thought.

"While watching the grave from the dugout where he sat," Cosgrave wrote, "Col. McCrae admired the vivid red poppies that were beginning to bloom among the graves. . . . McCrae commented on the surroundings out in the battlefield and then went out and wrote 'In Flanders Fields.'"[42]

Cosgrave added that McCrae wrote the poem while seated in the back of an ambulance and completed a draft in twenty minutes. McCrae biographer Dianne Graves believes the poem, "written during one of the most bitter early battles of the war, enabled John McCrae to express his sorrow, anguish and desperate concern that the loss of so much life should not be in vain. . . . Its three brief verses captured the mood of the time and gave it a universal appeal that was to make it one of the best known poems of the Great War."[43] McCrae would rewrite the poem numerous times through the summer and fall of 1915, during which time he took a short leave to England, assumed his post as officer in charge of medicine with No. 3 Canadian General Hospital, and travelled with its entire staff back across the Channel to establish the facility at Dannes-Camiers on the northern French coast. Indeed, his No. 3 CGH colleagues knew of McCrae's skill with pen as well as scalpel, and together Lt.-Col. Birkett, Lt.-Col. Elder, and Maj. Archibald encouraged him to seek publication. The London magazine *Punch* would publish the poem anonymously in December of that year, but for McCrae's McGill medical comrades and their fledgling hospital, even the longhand version circulated among the Canadians provided additional focus and inspiration for their work tending the sick and wounded behind the Western Front.

"He looks very well and is just as jolly as ever. He says we're going to win by dint of having more fresh reserves," Archibald wrote of McCrae that spring in England. McCrae described the expeditionary force men as growing "exceedingly bitter. They cry, 'Lusitania,' and go right over [the Germans]."[44]

Showing more than just bravado in his comments and fervour in his poetry, however, McCrae offered Archibald and others with No. 3 insight as to the conditions among the wounded men they would soon face. He spoke about the impact that long exposure to repeated bombardment had on the front-line soldiers. He called it "shell shock"[45] and told Archibald that it "simply knocks a man right out, as regards his nerves, even if he's not hit. And the Germans are showing this break-up worse than we are; they frequently surrender in small groups."[46]

On June 17, 1915, the officers and staff—about 315 volunteers—of No. 3 Canadian General Hospital, as well as five hundred horses and mules for the Army Service Corps, sailed from Southampton aboard the small steamer *Huanchaco*. The Admiralty had loaned a pilot to steer the ship through a minefield and a boom of chains arranged to protect the harbour. Three destroyers, two submarines, and two hydroplanes escorted the small ship to the open Channel, where—under strict regulations of no smoking, no voices raised, and no torn paper thrown over the side—*Huanchaco* steamed for Boulogne, France, docking safely the next day.

Nearby in Etaples sat No. 1 Canadian General Hospital and several of the British general hospitals. Just inland, between the villages of Dannes and Camiers, stretched about a mile of sand dunes with fir trees and, adjacent to a railway track, an open stretch of flat land where the newly arrived Canadians found tents erected and hot meals waiting for them. Right away, several privates contributed to the welcome by constructing a McGill crest made of bricks, coal, and seashells in the dirt.[47] Within days, roads were built into the site. As well, 19 Neilson tents, 159 bell tents, and 55 marquees went up; each marquee had outer and inner shells with three feet of air space in between, and each could house 50 to 60 beds. Everything was fine until the wind picked up. "We eat dust. We have no tent floors yet and we live in our valises, (No trunks! They had to be left in England,)" Archibald wrote. "And a good many bugs crawl around and the flies are beginning to come."[48]

The meticulous newcomer may very well have counted the insects, so careful was he in his observations of life, the world, and attending to the wounded. He wrote letters to his parents and wife, Agnes, almost daily. He organized his case notes, assembled a book of medical notes, and even jotted down pithy quotations and aphorisms he might incorporate into his journals, conversation, or correspondence to Canada. Often in his longhand letters he would pine for home, or a bathtub, or just a day to lie in bed. But Archibald never shirked his responsibilities, once complaining he often waited to go into action "like a scalpel on a tray, waiting to be used by the operator when the time comes, and just keeping sharp."[49]

The preparation continued through the heat and dust of the summer. In July a chaplain reported to the unit along with a matron and more nursing sisters. Prime Minister Robert Borden paid a visit to inspect. Then British medical officials stopped by to ensure that No. 3 had a proper water supply as well as nitrous oxide gas for anesthesia. In early August more dignitaries dropped by—including Minister of Militia and Defence Maj.-Gen. Sam Hughes and Lt.-Col. Sir Max Aitken—not to mention officials from the neighbouring No. 25 British General Hospital, No. 1 Canadian General Hospital, No. 1 Canadian Stationary Hospital, and No. 2 Canadian Stationary Hospital.

On August 7, No. 3 rehearsed with dummy patients as if they were arriving in a convoy of ambulances. The staff had rehearsed everything scores of times. As patients arrived on stretchers or on foot, they entered the admission tent, where a sergeant and two orderlies processed them. Gathering details verbally or from a tag attached to the patient, the orderlies completed a hospital card to accompany the patient into the ward. At a diagnosis table there, two medical officers made a provisional diagnosis, designating the patient as medical, surgical, or special case. At the final table, the registrar assigned the patient to a vacant bed to await treatment. With this final rehearsal complete, No. 3 awaited its first patient. At 8:30 p.m. that same day, thirty-six wounded arrived. By nine all were processed, including a Pte. MacMutchkin.

"I was wounded in the Salient," MacMutchkin wrote in his diary. "I arrived eventually at No. 3 Canadian General Hospital and will never forget my reception. As I was helped out of the ambulance, the Colonel took my hand, then three lieutenant-colonels took my pulse, four majors hurried to take my temperature, and some blighter took my watch."[50]

The *Toronto Star* covered No. 3's initial days. When the facility was up and running, correspondent Britton B. Cooke was invited to follow patients from reception to recovery. In particular, Cooke noted that ambulance after ambulance arrived and that as fast as they did, the hospital organization absorbed every wounded man with skill and precision. He suggested that the operating theatre rivalled any he'd seen in the Toronto General Hospital (TGH) and reported the exchange between a conscious wounded soldier and the doctor in an examination room.

"Where's the trouble, old man?" asked the doctor as the new patient was lifted under the x-ray machine. "Thigh?"

The man nodded, and Cooke noted that the soldier's Adam's apple seemed to protrude abnormally as he swallowed nervously while under the device.

"Righto," continued the doctor. "Won't hurt you a bit."

And a nurse, a kind of second lieutenant in the room, brought two wrapped plates. Orderlies gathered around and lifted the wounded man until one of the plates was in position. Then the x-ray machine was moved into place.

"Time me for fifteen seconds," the doctor said to the nurse.

The wounded man's eyes grew big with wonder, Cooke wrote, as he watched a sort of blue lightning in the darkness. And when the nurse had completed the fifteen-second count, during which time the second plate had recorded a picture of the hidden shrapnel splinter, the current was disconnected and the patient taken out to make room for the next one.

"There is no better place—in fact no place as good as this—for gaining a real picture of a battle," correspondent Cooke wrote.[51]

Still, as precise as some of the science at the hospital seemed, some of its success relied on instinct. Like his comrade Lt.-Col. McCrae before him, Maj. Archibald learned the surgery of wartime medicine not only via its mechanics but also by way of judgment calls made over the patient on the operating table on the spur of the moment. He recognized that in many ways every surgery was new surgery. When he coped with wounds caused by sharp-pointed rifle bullets, he noted that they rarely caused serious inflammation of the wounded tissue; he called these "humane projectiles of war." The same with round bullets from bursting shrapnel. But when he faced wounds caused by rough, irregular fragments of casings from high-explosive shells, he noted that they carried infection from the injured man's skin or clothing into deeper, wider lacerations and resulted in more serious damage. He called the bulk of his work "shrapnel hunting,"[52] using x-rays (from the hospital's department of radiology) and probes to locate bits of steel embedded in a wounded man's body before attempting to take them out.

Searching for and removing shrapnel became a great deal more complex with head wounds. Archibald's medical casebooks reflected the new reality that most patients with "direct injury through the head" did not survive. Fragments undetected inside the skull may well have caused catastrophic injury and infection even before a surgeon attempted to intervene. From his own post-mortem work, Archibald concluded that the adhesions around parts of the brain that protruded into openings caused by fractured bones in the skull should not be disturbed while making repairs. He cautioned against lifting scalp fragments in surgery that might break the adhesions and increase the possibility of contamination deeper in the brain.

Well and good on paper. On the afternoon of September 22, Maj. Archibald attended a patient who'd taken shrapnel to the head; he had to find and remove a piece of shell from an abscessed brain cavity. The intricacy of the removal procedure attracted interest from all over the hospital, and fellow surgeons slipped into the operating theatre to watch their colleague at work.

"[Archibald] located the fragment with a telephone probe," the No. 3 war diary stated, "and after much difficulty, brought it gently to the surface."

When the fragment appeared and the doctor ably brought it out, an audible "Well done" circulated through the operating tent.[53]

"Fortunately, with our excellent x-ray work, the best in this camp, we get the fragments localized," Archibald wrote, "and nearly always we can go right to the spot."[54]

The Battle of Loos, France, brought the first great hospital-wide test for No. 3. On September 25, 1915, as the Anglo-French offensive on the Western Front began, the McGill hospital staff received orders to evacuate nearly all its existing patients in anticipation of a flood of new wounded. In three days they transported 290 patients to England, while increasing bed capacity—in corridors, in the reading tent, in the chapel tent, and with stretchers and straw palliasses (mattresses) everywhere—by 500 to 1,560 beds. Under a moonlit sky on the next night, a convoy of 243 wounded arrived; among them were members of the Gordon Highlanders, one dead on his stretcher and another dying soon after his arrival. It was the beginning of a week that saw 1,000 patients admitted and treated, and almost as many evacuated to England.

An orderly recorded the frenetic pace of the week as "a confusion to me of blood, gaping wounds, saline, and bichloride," while the surgical staff, including Maj. Archibald, performed more than thirty operations a day.

On one of the mornings after, Archibald wrote to his wife that he'd had a "tragic case . . . of sudden death while I was giving a man an inoculation of serum . . . and it affected me badly,"[55] but not so much that it completely dispirited him or blunted his drive to do better.

Archibald never ceased documenting the medicine that he and his colleagues practised under canvas. Recorded in his numbered army books were the names, ranks, and serial numbers of each injured soldier, as well as the date of injury, when the patient arrived at No. 3, what kind of wound the soldier had sustained, and, if possible, the man's final disposition. He noted where a bullet or shrapnel had entered and exited a man's body, describing the foreign body responsible. He noted treatment, nature of surgery, and if there were any complications. And he recorded post-mortems in the event of a patient's death. And if the data weren't complete in his medical files, they could usually be found in his letters home to his wife, as in the case of his unique use of a fellow officer's blood on October 25, 1915.

"Dear Girl," he later wrote Agnes. "I have had a splendid case yesterday and today—a man who very nearly died of a hemorrhage and I gave him blood from [Capt.] Bill Howell's arm, and have probably saved his life. He was almost gone.

It happened yest[erday] morning, and all day I stuck close to him. Today, he is fine and rapidly recovering."[56]

In his army book notes and in the letter home, Archibald explained that during a recent attack on the front lines, the soldier was shot through one leg. The intensity of the battle and the inability of stretcher-bearers to reach him meant he lay on the ground in no man's land for nearly twenty hours. During that time, the man took another bullet, this time in his other leg. By the time he was delivered by convoy to No. 3, he had lost an enormous amount of blood. Doctors operated on his wounds and he seemed to be recovering, but several days later he had a hemorrhage from one of the wounds. That's when Archibald patched him up again and tried an experimental transfusion of blood—certainly the first at No. 3 Canadian General Hospital—from a donor in the operating theatre to the patient on the operating table. "It's a comfort to realize that we were able to pluck one brand [from the fire] anyhow," Archibald concluded.[57]

C.A.W. Gallagher, a member of the hospital's orderly staff and an undergraduate arts student from McGill, wrote about the work of the hospital being "curative" as opposed to "preventive," since so many of their patients arrived coated in the thick yellow mud of Flanders. Gallagher and several of his classmates assisting at No. 3 reinvented the McGill University newspaper as the *McGilliken* and offered stories from the daily grind of hospital cases. Gallagher described the cosmopolitan nature of the patients from around the Empire—all classes, all accents, all irrepressibly cheery, no matter the circumstance. "One case I remember especially," he wrote. "A poor chap with about half his head blown in called over to me one evening, 'I wonder if I might have a drink? I think I could sleep better if I had one. I hope you don't mind me troubling you.' Can you beat that for a fellow who has been through so much and yet who expects so little?"[58]

The military personnel at No. 3 seemed to thrive amid their outdoor surroundings at Dannes-Camiers. Nursing Sister Harriet Drake wrote to her family that she adored residency in her "little bell tent," praising its comforts and pretty view of cornflowers and poppies nearby, "not withstanding the absence of trees." She added, "The outdoor life does wonders for me. The air is so good and we are practically out of doors all the time,"[59] the exception being when she and the other nursing sisters took their meals in the mess hut.

Right after the hospital arrived and built its tent city, Maj. Edward Archibald also waxed eloquent to Agnes about No. 3's outdoor setting. As well as the pleasantly warm days and cool nights, he did note, however, that locals had explained that the place where the hospital tents were pitched originally was "continuously under water during the winter, the soil being more chalk and clay than sand; we talk of transferring the tents up on the slope of the hill, but up there we'll get the wind at its worst."[60]

The winds and rains of autumn did indeed find them in mid-October. They had swept in from the ocean the same day as the first convoy arrived from Loos, but continued for days. The stormy weather ripped tent pegs from the soft ground and tore the outer and inner layers of the India tents and marquees, and then the downpours flooded several of the wards, turning much of the hospital grounds into a quagmire with mud knee-deep in places. Maj. Archibald, so often upbeat and capable of handling the stress, was coming undone along with his tent, "flapping in the wind with an awful row, like the sails of a ship in a gale. . . . I begin to be a bit tired of tent life under present conditions."[61] The dishevelled state of the hospital in the grips of an autumn storm and the frustration most of the staff felt in the resulting conditions around them was amplified in Archibald's next letter home.

"It's been raining here for a solid week," he wrote Agnes. "I am a bit depressed this morning. My hemorrhage case . . . to whom I had given blood twice . . . died this morning. I had had such hopes [for] him. And then, after a day and a half of decent weather, the rain came on again last night. Today is a dull gloomy grey, cold and raw and wet and of course with more mud. And the wards are so dank and dark. And another of my patients is getting worse."[62]

Infection—the plague of every medical team in a theatre of war to date—continued to haunt even the most aseptically diligent of No. 3 hospital personnel. A noted bacteriologist of the time pointed to streptococcus as "the greatest enemy of the wounded . . . by reason of its frequency and its tenacious resisting power."[63] Following the flurry of work in September and October—processing nearly 3,500 patients—Capt. L.J. Rhea, the officer in charge of pathology at No. 3, ran a check of cultures taken from the operating room floor, which staff had attempted to cleanse with turpentine, linseed, and kerosene. Rhea's analysis found no pathogenic bacteria. Nevertheless, the doctors reported secondary hemorrhages in patients, which Lt.-Col. Elder suggested in his diary came from organisms infecting the wounds. The resulting smells proved unbearable, and in some cases "the tissues are so rotten with infection that portions of muscle tissue can be removed by the handful." For the record, Elder, the officer in charge of surgery at No. 3, applauded his surgeons and staff for completing 450 operations in the surgical wards, resulting in 21 deaths. He concluded, "I have never seen [results] equaled in civil surgery."[64]

On November 1, 1915, after 136 days on French soil and 86 days receiving military patients, No. 3 Canadian General Hospital had officially passed muster. Its medical staff from McGill had processed an average of forty patients a day and performed an average of five surgeries a day (those numbers would treble and quadruple in 1916). They had managed to salvage more limbs than they amputated. They had examined thousands of blood, urine, fecal, sputum, and gastric cultures, fighting infection with as much hygiene in surgery and on the grounds as aseptic procedures allowed. And since they remained an outdoor facility, they had fought off the elements into the first frosts of autumn.

But the ground rules, as it were, changed almost with the turning of the calendar. On November 2 the nursing sisters staged a masquerade party for the NCOs and men. As the festivities celebrating the unit's success concluded, a fall gale blew in with a vengeance, bringing down the sergeants' mess tents and several staff sleeping tents, and ripped many of the ward tents to ribbons, leaving patients, doctors, and nurses literally out of doors. Seemingly unflappable, No. 3's Nursing Sister Harriet Drake recalled one of those stormy nights when the commanding officer, with chaperone at his side, made rounds to ensure the safety of his staff. He happened on a tent door flapping in the wind.

"Sister, don't you want your tent closed?"

"No, thank you, sir," a sleepy nurse's voice came back.

"Sister, don't you want to be laced up?"

"Not at this time of night," came the reply.[65]

Sister Harriet soldiered on, saved by a pair of rubber boots borrowed from a soldier, along with donations from home, including "Mrs. Johnstone's bed socks, Mrs. Phillips's pillow, and Mrs. McMaster's slippers. I wear them constantly."[66] As stoutly as they pretended to take the daily grind, nearly all the medical personnel at No. 3 felt the tension of the first months in operation and the November gales that had nearly blown their facilities away. Fatigue had even overcome now veteran hospital surgeon Edward Archibald. Following the gales, the hospital learned that its second in command, Lt.-Col. H.B. Yates, had come down with bronchitis and was invalided to England; he died just weeks later.

Archibald—always prepared and ever able—was suffering. "We have been losing more of our patients than we did at first, and losing some that we hoped to save, and that too takes the starch out of me," he wrote to Agnes. "I want to get away from seeing brave men die—mere lads, many of them. It's terrible. After I get back, I shall be content to see some of my patients die, whose time it is to die.

"I thought I could bear the sight of death easier than with the hospital at home. I find I can bear it less. It is all so undeserved, so untimely, so contrary. It's a case of lockjaw, following on trifling wounds, that is hurting. He ought to have got his injection of anti-tetanus serum before he came down from the front, and he did not. . . . We have worked hard over here. But it seems useless."[67]

On January 3, 1916, No. 3 received orders to relocate indoors at the Jesuit College in Boulogne, providing respite for the challenges ahead.*

---

* Two years on, No. 3 Canadian General Hospital continued to treat Western Front wounded—thousands every month. Meanwhile, No. 3's experienced pathologist, John McCrae, had moved on; by January 1918 the First British Army had appointed him consultant physician, the first Canadian so recognized. That same month, McCrae contracted pneumonia and meningitis at No. 14 British General Hospital in Wimereux, France, where he died at age forty-five.

CHAPTER FOUR

"DO SOMETHING ABOUT THOSE SLACKERS!"

MY FATHER NEVER EXPECTED he'd come face to face with General George S. Patton, the commanding officer of the army in which he served during the Second World War. But it happened, in a manner of speaking. Alex Barris, a lowly sergeant in the US Third Army, met "Old Blood and Guts" in much the same fashion as depicted in the 20th Century Fox biopic released in 1970. The circumstances were eerily similar. The tone of the general's speech was much the same, and it contained a lot of the same expletives and phrasing as his pep talk to the US 6th Armored Division did, just ahead of D-Day. "No bastard ever won a war by dying for his country," Patton had begun his oratory on May 31, 1944. "You won it by making the other poor dumb bastard die for his country."[1] Patton was notorious for speaking his mind in such commentaries. But the one he delivered to the US Third Army eight months later, on January 30, 1944, certainly stuck with my father, especially because Patton was ultimately my father's commanding officer.

...

JANUARY 30, 1945—VECKRING, FRANCE

IT WAS NO SECRET that General George S. Patton could be a prickly commander if he didn't get things his way. With battle-field credits that stretched all the way back through the liberation of France, Italy, and Sicily to his first invasion success at Casa-blanca in North Africa in 1942, few could argue with his record of victories. Still, none of the good press about his battle honours could completely expunge Patton's infamous outbursts—slapping and verbally abusing two army privates during the Mediterranean campaign in 1943, when the men were apparently recovering from battle fatigue.* At the end of January 1945, "Old Blood and Guts" himself faced frustrating times. Gen. Dwight D. Eisenhower and Lt. Gen Omar Bradley seemed unsympathetic to Patton's plans to accelerate the Saar-Moselle Triangle campaign; what's more, they appeared to deny him access to further armoured support when he felt he could finish the job in Saar-Moselle and take the war to the Germans in the Fatherland.

Undaunted, Patton launched a tour to meet and address officers in his command, including members of the morale-depleted 94th Infantry Division. In their case, the general ordered an outdoor briefing at Veckring, about seventy miles to the rear of the front line in France. Barris, as a technical sergeant in the medical corps, was rounded up in a kind of dragnet to be part

---

* On August 3, 1943, at an evacuation hospital in Nicosia, Cyprus, Patton slapped and verbally abused Pte. Charles H. Kuhl, who was recovering from battle fatigue. On August 10, in similar circumstances, he slapped Pte. Paul G. Bennett. Following each incident, the general ordered the men back to the front lines and further issued orders to his subordinates to discipline any other US soldier complaining of similar difficulties.

of that ready-made audience for Patton. He remembered being hustled into a small valley, a natural amphitheatre full of colonels, lieutenants, and NCOs like himself, maybe 3,000 men in total. Four or five reconnaissance planes circled overhead, providing some sort of cover for what was about to happen on the platform holding a stand of microphones in front of the men. Fifteen minutes after all were present, a Jeep arrived with Patton standing erect, the sun glinting off his helmet and the pearl-handled revolvers he wore on each hip. He strode from the Jeep directly to the mic and, unintroduced, he spoke.

"You are soldiers in the United States Army," my father recalled him barking in a rather high-pitched voice. "When we take a piece of goddam land, it's the goddam property of the United States. And the way to take it, goddam it, is to get in there and stick 'em in their goddam guts. You don't win a goddam war by letting the sons of bitches push you back. [I] don't want any yellow bastards in this army giving up a goddam inch to the sons of bitches we're here to kill. It'd be better if the goddam cowards disgracing our uniforms were killed rather than be allowed to go back to America to breed another generation of yellow bastards . . ."[2]

About an hour later, when he was finished berating the assembled officers and NCOs, Patton retraced his steps to his Jeep and, again standing next to the driver, swept past a dumbstruck audience. My father recalled that as the general exited the amphitheatre he made "no attempt to meet the eyes of any of his fascinated spectators, but stared straight ahead, as if he were there only to be seen, not to see."[3]

The Veckring rant appeared to be the equivalent of slapping those two privates during the Mediterranean campaign in 1943—an attempt, perhaps, to embarrass the 94th's officers into better performance. In effect, he was shaming them all—commanders, infantry, corpsmen, everybody—as malingerers, idlers, cowards, and non-patriots. In private meetings held with Maj. Gen. Harry J. Malony, CO of my father's infantry division, Patton came close to relieving the general of his command, because, among other things, Patton claimed that the 94th was the only division in his army whose non-battle casualties exceeded its battle casualties. Patton had either been given misinformation or failed to recognize that the non-battle casualties—troops hospitalized with frostbite, trench foot, colds, fevers, pneumonia, and other debilitating side effects of endless days and nights outdoors in harsh winter conditions—were the fault of the Third Army command itself.

When word of Patton's diatribe trickled down to the rank and file, men such as the corpsmen and front-line soldiers felt betrayed and hung out to dry. Since the 94th had arrived at the front lines in the Saar-Moselle Triangle in early January, Patton's Third Army quartermasters had failed to supply its 94th Infantry subordinates with the appropriate winter fighting gear—insulated battledress and boots—or any kind of shelter. Such obligations were apparently not high on the general's priority list; when Patton wrapped up his meeting with Malony on January 30, he left these parting words: "You're doing fine otherwise, but goddammit, do something about those slackers!"[4]

It appeared Patton was blaming the effect and not the cause of the 94th's sad state. In three weeks of sustained but tentative attacks during the coldest winter of the war, the Ghost Corps had advanced in all sectors along the base of the Saar-Moselle Triangle. American intelligence showed that the 94th, despite being hamstrung, had reduced the Germans' panzer troops and armour effectiveness by as much as 50 percent. But casualties proved equally horrendous on the American side. On January 25, an attack against the German high-ground stronghold at Schloss Berg cost the life of a company captain and left a second lieutenant in command. As was often the case in this campaign, by day's end it was privates leading squads and sergeants leading platoons.[5] The war as viewed by those closest to ground level often looked vastly different from the war the generals saw.

JULY 21, 1861—BULL RUN CREEK, VIRGINIA

NURSES IN THE MIDDLE of American Civil War battlefields recognized that contrast too. One nurse attending to an artillery unit recorded in a diary that the day broke bright and clear, "bringing the two contending armies in plain sight of each other."[6] On one side of Bull Run Creek, near Manassas Junction, Virginia, just twenty-five miles from Washington, DC, the nurse with the 2nd Michigan Volunteers noted that the Confederate troops—some 20,000 of them—had dug themselves into high ground atop the southern bank of the creek. They had also felled trees to allow their gunners a clear view of Union troops—numbering 35,000—approaching from the north. When the 2nd Michigan settled into its place on the line in front of Bull Run, Franklin Flint Thompson, aged twenty, dismounted with the other Federal Army nurses and prepared their standard first-aid equipment: a haversack of lint, bandages, adhesive plaster, a water canteen, and, in some cases, a flask of brandy. Moments later, a Southern battery across the battlefield announced the start of engagement, and Nurse Thompson recorded impressions of the first major battle of the Civil War. It was July 21, 1861.

"A shell burst in the midst of the battery, killing one and wounding three men and two horses," Thompson wrote. "I stooped over one of the wounded, who lay upon his face weltering in his blood; I raised his head, and [saw Willie L.] was mortally wounded in the breast, and the tide of life was fast ebbing away."[7]

This scene was a microcosm of the way opposing armies clashed in the Civil War. Thompson's diary noted that nothing could be heard over the explosions of artillery shells, the clashing of steel swords and bayonets, and the ceaseless roar of muskets. The nursing group suddenly had its hands full. Only a junior nurse, Thompson was immediately sent to retrieve fresh supplies at Centreville, seven miles away. The nurse returned to a field of dead and dying soldiers and was next told to gather empty canteens, dash to a nearby spring, and deliver water to the wounded, who were by then ravaged by thirst. Thompson was haunted by images of a field of men flailing and shouting, limbs torn and mangled, bodies crushed and lifeless, and the ground stained with blood everywhere. As a Federal Army colonel dashed along the lines of the remaining Michigan troops, encouraging them to re-enter the fight, he was, to Thompson's horror, shot through the heart; with no time to carry him off, "we folded his arms across his breast, closed his eyes, and left him in the cold embrace of death."[8]

Back at Centreville, Thompson and the other nurses sought

refuge in a stone church, seconded by Federal medical staff as a field hospital. Outside the building, bodies, arms, and legs lay in heaps, while inside surgeons carried out amputations and impromptu suturing among rows and rows of wounded; the junior nurse counted twenty-one extracted musket balls lying beside the operating tables. With no skill as a surgeon, no haversack medical supplies left, and little water to dispense, Thompson could do little more than provide consolation, as illustrated in the diary when a wounded soldier lying on the floor beckoned the young nurse.

"What can I do for you, my friend?" Thompson asked, suddenly realizing it was the same Willie L. so horribly wounded in the chest at the start of the battle hours earlier.

"I wish you to take that," the man said weakly, pointing to a small package sitting beside him. "Keep it until you get to Washington, and then, if it is not too much trouble . . . write to my mother and tell her how I was wounded, and that I died."[9]

When Thompson drew nearer, the wounded man put his hand to his head to try to separate a lock of his hair with his fingers to send to his mother with the package. The two nodded in understanding, and as Thompson complied with this last request, the chaplain arrived and prayed for the man. Moments later, he died.

Thompson's diary, published in 1865, offered post–Civil War America extraordinary insights into the perilous life of a nurse on the front lines, from the First and Second Battles of Bull Run to Antietam and the Peninsula campaign, to Fredericksburg and beyond. Thanks to Thompson's vivid personal accounts of medical assistance given on now-famous battlefields and in Union hospitals, readers had probably never felt closer to the life-and-death struggles of soldiers wounded in war, unless they had experienced them first-hand.

But the memoir, *Nurse and Spy in the Union Army*, does not credit Franklin Flint Thompson. Following the subtitle— *The Adventures and Experiences of a Woman in Hospitals, Camps, and Battle-Fields*—it names the author as Sarah Emma Edmonds, a veteran of the American Civil War who, it was later learned, had successfully maintained two identities throughout the war, one as a woman, another as a man. Edmonds had ful-filled wartime service to the Union Army as a nurse, a soldier, and a spy. It wasn't until twenty years later that she admitted to deceiving her way into the army as a man.

What's more, Nurse Thompson, actually Edmonds, wasn't American. One of six children, she was born in 1841 and raised on a farm at Magaguadavic, New Brunswick, in eastern Canada. In that rural environment, Sarah became very com-fortable shooting firearms, riding on horseback, and, thanks to her mother's home remedies, attending to illness and inju-ries in the country.[10] However, when her father arranged for Sarah to marry a much older farmer, she ran away to the US; she settled in Connecticut and into a career selling Bibles.

In 1860 she moved to the Midwest, and the next year, when war broke out, she presented herself—disguised as a man adept in basic medicine—to a recruiter with the 2nd Michigan Volunteers. Since the entry medical exam tested enlistees only for basic vision and hearing, she passed easily, and when she notified the recruiters of her first-aid skills, she became a field nurse under the name Franklin Thompson.

Both she and the 2nd Michigan Volunteers with whom she served experienced their baptism of fire at Bull Run. For the next four years, Edmonds as Frank Thompson managed to navigate her way to the heart of a Federal Army regiment. She earned its trust as a nurse under fire, as a dispatch rider running messages to commanders along the front line, and later as a spy infiltrating Confederate strongholds in disguise—dyeing her skin, wearing wigs, and masquerading in men's clothing. At different times she impersonated an African American, a peddler, and a laundress, all to gather Confederate documents and military strategy.

In the final pages of her memoir, Sarah Edmonds paid heartfelt tribute to Civil War nursing, and in particular to the woman who "twists up her hair in a 'cleared-for-action' sort of style, rolls up the sleeves of her plain cotton dress, and goes to work washing dirty faces, hands and feet . . . writing letters for the boys or reading for them, administering medicine or helping dress wounds. And everything is done so cheerfully that one would think it was really a pleasure instead of a disagreeable task."[11] The memoir sold more than 175,000 copies, and Sarah Edmonds donated all proceeds for the relief of those wounded at the front.[12] To raise more money for a home for Civil War veterans, she wrote a second book and applied for a pension for her years of military service; but because records concluded that the "disappearance" of Franklin Thompson was due to kidnapping, death in action, or desertion, she had to campaign to prove her male identity. It took a government bill in Congress in 1884 to secure her a full soldier's pension, the only woman to receive such an honour at that time.[13]

. . .

APRIL 25, 1915—YPRES SALIENT, BELGIUM

SARAH EDMONDS HADN'T SEEN WAR up close until Confederate shells burst around her at Bull Run; Francis Scrimger didn't get his introduction until he arrived at an advanced dressing station (ADS) near Wieltje, Belgium. There, on April 22, 1915, he and fellow officer George Nasmith witnessed the Fourth German Army unleash poisonous gas against Allied troops in the Ypres salient. Even though his ADS was more than a mile from the creeping noxious gas, Scrimger, recently recovered from bronchopneumonia, soon felt his eyes tear up and his throat grow raw from the chlorine fumes. The following day, as both the German and Canadian sides dug in, then evacuated[14] and then dug in again, the front line became disorganized, putting added pressure on infantry and medics. According to protocol early in the Great War, the wounded went from front-line trenches via stretcher-bearers to regimental aid posts (RAP), farther back via wheeled stretchers to advanced dressing stations, and finally well to the rear of the fighting via motor ambulance to casualty clearing stations. That was the prescribed procedure.

On April 23, however, when Scrimger caught up to his 14th Battalion, Royal Montreal Regiment, he made his first foray into the front-line trenches to try to administer first aid to the wounded there. He noted that the trenches were muck-filled and abnormally warm. The odour of cordite from spent shells and even some leftover chlorine fumes filled his nostrils. And when the sun set, there was an enforced blackout all along the line, with no cigarette smoking in the trenches' exposed gaps. All the soldiers deployed here were hunkered down and speaking in low voices. For the thirty-four-year-old doctor, attending the wounded under such conditions seemed a long way from prescribed procedure.

"I was able to dress five badly wounded men under shrapnel fire without getting hit," he wrote in his diary, remembering in particular, "the sound of shrapnel is very nasty. It comes with a wicked swish and sing. . . . I got rapped on the heel by a [piece of] shrapnel this afternoon, and thought my time had come several times, but was able to dress a number of cases—too many—one wound through the brachial plexus; during the dressing, shrapnel landed three times in the lee parapet."[15]

Born in 1881, the second son of a Presbyterian minister, Francis Scrimger grew up in a modest and religious home in Montreal, but he didn't hear the call that his brother Tudor did to follow their father into the clergy. Instead, Francis studied violin, enjoyed learning to speak French, and graduated with first-class honours in biology at McGill University. About 1900, during a summer vacation, he joined a geological survey in Manitoba. As his summertime commitment wound down, the cook in the party fell ill with what was believed to be either typhoid or appendicitis.[16] Francis volunteered to stay behind and nurse the cook until he recovered. Francis came home suddenly intent on pursuing a career in medicine. In the first decade of the new century, Scrimger studied under such McGill luminaries as John McCrae and Edward Archibald, then spent four years at Royal Victoria Hospital and got his introduction to military medicine with the 2nd (Montreal) Heavy Brigade. When the Great War began, he joined the first contingent of the Royal Montreal Regiment and crossed the Atlantic with the First Canadian Division in October 1914.

Now in his first active command, in charge of the 14th Battalion's advanced dressing station, Scrimger faced challenges they'd never considered in basic training camp back at Valcartier, Quebec. At the Wieltje ADS on this particular April night in 1915, he had only six stretchers available to him, as several had been broken or lost. But that didn't matter, since the enemy shell and machine-gun fire seemed relentless. That meant no stretchers going out, no wounded being picked up, and none being evacuated farther back to casualty clearing stations. With nothing moving, no bearers were coming forward to replenish dwindling medical supplies either. Scrimger attended around the clock, with whatever he had on hand. In fact, he wrote in his diary that he'd worked forty-eight hours straight without sleep and hadn't noticed.

By his third day at the front, when shelling let up, Scrimger had moved back to brigade headquarters, where he finally managed to catch a few hours of sleep. He was probably wakened by the German reconnaissance aircraft that swooped low overhead, because he recalled that shortly afterward more enemy artillery shells and gunfire were suddenly pouring into their position. But Scrimger didn't have time to worry about it; he was on the move again to an advanced dressing station—just behind the front line that his battalion was holding—in a farmhouse nicknamed "Shell Trap Farm."[17] The place would quickly live up to its moniker.

The ADS farmyard consisted of an abandoned house and a dugout barn surrounded by a water-filled moat. One narrow roadway provided the only way in or out at ground level. But travel on the road proved too hazardous; it was well within the range of German guns, and any movement on the road immediately drew fire. A stretcher-bearer party sent down the road toward St. Jean had been lost in one German barrage.

On April 25, when enemy shelling intensified, Scrimger—as the senior officer on site responsible for thirty to forty personnel and wounded—decided the position was no longer tenable. He gathered the wounded in the safest room of the barn to await a nighttime convoy of ambulances. Among the wounded was Harold McDonald, a captain with the 3rd Infantry Brigade; he had been hit in the neck and shoulders. Moments after Scrimger dressed McDonald's wounds, a German shell hit the building and set it ablaze. Everyone had to vacate the barn on the double or be lost, and the only safe way for the wounded to escape was to crawl out of the burning building, slip down the sides of the moat, and swim to safety on the far side.

"The staff were forced to abandon the building [to] leave me there as an apparently hopeless case," McDonald told a reporter later.[18]

"I got the wounded out," Scrimger wrote in his diary, "among them a staff officer."[19]

"Scrimger carried me out and down to the moat fifty feet in front, where we lay half in the water," McDonald continued. "[He] curled himself 'round my wounded head and shoulder to protect me from heavy shell fire."

Scrimger later noted in his diary that the Germans poured in seventy-five six-inch shells, five of them within fifteen feet of the spot where he and McDonald lay hunkered down on the bank of the moat, and "we were half smothered in mud."

"[Scrimger] stayed with me until the fire slackened," McDonald said finally, "then the stretcher-bearers carried me to the dressing station."

With the Second Battle of Ypres ongoing and the tenuous situation all along the Ypres salient for weeks after the evacuation at Shell Trap Farm, it's little wonder that neither man considered the events of April 25 again until Col. R.E.W. Turner, of the 3rd Canadian Infantry Brigade, assembled the troops, including Capt. Scrimger's No. 2 Field Ambulance, behind the lines. It was raining that June day as Turner announced that Capt. Francis Scrimger would be awarded the Victoria Cross for his actions, including the evacuation of the wounded at the barnyard advanced dressing station near Wieltje.

When he heard the news, Scrimger's former teacher and now comrade-in-arms Edward Archibald tried to explain the man's actions: "Scrimger's behaviour during this time is not to be explained merely as that of a brave man rising to the occasion. It was a revelation of another side of his character," Archibald wrote. "There is in him a rigidity, a fixity of purpose which made him inexorable in going through with anything he had made up his mind to do. Nothing inspired him to effort like opportunity or difficulty. The German army might try to prevent him from doing his job; he would go on with that job until he had finished it or been blown to pieces."[20]

During the summer of 1915, Scrimger went on leave to England, to Windsor Castle, to receive his Victoria Cross. Remarkably, when the modest recipient of the Empire's highest military award emerged from the ceremony, he bumped into none other than Harold McDonald.

"There he is!" said McDonald, who was seated at a restaurant, in the midst of an interview with a reporter. "The man that saved me!"[21]

The reporter invited Scrimger to join them and got the scoop of his life—not only the story of a soldier-in-peril saved, but also of the medic-in-peril who saved him. They had both lived to tell the tale.

SPRING 1915—
THE ROAD FROM PARIS TO BOULOGNE, FRANCE

THE ACTIONS OF MEDIC FRANCIS SCRIMGER at Shell Trap Farm in Belgium exhibited the "fixity of purpose" of a medic bent on saving one life. The innovation of medical officer Cluny Macpherson behind the lines in France illustrated his dogged efforts to save many.

On an evening in late April 1915, a Daimler staff car and three touring automobiles threaded their way through military traffic moving away from the Western Front. The four British motorcars whizzed past the slower vehicles as if life depended on their quick passage. It did. At the steering wheel of the Daimler, on loan from the British War Office, was the thirty-six-year-old principal medical officer of the 1st Newfoundland Regiment. Capt. Cluny Macpherson pressed his four-cylinder automobile as much as he dared, given the lumbering wartime traffic around him and the top-secret cargo piled in the motorcar's front and back passenger seats.

"It was a real cutting-out dash," Macpherson wrote later. "[I] had [ten] great rolls of Tri-acetyl-cellulose film, each [roll] one-by-one-hundred metres long packed in wooden cases."[22]

Barely out of Paris and heading toward the seaside port of Boulogne, one of the three touring cars began to sputter. The chauffeur signalled to Macpherson that his vehicle wouldn't be able to continue and pulled off the road. Rapidly and gingerly, the medical officer in charge of this mini-convoy orchestrated a transfer of the cargo from the disabled car, redistributing the boxes equally between the other two touring cars. Not much farther along, another of the cars broke down; Macpherson took its wooden boxes and added them to his already laden Daimler. Darkness didn't slow the convoy, but the weight of the boxes full of precious cellulose eventually proved too much for the third car. It too pulled to the side of the road. With no space left in his car, Macpherson made specific note of the breakdown location of the third touring car, instructed its driver to remain with the vehicle to keep its contents secure, and carried on into the night.

"I made all haste for the coast in the Daimler," Macpherson wrote, "stopping only at Abbeville about 2 a.m. to wake up transport depot [staff] and have a lorry sent back to pick up the cases from the disabled touring car."[23]

At that hour of the morning, Capt. Macpherson faced a nearly impossible task. First, he needed to persuade the NCO night guard at the British ordnance headquarters in Abbeville to wake his superior officer to hear the plea of an Allied captain wearing Newfoundland Regiment insignia, which he'd likely never seen before. And then he had to convince that ordnance CO to dispatch an empty truck back down the road into the Norman countryside in the middle of the night—all to retrieve a mysterious box of cargo that he, Macpherson, urgently needed delivered dockside at Boulogne for immediate shipment to England. Nevertheless, Macpherson succeeded. The lorry was sent and the captain got to Boulogne with his precious cargo. He and all ten boxes, safely stowed aboard, left on the morning steamer for Folkestone.[24] The clandestine operation had taken a couple of days, but it had given Allied commanders the chance they needed to organize a response to the German army's sudden breakthrough along the Ypres salient on April 22 and 24, 1915.

Just days earlier, Cluny Macpherson, newly dispatched by the governor of the Dominion of Newfoundland to offer his medical services to the Royal Army Medical Corps, had arrived on the Western Front. As a member of the St. John Ambulance Brigade, he'd been asked to visit base hospitals in France to assess ambulance transport in the vicinity of the fighting near Ypres, Belgium. At one of the base hospitals, he'd shared a meal with two British professors working nearby at the Imperial College of Science and Technology. The German chlorine gas attacks on April 22 and 24 dominated the conversation. Medical personnel and scientists on the Allied side seemed desperate to come up with a rapid and effective response.

"I'd be a good guinea pig for testing," Macpherson told the professors. "When we made chlorine in a test tube [at school,] I lost my voice for a week with laryngitis."[25]

It turned out that Professors H. Brereton Baker and William Watson had already begun work on an antidote to the murderous toxic gases, at their college laboratory. The confusion of the battle along the Ypres salient had delivered into British hands a German soldier involved in the gas attack. In addition to the information gleaned from the captured German, the RAMC had secured his primitive gas mask, made of veiling and cotton waste. Macpherson joined the two professors analyzing chemicals in the veiling in order to come up with a prototype defence for expeditionary troops. He found an equivalent veiling at a French millinery shop and, in addition, made an overnight dash to London and back to retrieve two steel cylinders of chlorine so that the three men could begin gas mask trials. The experiments nearly killed them.

The prototype mask mimicked the surgical mask that doctors used to prevent respiratory contamination during operations. But to provide adequate protection for breathing, the defensive mask had to be held against the user's face, using both hands to keep the layer of cotton firmly pressed over his mouth and nose. The mask gave no protection for the eyes. Despite these apparent shortcomings for use by combat soldiers, Macpherson, Baker, and Watson went to some trenches outside the town of St. Omer, donned the prototype masks, and released some chlorine. The results, Macpherson reported, were disastrous. Watson was so badly gassed they had to rush him to a nearby Canadian military hospital for treatment. When he visited Watson at the hospital later that day, Capt. Macpherson also saw some of the casualties of the actual Ypres gas attack. It was clear that the two scientists and the medical man would have to revise their design completely.

Macpherson had anticipated the problem, however, and offered an idea he had toyed with on his trip to England to get the chlorine cylinders. He had drawn a pattern for a mask that didn't just cover the soldier's face but his entire head, like a hood. Made of Viyella cloth, the design called for a mica window to allow the soldier to see and a breathing tube through which he could exhale. Indeed, while visiting Watson at the Canadian military hospital, Macpherson had persuaded a nurse matron to cut out the pattern and sew the mica window into the resulting hood. When all seemed lost at the lab that day, Macpherson pulled out his alternative prototype. "Try this!" he suggested to his colleagues. "An anti-gas *helmet*."[26]

Eager to try anything that might solve the problem, they then impregnated the cloth hood with the chlorine antidote—hyposulphite of soda—and gave it to a Royal Engineer, a Col. Harvey, to try it on. At the end of the laboratory, the scientists had prepared a small, glass-partitioned booth for further experiments. Harvey volunteered to be the guinea pig; he would wear the helmet inside the chamber while Macpherson and the professors released chlorine gas around him. With the hood firmly placed over his head and tucked into his tunic, Harvey entered the chamber and walked about as the poisonous gas was introduced. After five minutes, Harvey called out to the professors, asking why they hadn't yet released the gas. And with that, he pulled off the hood.

Capt. Macpherson dashed to the door of the chamber, threw it open, and immediately sprayed the bare-headed Harvey with hyposulphite of soda. Moments later, when he'd recovered from the shock, Harvey explained what had happened. While inside the chamber with the helmet on, he said, he'd only been aware of a slight smell of chemical. That's all. Harvey volunteered for a second trial. Inside the chamber again with the helmet firmly secured on his head and chlorine gas flowing around him, Harvey worked at a bench and walked around in the enclosed area for thirty minutes, apparently unaffected by the gas.

The successful trial caused great excitement around the lab.

Suddenly the military brass arrived, including Charles Foulkes, Britain's chief advisor on gas warfare; William Robertson, the chief of the Imperial General Staff; and Arthur Sloggett, the director general of medical services (DGMS) in the field. Sloggett watched a demonstration of the helmet in awe. "Why, man, one could fight in that!" he exclaimed and asked where the helmet had come from.

"That officer gave it to me," Professor Baker said, pointing at Macpherson.[27]

"Where did you get this?" Sloggett queried Macpherson.

The Newfoundland medical officer retraced his helmet's evolution—a drawing on the trip from London, the nurse matron's sewing the prototype together, and the trials in the chamber with Col. Harvey. Macpherson added that his experience transporting patients with similar headgear as protection against cold weather in Labrador illustrated that the material could be breathed through while preventing penetration by the chlorine. This sparked a confab among the brass, and just as quickly curt instructions from Sloggett.

"Young man, you're for London," Sloggett told Macpherson. "Quick with your packing!"

His new orders came with such priority that Macpherson was transported across the Channel in a Royal Navy destroyer. With him Macpherson carried a letter to the DGMS within the UK, Sir Alfred Keogh, in London, requiring the medical service to give Macpherson all necessary assistance to mass-produce the helmets with all possible haste. The Committee on Gas Protection was organized under British Army surgeon Col. William Horrocks, with Capt. Macpherson suddenly in sole charge of turning out the helmets.

"They sent me to perhaps the most red-tape-bound institution in the [British] Army, the Royal Army Clothing Factory," Macpherson wrote later. "[They] asked for a 'sealed pattern,' of which I had never heard. I just went 'round London and cornered the market in several commodities and poured them into [the] factory."[28]

He bought up all the essentials—khaki Viyella, mica, ammonia vaporole, and hyposulphite of soda. It was over this last item that he butted heads with the tanning industry; without hyposulphite of soda the tanners couldn't treat the leather for army boots. But on Macpherson went. The work of cutting and sewing together the helmets soon outgrew the official production centre, so he expanded the process of dipping and parcelling the helmets at the three biggest laundries in London. Without consultation, he put out a call for women volunteers. Soon he had hundreds from every walk of life offering their services; he organized three eight-hour shifts of women working at each laundry, only paying the forewomen at each location. Macpherson had a task to accomplish, and accomplish it he would. Along the production lines, however, a serious problem emerged—a design flaw.

"We found mica [the goggle portion of the helmet] very hard to work with," Macpherson wrote. "It cracked and therefore leaked. . . . I begged to be allowed to replace the mica with photographic film, but [British Army] Staff Duties would not allow it, because film was explosive!"[29]

Macpherson calls it a coincidence, but one night while his anti-gas helmet production was in high gear, he took an evening off, responding to an invitation to attend a scientific lecture by his friend Harry Batterbee. The subject of the presentation was a new film product called triacetyl cellulose, or as Batterbee described it, "non-flammable film," for an entertainment industry that had experienced debilitating fires in movie theatre projection booths, where hot projecting equipment regularly ignited the nitrate-based cellulose film stock.

The non-flam film made Macpherson sit up. Here was the very solution to his cracking mica problem. And who manufactured this miracle material? Eastman Kodak in the United States and two companies in France—one in Lyons and the other, Pathé, in Paris. Overnight, Macpherson was back across the Channel, knocking on the doors of the two French firms manufacturing triacetyl cellulose.

At the Paris operations of the Lyons firm, where Macpherson and an interpreter, Col. Keddie, arrived the next day, they learned that the French War Office had just assigned the firm's entire output of non-flam film to the production of dope (waterproof varnish) to cover the wings of French military aircraft. Even as Macpherson examined samples of the product, French air officers entered, challenged the Newfoundland captain and his aide, and ejected them from the plant. Next, at Pathé, company officials told Macpherson they could offer him nothing. When Macpherson and Keddie threatened to go over their heads to the French War Office, the Pathé people asked how much film the captain would need. Macpherson and Keddie consulted in a corner.

"[Alfred] Keogh has authorized me to get enough for 200,000 helmets only," Macpherson told Keddie, adding, "Even though the helmet is at the experimental stage, I have every faith in it." And so Macpherson suggested they request enough film for a million helmets.

"You're new to this business," Keddie warned Macpherson. "[Changing the order] could have dire consequences."[30]

"I'll take the responsibility," Macpherson said. "Let's ask for enough for one million."

Pathé accepted the order, and by five o'clock that afternoon the plant had the ten unlabelled wooden cases ready for loading. Thus Capt. Cluny Macpherson found himself at the wheel of a Daimler leading a convoy of touring cars, all heavily laden with boxes of non-flam film and motoring northward with dispatch into the night, toward a rendezvous with a steamer waiting in Boulogne harbour. The next day, safely back in London with his top-secret cargo, Macpherson went right to his desk to write up a full confession for his immediate superior. Col. Horrocks was appropriately appalled by Macpherson's temerity and sent him up the line to DGMS Keogh to explain his activity in France and his unilateral decision to alter the size of the non-flam film order.

"And did you manage to get enough for the whole 200,000 helmets?" Keogh asked.[31]

"When I found out how difficult it was to get any," Macpherson answered, "I thought it better to get enough for one million."

"How dare you do such a thing?" Keogh exploded.

"I thought it in the public interest," Macpherson said, and before his superior could say another word, he added, "Let me answer that question in a week's time."

"All right then. I'll see you in a week's time."

In the week Keogh had granted him, Macpherson took over the Great Hall at St. James's Palace in the City of Westminster. With record speed, he directed his factory staff to build wooden stands and rollers to receive and dispense the rolls of triacetyl cellulose. Then his army of women volunteers organized to cut the film to the exact size required to replace the mica and fill the visor in each anti-gas helmet with the new non-flam film. As his workers began to stockpile the new military gas masks, Macpherson said the entire palace reeked of acetone. Seven days later, he returned to DGMS Keogh's office.

"Well, Macpherson, what can I do for you today?" he said.

"My week is up today, sir, which you so kindly granted in which to answer your question about the one million eye pieces," Macpherson explained.

"You go to hell, Macpherson!" Keogh laughed.

Sensing the meeting at an end, the Newfoundland captain saluted his superior officer and turned for the door. But Keogh called him back. "Why the devil didn't you get five million?" he asked sarcastically.

Capt. Macpherson's strong belief in the invention, his fearless approach to manufacturers of top-secret materials, and his audacious willingness to plunge ahead no matter the rules or bureaucratic barriers had generated a life-saving device in the middle of world war. All were calculated risks that, in his view, were well worth taking. "My helmet," Macpherson wrote later, "had well proven its value in the week."[32]

As if his globetrotting between Britain and the Continent during those few critical days after the German gas attacks weren't enough, Cluny Macpherson made numerous additional trips back and forth, establishing two impregnation depots for the helmets in Abbeville and Calais, France. Next, the eager captain took on the challenge of finding protection for Allied soldiers against flame-throwers that Allied intelligence anticipated the Germans might introduce along the Western Front. But Macpherson wasn't allowed to stay in the region long enough to see these devices developed; he was soon deployed to Gallipoli to rejoin his Newfoundland Regiment, just as the Allied evacuation there ended. But the stress, sleeplessness, and strenuous pace had taken their toll. In October 1916, Macpherson was sent home to Newfoundland to assume responsibilities as director of medical services in the army; at age thirty-seven, he was the youngest DMS ever.

Over the course of the Great War more than twenty-two million of Macpherson's anti-gas helmets were manufactured. Had he patented his device or sought publicity for it, both the medical and military worlds might have paid greater attention to him. But, as the long-time physician quickly pointed out in his notebooks of the day, "[I] belong to a profession which does not register nor patent its discoveries, but gives them freely in the cause of humanity."[33] Dr. Macpherson received numerous other honours and distinctions during his medical career, among them Companion of the Order of St. Michael and St. George, Honorary President of the Newfoundland Council of the St. John Ambulance, Honorary Vice-President of the Newfoundland Council of the Canadian Red Cross, Fellow of the British Royal College of Surgeons, and on and on. Especially important to Macpherson, however, was an acknowledgement from fellow surgeon and British officer John Rees.

"Put a young Colonial who knew nothing about London or Army or manufacturing in charge of a job where speed of production was all important, and it worked," Rees said. "That young chap knew nothing about red tape except how to cut it when it tangled him."[34]

Historians and military peers further agree that Dr. Cluny Macpherson's innovation, born as a sketch in desperate pursuit of a life-saving solution, not only short-circuited military bureaucracy at a time when a solution was most needed but also delivered a far greater dividend—the stuff of legends, best-selling espionage novels, and blockbuster movies. They suggest that his anti-gas helmet design and its quick production "saved the Channel ports which the Germans fully expected to occupy as a result of their surprise gas warfare."[35]

AUGUST 10, 1944—GRAINVILLE-LANGANNERIE, FRANCE

EARLY IN THE TWENTY-FIRST CENTURY, the family members of Second World War veteran Bob Ross gathered at the family home in southwestern Ontario to commemorate the sixtieth wedding anniversary of Bob and his wife, Jean; in doing so, however, they also ended up celebrating the initiative of another quick-thinking medic in the battlefield.

Among the invited guests for the anniversary celebration was Bob's lifelong friend and army buddy Jim Brittain. But Brittain wasn't just a casual participant that day; the Ross family requested his presence as the guest of honour. Indeed, during one of the tributes to their parents, the Ross offspring said, "If it weren't for Mr. Brittain, we wouldn't be here." It was true.

In August 1944, the Allied armies of Canada, the United States, and Britain had gained a significant toehold in France.

The Normandy invasion had advanced from the D-Day beaches inland toward the city of Caen. At the time, Privates Ross and Brittain were serving with the Lincoln and Welland Regiment (L&WR)—the former as a rifleman and the latter as a medic. The regiment had roots in southwestern Ontario going back to the formation of local militias during the War of 1812, so when it mobilized in 1939, many of its enlistees knew each other as neighbours or were in fact related. Gord Brittain, Jim's young brother, joined the L&WR two days before he did; they both lied about their ages, but Gord didn't like his potential assignment as a medic, so when Jim joined, with a resumé displaying some St. John Ambulance training, brother Gord convinced him to take his spot.

"I'd like to be in the medical corps," Jim Brittain announced to the medical officer in charge.

"We just lost a volunteer," Capt. George Lewin said.

"That was my brother," Brittain explained.

Lewin, who'd been a doctor in private practice before enlisting himself, looked over the new volunteer's papers, noticed the St. John training, and concluded, "You're in."[36]

Training at Niagara-on-the-Lake proved pretty basic—inoculating troops, cleaning and dressing cuts, setting broken arms and legs, and processing urine samples. After a stint on the Pacific coast, the regiment landed in Newfoundland; while stationed there, Brittain and his medical squad not only attended to the needs of the eight hundred troops in the Lincoln and Wellands but also provided basic health care to civilians at the neighbouring outports Gambo, Dark Cove, and Middle Brook. One of Pte. Brittain's first tasks was helping a family bury a stillborn baby in a shoebox.

On December 12, 1942, when the regiment was stationed at the Lester's Field barracks in St. John's, the L&WR medical unit responded to an emergency at the Knights of Columbus Hostel. The downtown facility, used by servicemen as a sleeping, dining, and recreation centre, was ablaze. Brittain attended to the burns of some who'd barely escaped and helped bury some of the ninety-nine who died. "In a way, it prepared me for what was coming," he said.[37]

Overseas, Operation Totalize—the early August push through Caen to cut off the German retreat at Falaise—had positioned Brittain's battle group near the town of Grainville-Langannerie. On August 10, 1944, the L&WR conducted a recce operation onto higher ground—Hill 195—just outside the town but well within range of enemy artillery fire.[38] Brittain couldn't recall which was hotter, the blistering sun or the German fire from mortars, machine guns, and 88 mm artillery. Brittain remembered an incoming shell striking an L&WR Bren-gun carrier. When the smoke cleared, four men on the carrier had severe head wounds, and off to one side he spotted Pte. Ross next to the wall of a building. "People were rushing by him," Brittain said. "I thought he was standing upright in a slit trench. But no, his leg was off at the knee."

There were stretchers leaning up against the building nearby, but the shell blast had shredded the canvas and shattered the stretcher arms, so Brittain grabbed a stick to use as a tourniquet and applied it to Ross's groin as tightly as he could, to stem the bleeding from a main artery. "I remember having to get a door and laying him on it. I remember him wanting to have his [detached] leg on the stretcher with him," he said. "Which I did."

Shelling in the area continued for several days. Those fighting on the hillside recalled running low on ammunition, food, and water. L&WR troops who survived the engagement afterward referred to Hill 195 as "Butcher Hill." Medics such as Pte. Brittain just remembered the carnage—eight killed in action, more than forty wounded, and two more who died of their injuries later. But not Bob Ross. When the shelling ceased, he was safely evacuated, treated, and shipped home. But Jim Brittain's service as a medic had just begun. The Lincoln and Welland Regiment remained at the sharp end of the fighting with the 10th Infantry Brigade, 4th Canadian Armoured Division, all the way through Belgium and northeastward, pushing German troops closer to the River Rhine.

During Operation Basher, on March 10, 1945, the L&WR reached the south side of the German town of Veen. Pte. Brittain was attending to wounded in a tent. "A shell landed and shrapnel came through the canvas and got me," Brittain said. The hot steel tore into his shoulder and created a sucking wound, "where the air goes in and out of the chest and your lungs collapse. . . . But I was in a medical area, and they laid me on my back with bandages."[39]

Within hours Brittain had taken his first ride aboard a DC-3 transport aircraft, which airlifted him back to south England; after surgery and convalescence, he was transported home aboard the hospital ship HMCS *Letitia*. Since, among other skills acquired in the army, he'd become the regiment's chiropodist, after the war, Brittain used a veteran's allowance to attend podiatry courses in Cleveland, Ohio. He then returned to Ontario, where he built a peacetime practice in Oshawa and eventually St. Catharines. He kept in touch with wartime comrades, including his medical platoon mates and the officer who led the medical unit, Dr. George Lewin (who later delivered Brittain's son, Ron).

For his part, Bob Ross, who recuperated from the loss of his leg in France, never forgot Jim Brittain, the medic whose quick action had saved his life. And nothing less than guest-of-honour status seemed appropriate at the Rosses' sixtieth wedding anniversary party.

AUGUST 19, 1942—DIEPPE, FRANCE

KNOWING—AND ACTUALLY MEETING AGAIN—a patient who had survived by your hand no doubt helped overshadow memories of those who did not. The success of having saved Harold McDonald from further injury and possibly death at Shell Trap Farm would almost certainly have helped Francis Scrimger soldier on through the crushing loss of so many others at Ypres in 1915. Learning, long after Falaise, that Bob Ross had survived evacuation and surgery likely buoyed Jim Brittain during his own recovery from wounds sustained at the Rhine in 1945. It's difficult to imagine, however, that the medical personnel who came through the crucible of Dieppe found any solace in those they saved, since there were nearly a thousand they could not.

Wesley Clare, a medical officer with the Royal Hamilton Light Infantry (RHLI) during the August 19, 1942, raid, probably knew the grim numbers before anyone else. As a prisoner of war by midday, he saw most of the casualties strewn across the

Dieppe hospital grounds under German guard that evening. "I would find out that 545 soldiers from our brigade had died that morning," he wrote, "[including] 197 from my regiment, the RHLI."[40]

After completing a medical program at Queen's University in June 1940, Clare enlisted in the army the day he finished his last Medical Council of Canada exam. Less than two months later, he'd finished basic training and was en route to England, arriving in time to witness the final days of the Battle of Britain. During his first year overseas, he served with field ambulance units in south England. Then, in March 1942, the 4th Canadian Infantry Brigade needed unmarried medical officers to replace three who were married. He qualified and was posted to the RLHI for two months of dawn-to-dark commando training—climbing cliffs, marching double time, and making assaults from water to land—on the Isle of Wight. In June the officers, including Clare, learned that the objective was the French seaport of Dieppe. For the rank and file it would remain a secret; meantime, Clare tried to keep his medics on their toes.

"I held a surprise inspection of the medical kits, checking the shell and first-aid dressings, triangular dressings, etc.," he wrote. "We had been issued two hundred syrettes of morphine for more than five hundred men, which had to be divided among twelve stretcher-bearers. As this was to be a raid—in at dawn, out at noon with the tide—we were taking minimal supplies."[41]

However, it wasn't until after all the members of Operation Jubilee—about 5,000 Canadians, 1,000 British troops, and 50 US Army Rangers—had boarded their respective ships for the crossing that ammunition, supplies, and actual maps of the target were issued. The surprise attack was compromised when some of the Dieppe-bound assault vessels engaged an armed enemy convoy, alerting German coastal defences. The in-and-out raid had a series of less obvious objectives,* but the overt action intended to seize, occupy, and then withdraw along about a mile of open beach in front of the town. Clare's medics came ashore with the RHLI at a stretch of ocean front code-named "White Beach."

"We landed late, after daybreak," he pointed out, emphasizing that all the RHLI landing craft were one to two miles out at sea when they were launched and were therefore visible and exposed all the way in. "We landed in chest-deep water and had to crawl up a rough beach under heavy fire."[42]

The armoured support also landed late at White Beach. Strategy called for the Calgary Tanks to land on "Red Beach" simultaneously with the RHLI and the Essex Scottish to silence pillbox guns and help the infantry breach the sea wall in front of the town. The delays at sea threw off the timing, and the daylight at about 6 a.m. put inbound tank landing craft (TLC) and infantry landing craft (ILC) in plain view of the German shore batteries well before the Canadians reached the beach.

Aboard his landing craft with C Squadron in the third group of landing Calgary Tanks, Capt. Laurence Alexander prepared his two medical vehicles and staff of four—Cal Halmer and Carl Morrison operating the Blitz ambulance; Sgt. Lea

---

* In his 2013 book, *One Day in August: The Untold Story Behind Canada's Tragedy at Dieppe*, David O'Keefe re-examines the raid to show that during the main Dieppe assault, Royal Marine commandos were to penetrate the inner harbour and capture a four-rotor Enigma machine at the Hôtel Moderne, as well as code books aboard German trawlers moored along the wharf. The Marines were repeatedly thrown back by heavy German fire at the entrance to the harbour.

Rutledge, Capt. Timmy Cameron, and Alexander himself on the carrier. Both vehicles' motors were running. They just had to wait their turn to disembark behind two tanks and then they could join the assault.

C Squadron's troubles began the moment TLC No. 8 purposely ran aground on the shore and dropped its front unloading door. The first Churchill tank down the ramp immediately got stuck in the deep chert rock: when a tracked or wheeled vehicle tried to climb the chert slope, it soon dug itself down, literally stopping in its tracks.[43] It couldn't go forward or backward. Worse, it prevented anything else from exiting the TLC, so all four vehicles began taking direct fire. Three engineers who leapt from the landing craft to help the tank crew were mowed down by machine-gun fire. Some first-wave tanks had managed to surmount the chert, but most suffered the same fate as the C Squadron tank crews—sitting ducks on a wide-open beach. TLC No. 8, with its one tank and two medical trucks, was ordered off Red Beach to find a better landing spot; it moved west to White Beach to try to disembark the tank and trucks in front of the Dieppe Casino.

"As we drew nearer we were caught in a terrific hail of fire from shore batteries, field guns and a constant hail of machine-gun fire and bursting shrapnel," Alexander wrote later. "When we were within fifty yards of shore, all hell broke loose. The call for stretcher bearers was heard in all directions."[44]

Alarming though it was, the call was not foreign to Capt. Alexander. Just sixteen when the Great War drew Canadian troops to Flanders in 1914, he had volunteered as a stretcher-bearer and suffered respiratory damages in gas attacks during service along the Western Front. Nevertheless, Alexander had fulfilled his wartime commitment and had returned to obtain his medical degree in Manitoba. He had married and settled in Saskatoon to establish a medical practice with his brother. Before the Second World War, he had moved to Calgary on his own, providing medical care at city hospitals and at the Stoney-Nakoda First Nation reserve. So, when war broke out in 1939, he had both wartime and peacetime medical experience to offer. In 1941, at age forty-three, he became a medical officer with the 14th Canadian Army Tank Regiment, the Calgary Tanks.[45] In front of White Beach now, and with motors running again in his two vehicles waiting to get to shore, Alexander left his carrier to respond to the call for medics aboard TLC No. 8.

"On reaching the upper part of the [landing craft], a shell exploded," Alexander said. "[It] knocked me back to the bottom of the boat, but I was unhurt. I climbed again, when another shell hit and blew me the opposite direction—right off the boat."[46] Airborne, he somehow grabbed hold of an engineer, who pulled him back aboard. But the effectiveness of the entire TLC was now in question. As the ship's crew released the front unloading door to deliver its cargo of the tank, Blitz ambulance, and carriers, an enemy shell blew apart the door cables and rigging, effectively jamming the door beneath the bow. Like so many of the tanks stuck in the chert onshore, the landing craft became a stationary target for the German shore batteries. TLC No. 8 then took a third direct hit; there would be thirty more in the minutes that followed, either killing or wounding the entire ship's crew. Among the wounded, the captain issued an "abandon ship" order and jumped into the water. By this time Alexander had managed to pull himself into what was left of the superstructure near the bridge. From there he heard calls from below to reverse engines.

"No living people above the deck," Alexander shouted to the tank and naval crew below. Then he heard a cry for help from a nearby catwalk; he ran toward the voice, only to discover the catwalk "crowded with dead and dying men—all wounded, not one uninjured man."[47]

All this, and the chief medical officer hadn't even stepped off the landing craft to attend to the men in his own outfit, the Calgary Tanks, or the infantry taking fire on the beach. No doubt torn, he continued to attend to those around him on the TLC as it swung around and floated sideways onto White Beach. He later wrote that machine-gun bullets beat "a constant tattoo on the boat" and that inside the boat "was a sheet of flame." He continued feverishly binding the wounds, only to find his patients killed moments later by the next volley of incoming shells. It was approaching 8:30 in the morning. In the moments when he was able to survey the scene outside the vessel, Alexander spotted the tank of his squadron leader, Lt.-Col. Johnny Andrews, sinking in the surf between the TLC and the shore; the cover of its turret was gone and survivors were attempting to get to smaller boats or wade through the surf to join the infantry assault, but they were all cut down by sniper fire.

Of the Calgary Tanks that did make it onto the beach, a handful from B Squadron in the second wave were scattered between the shoreline and the sea wall, where the Germans had constructed an anti-tank ditch. Stephen Bell, the wireless radio operator in a tank labelled "Backer"—the second

Churchill tank to leave TLC No. 4—said the incoming tracers and shell explosions looked "like the fourth of July." His tank received a direct hit coming down the ramp. The concussion knocked out Bell's radio, blew the lids off the tank's turret, and left three of the five-man crew in the turret temporarily unconscious. Driver Earl Snider managed to move the tank forward only about twenty feet from the water's edge before it, too, got bogged down in the chert. Bell counted at least fifteen enemy shell strikes on their tank; one lifted the sixty-ton vehicle into the air and dropped it back down again.

Backer's crew had no alternative but to evacuate the tank and join the fight outside. Bell set up the tank's Besa machine gun, using the stalled tank to shelter his one side; he and another gunner took turns returning fire from German positions. But the disabled vehicle simply drew more artillery shells that ricocheted off the tank body into its crew. Bell took shrapnel in his back and was bleeding from his ears, so he stuck pieces of field dressing in each ear. Gunner Bill Willard took hits across his foot, knee, and shoulder. Gunner Charlie Provis died from a bullet wound to the head. Then a mortar bomb exploded on their position.

"Willard got opened up right from his breastbone right down to his crotch," Bell said. "All we had was a first-aid kit, so [driver] Earl Snider and I got a couple of safety pins. We stuck everything back in and pinned him up."[48]

With little ammunition left in the machine gun and recognizing the need of others around them, Bell and his tank commander, Dick Wallace, began dragging the wounded from the beach behind them to what little shelter the tank offered. One man couldn't be dragged because his arms were so badly wounded. Wallace told Bell to get a blanket, but by the time Bell returned the man was dead. By eleven o'clock some of the navy vessels attempted a return to the beach to retrieve the wounded, but many of them were hit and sunk as they came in. Despite every effort, nothing could be done to fight, to retreat, or to save lives.

For the rest of his life Stephen Bell was haunted by what he saw that morning. "You could ask anybody who was on that beach and they'll tell you. The water was like red ink with blood," he said. "Bodies? You have no idea. Like cordwood, just floating, arms and legs and guts and heads. It's unbelievable. The water coming in was foaming red with blood."

Capt. Laurence Alexander never did manage to leave TLC No. 8. Eventually an infantry officer managed to restart the landing craft's engines and free it from the stones on the beach. A French hospital ship pulled alongside, allowing Alexander to offload his casualties. Shells from shore batteries, mortar positions, and German dive-bombers continued to explode around the crippled landing craft until, finally, HMS *Alresford*, a Royal Navy gunboat, nudged the landing craft out to sea and helped steer the battered vessel back across the Channel to England.

Ashore nearby on White Beach, RHLI Capt. Wesley Clare and his aid men could do little more than crawl their way over the chert to the scores of wounded in front of the sea wall. Eventually one of the abandoned TLCs drifted ashore, and Clare gathered his medics and wounded in the lee of the vessel to carry on the task of saving lives. A number of smaller landing craft attempted returns to pick up the wounded; most were either deterred or destroyed by heavy bombardment from the shore. Now Clare faced an additional threat—sea water was lapping farther up the beach with the morning tide and engulfing his position. It was just after 11 a.m. when Clare made a final decision.

"There were eighty to a hundred men huddled behind our now burning landing craft, and as the tide came in, it became obvious that we had to surrender before the wounded drowned," wrote Clare, the senior officer in the position. "I tied a triangular bandage to a rifle, and we surrendered."[49]

Though nearly two hundred men from his Royal Hamilton Light Infantry regiment had died in the Dieppe raid, Capt. Clare couldn't let that thought interfere with the job at hand. In his first hours of captivity, he triaged some of the wounded who soon filled both the nearby Dieppe and Rouen hospitals. Stephen Bell and Earl Snider assisted Clare in getting wounded comrades the treatment they needed; they managed to get Bill Willard, whose torso they'd stitched up with safety pins, into a hospital bed; Bell said when they pulled off his shirt, one shoulder was a mess of compound fractures.

Meantime, the rest of the Dieppe prisoners of war—nearly 1,300 men—were transported to a prison camp outside Paris. Among the POWs were 250 walking wounded, but with all of their medical equipment confiscated, Capt. Clare and two other medical officers from the 4th Brigade had to make do with paper bandages, paper dressings, and a few makeshift instruments. Several weeks later they would all be transported to a German prison camp in Ober Silesia to face an entirely new set of medical challenges, in what would be nearly three years of imprisonment at Stalag VIII-B.

Back in England, at 11:30 on the same night as the Dieppe raid, Capt. Alexander and the survivors of what was left of

TLC No. 8 were towed to a berth at Newhaven. "Oil, water and blood were over everything," he wrote in his journal, "and the days following were full of gloom."[50] Of his original assault group of 117 military men and thirteen naval men, Alexander's unit returned to England with only thirty military and three naval men alive, and most of them were wounded. Alexander himself had shrapnel wounds on his ankle, an injured tailbone, and a cracked jaw. His two ambulance medics, Carl Morrison and Cal Halmer, had arm and leg wounds but would survive.

Meanwhile, hospitals around Newhaven worked for two days and two nights—the surgeons at one hospital worked non-stop in its operating theatre for forty hours; another hospital attended to 401 wounded, 80 of them requiring surgery.[51] Despite the horrific overall losses—3,367 of the 4,963 Canadians in action became casualties—Alexander wrote that he could take some solace from knowing that twenty-eight tanks had made it ashore, albeit to be ultimately captured or destroyed, and that "we had succeeded in landing at an impossible point."

On October 2, 1942, the *London Gazette* published details of two investitures planned for Buckingham Palace later in the month. For their actions during the Dieppe raid, Capt. Laurence Alexander would receive the Military Cross (MC) and Lt.-Col. John Begg the Distinguished Service Order (DSO). In a rather clinical entry in his diary, on October 27 Alexander recounted that he and Begg walked across Green Park to the palace and, joining a number of other medal recipients, were led into different rooms according to the type of decoration.

There a set of hooks was attached to each man's tunic to receive the medal. Beginning at 11 a.m., the award winners were processed—marched to a raised platform in front of an audience, there to await the King, and then called forward by name. They were expected to bow and to step forward to have the award hung on the hooks by the King.

"Which beach did you land on?" King George asked Alexander as he placed the MC on his chest, "Red or White?"

"Both," Alexander said.

The King asked about the casualty numbers and if Alexander had managed to get them all away safely. Then, apparently, Lord Louis Mountbatten whispered something to the King about what had happened to Alexander's tank landing craft. Finally the King asked what had become of the casualties.

"Many were blown overboard."

"It was a dirty show. Good work. Congratulations," the King said.

They shook hands. Alexander walked off the platform, and as he exited the presentation hall, a royal assistant removed the medal from the hooks on Alexander's tunic, put it in a case, and handed the case to him. To complete what felt much like an assembly line, a photographer had Alexander and Begg pose outside the palace gates and took their picture. Capt. Alexander continued to serve in the medical corps right through the liberation of Sicily, Italy, Belgium, and Holland in 1945. He would receive further decoration for his innovative use of Jeeps as ambulances. It was all appropriate recognition for saving lives in the battlefield.

But Laurence Alexander might suggest that he enjoyed an even greater reward than any medal or citation ever delivered.

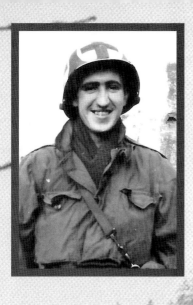

During the Battle of the Bulge, in 1945, these wooded areas just inside Germany hid a network of anti-personnel weapons—land mines, booby traps, and dragon's teeth (BOTTOM LEFT). When US infantrymen triggered them, it was up to medical corpsmen to bring out the wounded. Medic Alex Barris (TOP LEFT) directed stretcher-bearers with wounded to an aid station, and from there medic Tony Mellaci (BOTTOM RIGHT) arranged for motor ambulance transport. Both served in the 319th Medical Battalion with the US 94th Infantry Division.

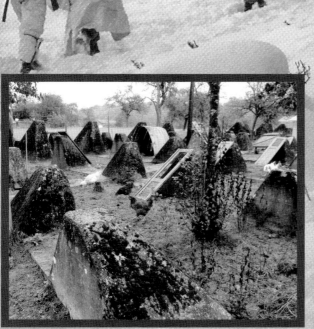

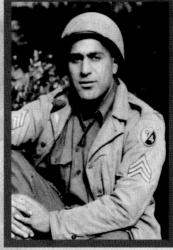

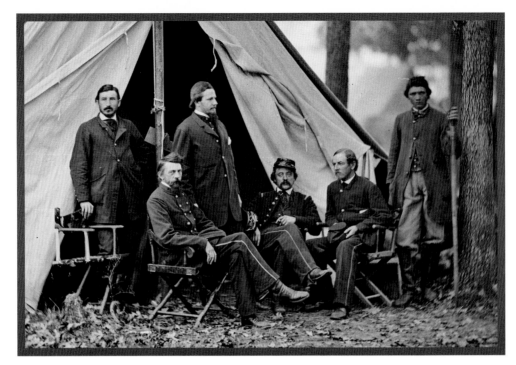

In the US Civil War, as many as 750,000 combatants died. As an example, casualties in the Battle of Marye's Heights at Fredericksburg, Virginia, on December 13, 1862, were typical—nearly 13,000 Federal soldiers killed or wounded in one day's fighting. It might have been worse on the Union side if not for the introduction of the field ambulance (BOTTOM) and a well-organized support system of ambulance trains to retrieve, triage, and treat the wounded. The concept was introduced at Fredericksburg by Jonathan Letterman (TOP, SEATED IN FRONT), medical director of the Union Army of the Potomac. He was later described as "the father of battlefield medicine."

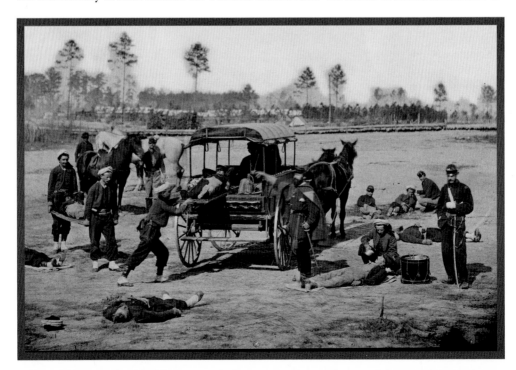

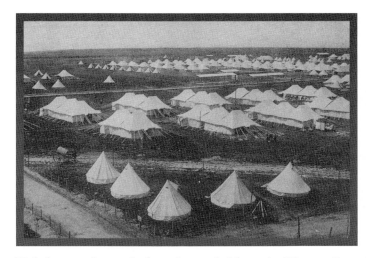

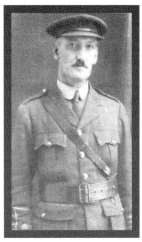

To help treat the steady flow of wounded from the Western Front in early 1915, McGill University as well as the Montreal General and Royal Victoria Hospitals transported 1,700 volunteer students, doctors, and nurses to France. Housed in tents (TOP LEFT) on open terrain along the French coast, No. 3 Canadian General Hospital (CGH) would initially provide 315 volunteer staff to support 1,040 beds tending the wounded.

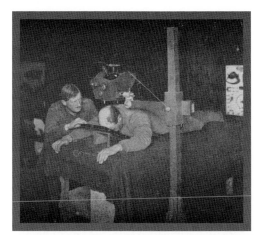

The facility at Dannes-Camiers, in France, included an admission tent, diagnosis tables, registration facilities, an x-ray machine (LEFT), operating theatres, recovery areas, and recreation huts. Among No. 3's most experienced surgeons was Edward Archibald (TOP RIGHT AND BOTTOM LEFT, FOURTH FROM LEFT), known for his work "shrapnel hunting" in body and head wounds. As well as daily convoys of wounded, No. 3 CGH welcomed Minister of Militia Sam Hughes, creator of the Canadian War Records Office Max Aitken (Lord Beaverbrook), and Queen Mary (BOTTOM RIGHT) on July 3, 1917.

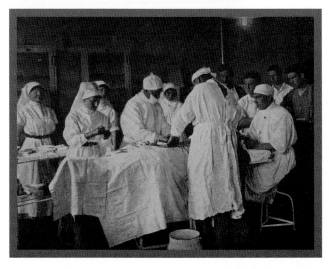

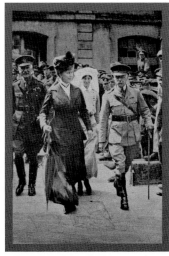

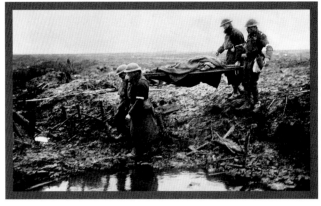

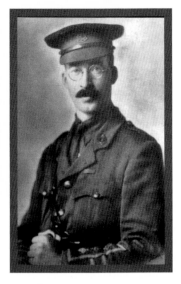

In April 1915, medical officer Francis Scrimger (RIGHT) evacuated forty wounded from the appropriately named "Shell Trap Farm" advanced dressing station in Belgium, shielding one man with his own body; he was awarded the Victoria Cross.

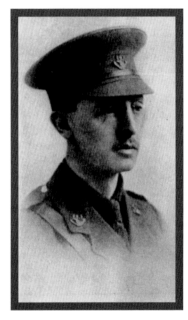

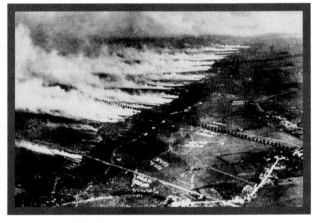

On April 22 and 23, 1915, German troops advanced behind a wall of chlorine gas (ABOVE RIGHT) against Allied trenches near Ypres, Belgium. Cluny Macpherson (LEFT), a medic from Newfoundland, then faced the task of finding a defence against the toxic weapon.

Remembering headgear he had employed to protect patients in transit from the cold in Labrador, Macpherson created a prototype helmet (RIGHT) combining a Viyella cloth hood, a breathing hole, and a visor made of non-flammable film; then he marshalled workers in the UK to manufacture a million gas masks before the Germans launched yet another gas attack. Not seeking fame or fortune, Macpherson gave his invention "freely in the cause of humanity."

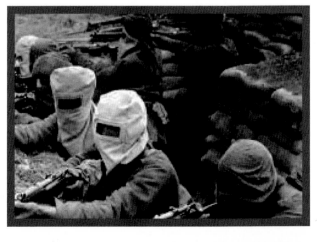

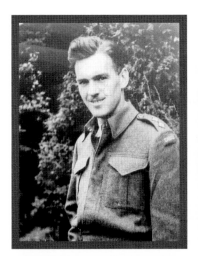

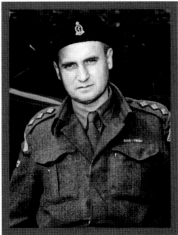

During the Dieppe raid in August 1942, medical officer Laurence Alexander (TOP RIGHT) attempted in vain to get ashore to attend Canadian wounded there; aboard a burning landing craft (MIDDLE), he dealt with dozens of casualties and listened to "a constant tattoo" of enemy machine-gun bullets pounding the vessel. Meanwhile, on the beach, medical officer Wesley Clare (TOP LEFT) faced the reality that eighty to a hundred wounded men huddled in the lee of a landing craft would have to surrender or drown in the rising tide. They would spend the rest of the war in German POW camps.

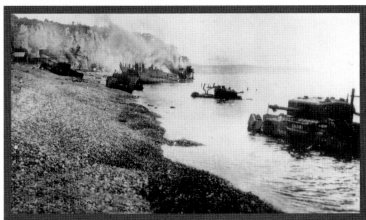

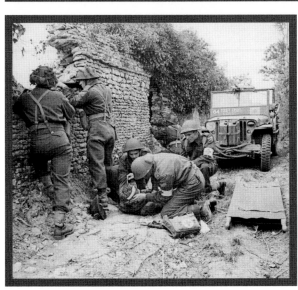

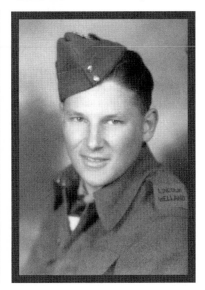

In Normandy during the invasion (ABOVE LEFT), medics coped with casualties alongside infantry firing on enemy positions. At Hill 195 in August 1944, medic Jim Brittain (ABOVE RIGHT), with the Lincoln and Welland Regiment, wasn't sure which was hotter that summer: the blistering sun or the continuous fire from German mortars, machine guns, and 88 mm artillery.

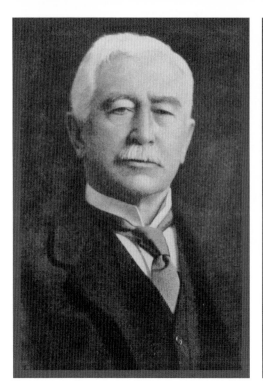

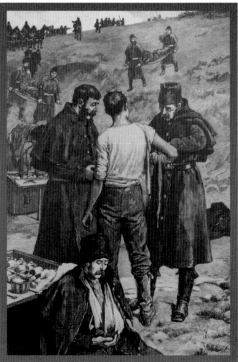

During the 1885 Riel Uprising, urban surgeon Thomas Roddick (TOP LEFT) had to adapt to conditions of a frontier battlefield in western Canada. Under canvas and out in the open near Batoche (TOP RIGHT), his medical corps conducted fifty-three surgeries, extricating bullets and treating fractures while keeping germs at bay.

Alannah Gilmore (BELOW) brought all the medic skills her deployment to Afghanistan in 2007 demanded; just as often, the crew commander of a Canadian Army Bison ambulance also relied on her trained "muscle memory" in emergencies and a keen sense of "situational awareness" to anticipate the unexpected.

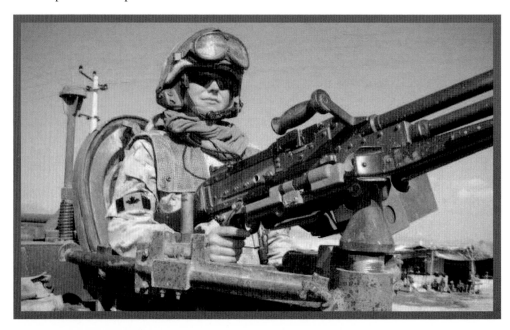

In 1916, rather than take a posting to train field ambulance recruits in England, Montreal volunteer John Kennedy (TOP RIGHT, ON LEFT) took a pay cut—from $1.50 a day as a sergeant to $1.10 a day as a private—to join No. 9 Field Ambulance in the Canadian Corps on the Western Front. He helped boost the morale of stretcher-bearers by getting their commanders to find qualified cooks to provide better food for ambulance crews.

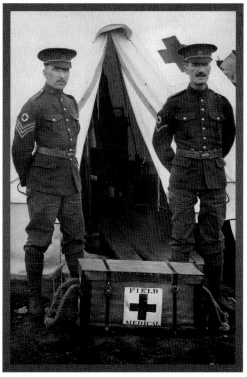

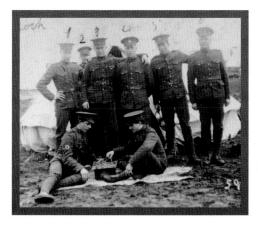

Characteristic of British Empire enlistees, Frank Walker (ABOVE LEFT, STANDING AT LEFT END) served on the Western Front with No. 1 Canadian Field Ambulance among volunteers who came from the same town or province, in his case Prince Edward Island. Field ambulance crews in the Great War had a casualty rate of 8 percent and a fatality rate of 4 percent. While more distant from the front lines, ambulance drivers such as Grace MacPherson (BELOW), with the Voluntary Aid Detachment of the British Red Cross, delivered wounded to military hospitals on the coast of France, where they became targets of German bombers in the spring of 1918.

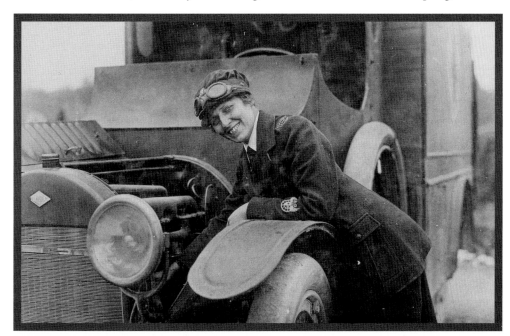

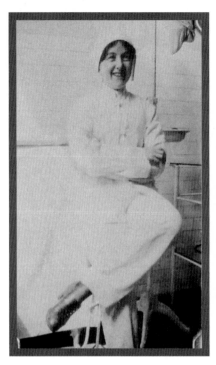
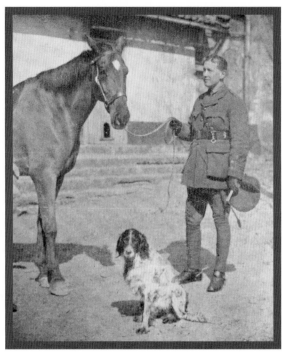

Medical staff in the Great War understood the risks of service close to the front. Field surgeon John McCrae (TOP RIGHT), shown with his horse Bonfire and dog Bonneau, operated on patients well within range of enemy machine guns and artillery. Working at military hospitals along the coast of France, forty miles behind the lines, offered Katherine Maud Macdonald (TOP LEFT) some sense of security. . . until May 19, 1918. During two hours of airborne attacks that night, German aircraft dropped 116 bombs on Allied hospitals; Macdonald, two other nursing sisters, and eight patients died of their wounds. Damage, as at No. 7 Canadian General Hospital (BELOW), was extensive. Of 3,141 women serving in the Canadian Army Medical Corps in the Great War, forty-six died of enemy action or disease while on duty.

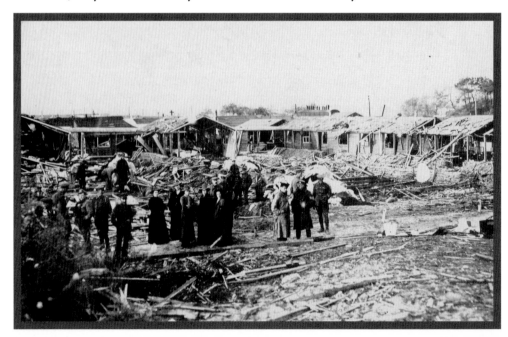

After the war, when Doc Alexander returned to Calgary to restart his civilian private practice, some of his army comrades pitched in. Former Calgary Tanks trooper Raymond Gilbert, captured and imprisoned after the Dieppe raid, came home to Alberta wondering what had happened to his regiment's one-time MO.

"[Doc Alexander] called me up and said, 'Ray, I'm opening an office. I need some patients,'" Gilbert said. "He [brought] my first [child] into being, and my second.'"[52]

Tough for a military medal to match that.

CHAPTER FIVE

"WHERE THE BULLETS FELL THICKEST"

BESIDES THE MEDAL HE SHOWED ME, my father kept one other memento from his time in the army and his service overseas during the Second World War. For some years into my adolescence, Dad kept his US Army jacket. It was made of wool, with some inside lining and a tight-fitting waistband and cuffs. Fashioned after the British battledress jacket, the equivalent coat in the US Army was intended as a field or combat jacket; later, because the chief of the Supreme Headquarters Allied Expeditionary Force had worn one, it became known as the "Eisenhower" jacket.

I learned later that my father's brother, Angelo, who had a knack for sewing, had tailored the jacket to make it closer fitting in the upper body. Anyway, my dad kept his Eisenhower after the war as a kind of fall jacket. I don't remember seeing any insignia on it. It did have that uniform "olive drab" colouring he always talked about. And I remember that he wore it a few times when we were outside during the first crisp days of autumn. As a teenager, when I considered some things associated with the war as "cool," Dad let me wear the jacket a few times. Occasionally I snuck into his closet to try it on. The wool was still neat, but scratchy around the collar, and the chest and arms were tight-fitting where I guess they were supposed to be. After putting it on in front of a mirror and stopping to look for a moment, I always made sure it went back onto the hanger and into the closet exactly the same way I found it, so he wouldn't suspect I'd disturbed it.

The reason those moments at the mirror stay with me is that I completely misunderstood the significance of that jacket. I eventually recognized that this kind-of-stylish olive-drab fall-weight jacket was not in my father's wardrobe for its looks. He didn't care whether they said it was British or American, or if it had any connection to Eisenhower. When he wore it, during his time serving in the US Army at the battle of the Saar-Moselle Triangle in the winter of 1945, nobody was around to compliment him on its stylish fit. That jacket—I suspect worn over several layers of shirts and under a heavier overcoat, if he could find one—helped to keep him from freezing to death during those inhospitable days and nights when he was the runner for the 319th Medical Battalion with the 94th Infantry Division.

That jacket was no fashion statement. It was wrong-season clothing the army had issued to him and all of his comrades-in-arms going into the Battle of the Bulge, and it would be only as functional as his improvisation skills allowed. In the 1960s I never bothered to check—I was too busy looking in the mirror at how cool it looked—but if I had stuck my hands into the pockets of his "Eisenhower," I might have found a few pine needles or dry flecks of mud that had come all that way (and all those years) from Campholz Woods. And if I had asked, he might have set me straight that his decision to hang on to this battle jacket had little to do with the way it made him look, and more to do with remembering how it helped him survive that horrid winter of 1945.

FEBRUARY 22, 1945—RIVER SAAR, GERMANY

ADDING LAYERS OF CLOTHING to protect against the sub-zero temperatures of the Saar-Moselle Triangle wasn't the only bit of improvisation my father and his fellow corpsmen generated that winter. Every day they had to find ways to extricate wounded from battlefields and keep them alive. So they scoped out vacant buildings in German villages, converting them to those hash-house shelters behind the lines to keep their patients from freezing to death. They liberated linen or white curtains to help camouflage the soldiers' battledress in snowy conditions. And they tried to streamline the transportation of wounded away from the fighting. The 319th Medical Battalion knew the evacuation protocol well. By the book, at least, the model for evacuating casualties consisted of five echelons, starting at the unit level. Sick or wounded from front-line units were transferred, usually by litter, to the first echelon—the aid station. From there, ambulances or other motorized vehicles moved patients farther back to the second echelon—a collecting station or a clearing station. And then, well behind the front lines, wounded were delivered by rail, water transport, or air evacuation to the third echelon—mobile hospitals. Finally, using similar transport, they would be delivered to the farthest point away from the fighting, the fourth echelon—a general hospital.

By the end of the twenty-first day of February 1945, American forces had taken the previously impregnable Saar-Moselle Triangle from its German defenders. The so-called strategy of attrition had delivered the anchor of the Bulge back into US Army hands. In the final three days of overrunning the Triangle, 94th Infantry Division troops seized five times as much ground as they had managed during the first full month of fighting, including the clearing of Campholz Woods, that stretch of the Triangle where my father had retrieved the wounded litter-bearers. Casualty rates during that advance, however, had been dear—611 wounded put through the clearing station on February 19, 344 treated and transported on February 20, and another 173 on February 21.[1]

Based on my father's experience at Campholz Woods—and borne out by the statistics—many of the casualties resulted from *Schü* mines that blew off feet or shattered them so severely they had to be amputated. As a staff sergeant in a reserve platoon at Campholz Woods, Jerome Fatora had to cope with the results of those *Schü* mines. With battalion medic Howard Ellinson, Fatora worked frantically retrieving GIs who'd tripped wires or triggered mines covered by the snow.

"We picked up this kid and all he had left was the patella [kneecap] hanging there; the rest of his leg was gone," Fatora said. Ellinson applied a tourniquet and the two carried him back. "He was laughing, he was in such shock. The bleeding was so bad, by the time we got him to an ambulance he was dead."[2]

On February 22, Fatora and Ellinson had to face demons of a
different sort. Having pushed the German defenders eastward
across the River Saar, the easternmost leg of the Saar-Moselle
Triangle, it was now up to the 94th to cross the river themselves
to pursue their enemy. Of course, the Germans had destroyed
all the bridges, so the Americans faced a nighttime crossing of
the Saar near Taben, Germany, in sixty assault boats. Medic
Ellinson had been a championship swimmer back in North
Dakota, but rifleman Fatora had grown up in Pennsylvania
fearing water; he'd never learned to swim. Nevertheless, Patton's orders were to "cross at once."[3] So, with twelve per boat,
the flotilla of GIs began the crossing at 4 a.m. But the Saar was
in flood. The seven-mile-an-hour current and undertow were
strong, and Fatora's boat capsized.

"The boat sank. I was up to my neck in water, and I can't
swim," Fatora said, but pillars and railroad ties left from the
sunken bridge gave the men flailing in the water something to
grab. Somehow Fatora made it to shore, and from there he
looked back to see his friend Ellinson pulled under by the current. "The man was a state champion swimmer from North
Dakota," he said. "I just think it had all gotten to him—the
war, all the men he'd tried to save. He just plain gave up."[4]

Ellinson was one of four men who drowned that morning
on the river.[5] By the end of the day—February 22—infantry
of two 94th Division regiments had established firm bridgeheads on the east side of the Saar. As they did, two battalions
of combat engineers managed to install first a footbridge and
then a larger pontoon bridge, which allowed the 94th to move
men and supplies in vehicles back and forth across the Saar
with greater speed and relative ease.

For my father's medical group, the dry and direct link from the west bank of the river to the east meant a faster, more efficient evacuation of the wounded to the aid or clearing stations, and eventually to the surgeons in mobile hospitals and beyond. Along with this convenience, however, came the prospect of higher visibility while on or approaching the pontoons. With enemy artillery and mortar units still dug in across the higher ground atop the east bank of the Saar, the possibility remained extremely high that US vehicles rushing to and from the bridgeheads might come under fire. That hazard didn't seem to occur to one of my father's commanding officers. Sometime before crossing the Saar, this particular CO, a major, had spotted eight or ten horses in a barnyard near the medical battalion's headquarters. My father noted that no one seemed to know where the horses had come from, whose they were, or how they had survived the fierce fighting that had gone on around them all that winter.

"But [the] Major suddenly had this idea," my father, a subordinate sergeant corpsman, wrote. "If we could bring the horses up to the Saar and across, we could hitch them to litters, which could be attached to a set of two wheels, and thus evacuate wounded men down the hill and to safety. I thought it a half-baked idea, but nobody asked me."[6]

Whether his advice was considered or not, the order to put the major's plan into action fell to T/Sgt. Barris. It was up to him to find volunteers among his corpsmen—preferably those who knew something about horsemanship—to round up the horses from their cozy little pasture on the west side of the river, and to bring them forward and across the river to await the next call for medical transport back to the rear echelons. My father noted that the first problem, finding able volunteers, nearly scuppered the entire operation: all the men in his litter platoon came from US cities; none of them had any experience leading a horse on a shank, much less riding one with a set of reins in his hands. And, of course, as my father pointed out, there were no saddles available either; inexperienced riders would be riding untrained horses—bareback—in an outrageous scheme to transport the wounded. At any rate, on the day chosen to move the horses forward and across the river, T/Sgt. Barris led the way in a Jeep—with a red cross flying—with about ten frightened soldiers riding or leading an equal number of skittish horses. And sure enough, a German tank hidden in the hills got wind of the convoy and opened up with its 88 mm gun.[*]

"The horses freaked and bolted and three or four guys were injured," my father wrote. "One poor guy cracked under the strain and later had to be evacuated, as much a casualty of war as those with physical wounds. Those of us who were lucky enough to escape harm, were kept busy bandaging the wounds of the injured, administering morphine to lessen their pain, and then getting them the hell out of there."[7]

The scheme my father dubbed "the mounted medics" was never revisited by his superior officer, or anybody else. However, T/Sgt. Barris still had to complete his report on the incident that had put half a platoon of litter-bearers out of action, killed at least one of the civilian horses, and forced the 319th Medical Battalion to return to its more traditional,

---

[*] Historian Nathan N. Prefer notes in *Patton's Ghost Corps* that even as they prepared to cross the River Saar at Taben, trucks of the 319th Combat Engineers carrying the bridge sections had to run the gauntlet of long-range enemy fire.

if no less traumatic, means of transporting the wounded. In my father's medical unit, that meant turning to his equal in the medical motor pool, S/Sgt. Tony Mellaci, and his fleet of three-quarter-ton Dodge ambulances. The 319th had twenty of them, all built with a metal chassis and bodies made of steel panels and plywood, and with room in the box behind for four litter cases and up front in the cab for two ambulance orderlies. While more powerful and manoeuvrable than their half-ton predecessors, the motor pool's ambulances could still give occupants hair-raising rides, as Mellaci learned in the last days of February.

During one of the first nights when troops of the 302nd Infantry Regiment were securing the town of Serrig, on the east side of the Saar, Mellaci got the call for an ambulance and as much plasma as he could carry. He and two other medics drove the ambulance from the aid post at Taben, across the pontoon bridge, and along a series of switchback roads up Hocker Hill to the infantry position at Saarfels Castle in Serrig. Mellaci arrived at the command post in the castle to find a young rifleman, who'd just joined the 302nd that day, writhing in pain on a stretcher.

"My legs!" the young soldier kept screaming. "My legs!"[8]

There happened to be a medical officer on the scene, a doctor forward at the front line with the platoon, and Mellaci remembered him repeating, "Don't worry about it, son, we're going to put leg splints on."

Mellaci watched as they put make-believe splints on the soldier, because his legs "were just skin and everything else looked like powder, both legs." Mellaci then applied tourniquets to the stumps of the man's legs. As he did, the wounded soldier grabbed his hand and wouldn't let go. Someone, likely the doctor, had already given him morphine, but Mellaci was instructed to insert an intravenous line for plasma.

"You'd better go back with him," the doctor told Mellaci, "to keep him calm."

So S/Sgt. Mellaci, with the wounded reinforcement still clinging to him, got into the back of the ambulance for the return trip through the dark, from Saarfels Castle, down the switchbacks of Hocker Hill, and across the pontoon bridge on the Saar. But the noise of the ambulance attracted the attention of German gunners and they opened fire. Mellaci thought his number was up. "I'm standing up in the back of the ambulance holding this bottle up so the plasma would still flow and this kid's hanging onto me." The driver kept going as fast as he could, dodging the shells falling around them, until they met vehicles travelling in the opposite direction. Unable to leave his patient, Mellaci told the other medic in the ambulance to clear a pathway through the convoy headed for the Saar. Finally the ambulance crew reached the aid post and was able to get its patient to triage and treatment. It had taken only minutes, but to Mellaci it felt like an eternity.

"We were all medics, but some guys never saw a needle or a bandage. I was a motor pool guy," Mellaci said. "This poor kid. I don't know if he lived through it or not. You could see the outline of his legs, but they were smashed. When I think about it, it makes me sick."[9]

...

MAY 9, 1885—BATOCHE, BRITISH NORTH-WEST TERRITORIES

TRANSPORTING WOUNDED TROOPS posed an entirely different set of challenges at the start of Louis Riel's campaign of resistance in 1885. That year, when the Métis leader made his second stand against the Government of Canada from his stronghold in Saskatchewan territory, Gen. F.D. Middleton, in command of the national militia, received orders to lead a force west to quell the resistance. The logistics of both geography and supply proved to be the initial problems facing the strategists supporting Middleton's operations. First, the armed force of 5,000 troops sat in Winnipeg, Manitoba. Meanwhile, the source of supply sat in Ottawa, nearly 2,000 miles away. And add to that the fact that the young nation—founded just eighteen years earlier—had "no fixed Departmental Medical Staff, no Field Hospital, or Ambulance Service, no organized Corps of Nurses."[10]

Canada's Surgeon General, Dr. Darby Bergin, turned to one man to organize the medical teams, supply them with necessary provisions, and launch the entire service quickly enough so that it could leave eastern Canada and catch up to Middleton's main combat columns before or as they confronted Riel's forces. Bergin chose an urban clinical surgeon and professor at Montreal General Hospital for the job. His name was Thomas Roddick. "One of the most distinguished of Canadian Surgeons," Bergin said of Roddick, "[he is] young, full of vigour, of powerful physique, knowing no fatigue, a first-class horseman, I [look] upon him as just the man for the place."[11]

To be sure, Professor Roddick appeared to have all the qualifications required to support Gen. Middleton's militia forces in the North-West. Born in Newfoundland and educated in Scotland and Canada, Roddick had become a star student at McGill University in the 1860s with his penchant for bedside surgery and fracture treatment and bandaging that was "a work of art."[12] In addition, by age thirty-eight he had accumulated as many military credentials as Surgeon General Bergin felt were necessary. While assistant house surgeon at Montreal General Hospital, Roddick had also served as assistant surgeon to the Grand Trunk Artillery, and just before his appointment at the outbreak of the resistance, he'd become surgeon for the Prince of Wales Regiment too.

Though Bergin didn't appear to note it in his recommendation of the Montreal professor, Roddick had an additional credential that proved extremely valuable in battlefield medicine. In 1872, while on a holiday in Great Britain, Roddick had visited the Glasgow Royal Infirmary to witness the work of medical trailblazer Joseph Lister. While others blamed bad air in hospitals for infections following surgery, Lister accused surgeons who didn't wash their hands and the unsanitary conditions of patients' wounds themselves for high rates of infection and mortality. Lister's methods of preventing germs from entering the body involved the use of carbolic acid— cleansing the wound with it, soaking the dressings with it, and eventually creating a mechanism that sprayed a continuous mist of the chemical over the operating area as surgeons worked. After several visits to Dr. Lister's labs and surgeries, Thomas Roddick became a "Listerism" disciple and returned to Montreal with a complete Lister antiseptic kit.

Fellow surgeon F.J. Shepherd assessed Roddick's impact on Canadian surgery. "It was he who first introduced the antiseptic methods of Lister in Montreal, and I fancy into Canada," Shepherd said. "It revolutionized the surgery of the [Montreal] General Hospital and banished erysipelas and hospital gangrene from the wards and reduced the mortality of operations to a minimum."[13]

Thus Thomas Roddick brought a full medical bag's worth of talents to his new position as chief of medical staff in the field. But perhaps his greatest skill in organizing the medical service near the battlefields in Saskatchewan territory had nothing to do with his horsemanship, his service in uniform, or even his newfound commitment to hygiene in the hospital operating theatre. Roddick had an administrative and logistical sense that Surgeon General Bergin recognized as being up to the task. And the first task required building a staff. Bergin and Roddick went to what might seem an obvious reservoir—the students and instructors of the medical schools at the University of Toronto and McGill, where first aid and stretcher drill were a regular part of medical school life. When word got to the schools, the Surgeon General's office was flooded with volunteers. But Bergin and Roddick determined there would be no unpaid volunteers; men, not freshmen, were chosen and would be compensated. So were nuns and women from ladies' aid societies and a Red Cross corps. Meantime, with no official army medical corps or, therefore, any medical officers to call upon, Roddick organized two field hospitals, each served by a surgeon major, six surgeons, eighteen to twenty dressers, and five orderlies.

After a snowstorm delayed its departure from Montreal, on April 7, 1885, No. 1 Field Hospital proceeded by rail to

Chicago, then to Minneapolis, and arrived five days later in Winnipeg. No. 2 Field Hospital would arrive a few weeks later. But Gen. Middleton's campaign was two weeks and four hundred miles ahead of Roddick on the Prairies. To expedite things, in Winnipeg Roddick had the Canadian Pacific Railway reconfigure a caboose and a passenger coach to take sick and wounded, and a boxcar for supplies and medical gear. With the rail cars stripped back to the walls, Roddick ensured that each was cleaned and prepared for hygienic work ahead. The result was Canada's first "hospital train," which quickly transported officers, surgeons, and orderlies to Swift Current. There the hospital train was placed on a siding, and on April 17 its staff immediately set to work receiving and treating the first wounded—four men suffering from cold and exposure, and a fifth with pneumonia.

Following military engagements at Fish Creek on April 24 and Cut Knife Hill on May 2, and a looming major assault on Batoche likely in a matter of days, the focus of the military action shifted north to Middleton's field headquarters outside Saskatoon. Roddick arrived in town on May 3 to accommodate the growing number of casualties and to prepare for even more. He requisitioned the three largest houses in the town to become hospital facilities. His General Orders required "the immediate removal of all excreta and foul dressings, and privies were constructed at convenient distances from the buildings. A man was detailed to apply dry earth frequently, so that the discharges were never left uncovered for longer than a few moments; water was abundantly supplied from the [South Saskatchewan] river for cleaning purposes, while delicious drinking water was obtained from a spring two miles from the village."[14]

As the climax of the campaign, the Battle of Batoche, began on May 9, 1885, Roddick dispatched Surgeon Major James Bell to move with Middleton's troops and to establish a field hospital as close to the engagement as possible. Roddick's system had all the precision of the Jonathan Letterman model introduced in 1862 at the Battle of Fredericksburg during the US Civil War. An ambulance train of twenty wagons joined the march. Each ambulance corpsman aboard carried a haversack with iodoform, bandages, absorbent cotton, and Esmarch's rubber bands. During the battle, Bell's ambulance corps occupied a church. It treated the wounded there until the church came under fire and then moved the wounded to a shallow gully, where the medical corps erected a hospital tent and several bell tents in which to carry on the triage and surgeries among fifty-three casualties. But even there several bullets passed through the tents as the surgeons worked.

Dodging projectiles, Bell's corps carried on its intricate operations: removing fragments of a jaw bone shattered by a bullet; treating a tibia fracture with a blue clay splint; extracting a bullet from the temple of a man shot through the eyeball; and removing a bullet that had entered a soldier's back between vertebrae and lodged in his chest. Among the final surgical procedures reported after the Battle of Batoche, however, one in particular revealed both the deft skill of the surgeons in the field and the impact of Roddick's newer, more hygienic field hospital protocols:

"Private Barton, 'Midland Battalion.' The right testicle was carried out of the scrotum, a Winchester bullet passing completely through it. The diseased tissue was pared away, and the testicle returned to the scrotum, having been cleansed with carbolic lotion and the scrotum brought together with sutures, leaving capillary drainage."[15]

But the chief of medical staff in the field added a final exclamation point to the list of his medical corps' contributions that summer. Thomas Roddick had to evacuate the wounded hundreds of miles back to Winnipeg. Wagon transport over dusty, rutted roads was not an option. So he evolved a plan to barge the wounded home. With the help of 7th Fusiliers captain Thomas H. Tracy, engineers from the regiment renovated three barges, scrubbing and whitewashing them for cleanliness; each was covered in canvas to deflect summer heat or rain, but with ample openings for ventilation at each end.

On July 3, 1885, the steamer *Alberta*—carrying a staff of medical dressers and nurses—steamed downriver from Saskatoon with a hospital barge on one side, a double barge on the other, and a final barge in front holding additional supplies and fresh vegetables. It took eleven days for the crew and eighteen wounded to cover the 1,100 miles via the Saskatchewan River and Lake Winnipeg, arriving at Winnipeg General Hospital on July 15. Thomas Roddick's impromptu military medical corps had exceeded all expectations, at least in the treatment of wounds and sickness.*

"Hopeless cases recovered. Dead men were brought to life," commented one of Roddick's medical colleagues. "Compared to the results which they had been accustomed to secure in the

---

* Sir Thomas Roddick, in addition to his remarkable aseptic medicine on the battlefield, served as dean of McGill's Faculty of Medicine from 1901 to 1908 and was instrumental in the creation of the Medical Council of Canada. He was knighted in 1912 and died in 1923. To honour his memory, in 1924 his widow, Lady Amy Redpath Roddick, had commemorative gates erected at the entrance to the McGill campus; she pointed out that Sir Thomas believed in punctuality, so clock towers appropriately adorn each end of the gates.

Montreal General Hospital in similar cases they were amazing.
. . . This was evidently due to the aseptic atmosphere of the tent
hospital. There were no germs there, while the Montreal General Hospital was saturated with them."[16]

In his summary report to the government in May 1886, Surgeon General Darby Bergin offered his assessment of medical operations during the North-West military campaign. In the multi-faceted document, Bergin complimented the purveyors, who supplied the field force, and the medical staff—from surgeons to ambulance corps, from nurses to transport, and from the Red Cross corps to the ladies' aid societies. But the chief medical administrator for the 1885 military expedition saved some of his most glowing praise for those he called "orderlies and dressers." Since the country had no trained ambulance corps or bearer companies at that time, Bergin had recruited volunteers from hospitals and medical schools mostly in eastern cities. He reported that almost every medical student in the Dominion, without exception, had volunteered his services. And for minimal pay, they exceeded Bergin's expectations.

"Many of these young men did noble work, regardless of danger," he wrote. "Where the bullets fell thickest . . . they were to be found, removing the wounded and the dying to places of shelter and of safety in the rear. . . . Amongst these non-combatant lads . . . are some of the greatest heroes of the war."[17]

JULY 1, 1916—SOMME RIVER VALLEY, FRANCE

MILITARY MEDICINE in the British Armed Forces received its royal designation as the Royal Army Medical Corps in 1898, just as the Empire was about to go to war in South Africa. As well as acknowledging the official roles fulfilled by medical officers, the proclamation included medics, orderlies, and stretcher-bearers, who all served under the general heading of "field ambulance." As was the case in Jonathan Letterman's Union Army field ambulance in the US Civil War, and Thomas Roddick's orderlies and dressers during the Riel resistance, field ambulance units were not as much vehicles as they were a large and diverse group of people completing a wide variety of medical tasks just behind the front lines.

By the time of the Great War, a field ambulance might include ten officers, fourteen NCOs, and 168 rank-and-file personnel. Add to that as many as fifty-seven Army Service Corps troops handling twenty-eight horse-drawn vehicles, and a total of 250 men and sixty horses might comprise a single field ambulance unit.[18] But the job of every field ambulance began where the fighting was—at the sharp end—where members of the team physically carried a wounded soldier away from a battlefield on a stretcher. And the stretcher-bearer exhibited at the very least a specialized skill, if not a unique brand of courage.

Herbert Horton wasn't the only stretcher-bearer to demonstrate such capability and calmness under fire at the Battle of the Somme in 1916, but he was among the few who offered his actions and reflections in a daily journal. The battle lasted five months—from July 1 to November 18—and killed or wounded over a million men. The big picture involved jockeying for acquired ground and moved opposing armies along the river valley from Albert, Beaumont-Hamel, and Bray to Pozières, Bazentin, Guinchy, and Courcellette. Horton summed up the Somme battlefields as "a man-made desert stretching to the horizon."[19] More important to a stretcher-bearer such as

Horton—originally from Birmingham, England, and serving with the 1st South Midland Field Ambulance—was the casualty case he was carrying and the ground between him and an aid post where his wounded patient could get the attention he needed to survive.

Bearers attached to the British and other Empire expeditionary forces often worked in teams of four. They were generally on call twenty-four hours a day; however, most calls came into their bunkers at night, such that they might catch as little as two hours of sleep before responding to a call for "Next squad out." Newly arrived at the Somme, nineteen-year-old Pte. Horton recalled the abrupt wake-up calls that summer. There was the discomfort of throwing off a bedroll blanket, quickly gulping down a cup of tea, and joining his three fellow bearers up the dugout steps and out into the cool night air of no man's land to retrieve a wounded man. That man weighed an average of 160 pounds, another twenty pounds with his boots and equipment, and even more if he was wet.[20]

"We lay [the wounded soldier] on our stretcher with a blanket over him, and start our journey back," Pte. Horton recorded in his diary. "Carrying in trenches we naturally have to take turns, with one man at each end of the stretcher and the remaining two disposed in front and rear ready to help lifting it, when necessary, head high to negotiate difficult corners."[21]

With practice and a sense of urgency each time they went out, the stretcher-bearers of most field ambulances learned how to alternate positions on the fly. They also worked out intricate ways to rig slings over their shoulders to relieve the pressure and weight on their arms, wrists, and hands while they strode as quickly as possible to an aid station to deliver their patient. Their route might be so routine that the bearers, without benefit of light, could feel their way along duckboard walks in communications trenches, or past discarded bombs or bodies along the way. To accelerate their run, ambulance men could also discard slings and packs or put a bearer on each corner of the stretcher.

"So, we deliver our charge at the dressing station to be examined and treated in the bright light of acetylene lamps—the smell of which, combined with the fumes of iodine and other chemical and human odours, remains a lasting memory."[22]

The race to save lives was equally hectic for the No. 1 Canadian Field Ambulance at Pozières Wood in late September. Frank Walker's bearer team received orders to clear out the aid posts in the area and move the wounded farther back. That's when the Germans began shelling the rear echelons of the Allied positions, making each run "a series of Marathon races"[23] between the forward aid station and the dressing station more distant from the fighting. In eighteen months of service along the Western Front, Walker's field ambulance group had sustained more than twenty casualties and he had already seen some of his closest chums killed or wounded. September 30 would simply add to the misery.

"McNutt has been hit through the back," Walker wrote in his diary. "His squad was carrying right ahead of us when the shell came over. It burst full upon them, scattering them like nine-pins, and a crazy sort of laughter came from our lips when we saw the Patient leap from the abandoned stretcher and go tearing across country for the nearest trench."[24]

Walker's friend Mac McNutt also jumped and ran for a

trench, joining the others seeking shelter there. But since Walker's first obligation was to the case he carried on his stretcher, he continued running. When he reached the dressing station and delivered his patient, Walker reported to his medical officer where McNutt had fallen. The major jumped into a motorized vehicle nearby and drove directly to the spot to retrieve the wounded stretcher-bearer. But it was for naught. McNutt died of his wounds in the hospital at Amiens six days later. "He was game right to the end," Walker wrote finally in his journal. "It would be hard to find a nobler death than that of a Stretcher Bearer."[25]

Characteristic of so many volunteer groups in the expeditionary forces of the British Empire in the Great War, young men tended to enlist in bunches from the same towns, even the same streets in those towns. They often volunteered to serve in the same regiments and then trained together, travelled overseas aboard the same troopships, and even served on the Western Front alongside the men who'd been their hometown friends and neighbours. A high-school dropout, Frank Walker got a job as a machinist in a foundry in Charlottetown, Prince Edward Island, but always maintained a fascination with classical literature; he tried his hand at poetry. He also maintained his friendships, so when the war broke out, Walker found himself in a field ambulance corps with men from Blooming Point, Charlottetown, and other points across the island. Pte. Walker shared most of his front-line experiences with men he'd known most of his life. Recalling one dash with fellow bearer Bill Grover, Walker revealed the greatest problem that field ambulance medics faced in their jobs.

"We saw above us climbing the ridge, an ambulance wagon,"

Walker wrote. "As it approached the summit, a shell came over, killing two of the horses. The driver unhitched the remaining team, and beat it, leaving the wagon with its freight of wounded alone on the hill."[26]

As Grover and Walker got closer to the top of the ridge in their own attempt to get out of harm's way and into Courcelette, they watched a second driver arrive on the scene of the abandoned wagon with a fresh team of horses. Immobile and exposed atop the ridge, the ambulance had clearly become a target of choice for enemy gunners. The two stretcher-bearers on foot watched the new driver hitch the fresh horses to the wagon and then, hanging on for dear life, encourage the team to advance. More shells landed nearby, just missing the moving target, but presently the wagon disappeared over the hill to safety.

"We cheered, Bill and I, though the excited driver never heard us, or even noticed us as he drove madly by. It was like watching a movie show," Walker concluded. "But now we had to take the ridge ourselves. We shut our teeth and sprinted. Nothing happened. We felt a little cheap. Fritz would not be bothered wasting a shell on us; [but] he must have enjoyed our exhibition of speed. We reached the Aid Post without further mishap, and secured a drink of Rum."[27]

That eighth of a pint of rum, or "tot," began as a Royal Navy tradition dating back to the Napoleonic Wars at the beginning of the nineteenth century. Ships at sea doled out the precious liquid—officers receiving it neat, while ratings got it in diluted form. For men of the field ambulance to receive a shot of rum was more likely the choice of a unit commander than a regulation. However, it no doubt proved welcome inspiration after a night of retrieving wounded while isolated in the dark in no man's land. Despite the horrific fatality numbers in the expeditionary forces, mortality statistics actually favoured field ambulance crews. Generally, those who served on the Western Front had a one-in-three chance of receiving a wound and a one-in-eight chance of dying. If a man served as a combat soldier, he had a 60 percent chance of becoming a casualty. Field ambulance crews had a casualty rate of 8 percent and a fatality rate of 4 percent. Of the seven hundred Canadians who went overseas with Pte. Walker in the field ambulance corps, 160 were killed or died of disease.[28] In his poem *Packing Out (A Ballad of the Stretcher Bearers)*, Walker sums up his service:

> Back and back we go, 'til the battle-field is clear,
> (It's good to hear the wounded chaps giving us the Cheer!)
> Back and back we go 'til the bloody job is through,
> Then it's "Good old Stretcher Bearers!" and "A double
>   Rum for you!"[29]

During his front-line service along the Western Front, Pte. Frank Walker and his No. 1 Field Ambulance comrades from Prince Edward Island had some occasional down time. That's when they would try to bury some of the dead, and if they found a dry, covered spot near an aid post, they would sit and play bridge, euchre, cribbage, or poker. But they also complained about the meagre food rations, and that the cookhouse was a quarter-mile away. Partway through 1916, the No. 1 Field Ambulance bearers handed off their position to a replacement crew, the No. 9 Field Ambulance.

Among those incoming stretcher-bearers, orderlies, and medics was a lance corporal originally from Belfast, Ireland; because his family had emigrated to Canada, his enlistment papers identified his home as Montreal. John Campbell Kennedy was among the older volunteers, thirty-one when he shipped overseas in 1915 with the 60th Canadian Infantry Battalion. After gaining a year's experience in Belgium at the Ypres salient, Kennedy was informed by his commander that he was posting him back to England to instruct. He protested and took a demotion in rank and a pay cut—from $1.50 a day as a sergeant to $1.10 a day as a private—to join the No. 9 Field Ambulance in 1916, en route to the Western Front in France. Nine months later he was back to a staff sergeant's rank, and his commanding officer, a Colonel Bazin, wanted his overall impressions of the 9th.

"Sir, may I speak?" Kennedy began.[30]

"Why not?" the colonel said.

"I can't speak without your permission."

The colonel gave him permission and then popped the question: "What do you think of the 9th Field Ambulance?"

"As a Sunday school bunch, they are okay," Kennedy said without hesitating. "As soldiers they are a washout."

The colonel asked him to elaborate. S/Sgt. Kennedy said he recognized a problem common among many of the support units such as the field ambulance corps—poor food rations. Further, he said, the food wasn't properly prepared. Kennedy informed his commander that the man in charge of preparing food for his units of the Royal Canadian Army Medical Corps (RCAMC) was not qualified.

"You mean to tell me [Sgt. Richards] isn't a cook?" the colonel asked.

"How could he be?" Kennedy said. "He was a bricklayer in civilian life!"

The staff sergeant offered a solution. He told his colonel that there was a cooking school for the military in Bruay. He'd read about it in the army's daily orders. "You send your six cooks there this week [and] your unit will be better fed, happier and better soldiers."

Better food and better cooks had an even greater impact than the stretcher-bearers realized. In the final phase of the war, as the Canadian Corps prepared for what would be the final push against the Germans—the so-called Last Hundred Days in 1918—S/Sgt. Kennedy and the No. 9 Field Ambulance were hot on the heels of the troops as they raced northeast from the start line at Amiens. On the first day of the Allied offensive, when they overran an enemy aid post, Kennedy's field ambulance group captured a senior German army medical officer.

"He spoke perfect English," Kennedy wrote in a memoir. "[He] told us we looked well fed and that he'd been told we were starving. . . . He offered Errol [Amaron] and me his card to write him a letter after the war was over. We said nothing doing."

Sgt. Maj. Amaron received the Military Medal and S/Sgt. Kennedy the Croix de Guerre. The No. 9 Field Ambulance entered the Belgian city of Mons at 4 a.m. on November 11, 1918. The armistice was declared seven hours later.

...

APRIL 9, 1917—ETAPLES, FRANCE

IF INJURED SOLDIERS SURVIVED those death-defying dashes aboard field ambulance stretchers, the emergency treatment in casualty clearing stations, and the bumpy ride aboard railroad coaches from the Western Front sixty miles back to Etaples on the coast of France, what awaited them there was truly a sight for sore eyes. Off-loaded from the hospital train and transferred into motorized lorries, the wounded were attended by ambulance drivers in goggles, gauntlets, blue uniforms, black leather trenchcoats, and aviator helmets. And if those ambulance drivers peeled back the goggles and helmets for a moment, they would often reveal what one journalist described as a "clear, bold face coming out from between the leather flaps . . . the girls looked like splendid young airmen."[31] These were the women of the Voluntary Aid Detachment (VAD) of the British Red Cross. One of these VAD drivers, whom Allied scribes called "angels of mercy," was twenty-three-year-old Grace Evelyn MacPherson. "I didn't mind the hard work. That's what I went over for," she said. "We had to clean the inside of the ambulances . . . repair flats and pump up the tires by hand . . . We served an area of over 50,000 beds."[32]

Their proximity to the south of England, just across the Channel, made a number of ports along the French coast ideal entry and exit points for Royal Army Medical Corps personnel and patients. Le Havre housed half a dozen Red Cross, general, and stationary hospitals; Le Tréport and Le Touquet were home to another half-dozen hospitals while the flatlands around Dannes-Camiers housed a couple of hospitals under canvas; Boulogne had three hospitals; Wimereux housed four more; and Etaples serviced another eight—Nos. 1 and 7 Canadian General Hospitals, Nos. 23, 24, 26, and 56 British General Hospitals, and No. 46 British Stationary Hospital, as well as the St. John Ambulance Hospital. By 1917, Grace MacPherson—one of 110 women VAD ambulance drivers there—had become a fixture ferrying wounded along rutted country roads and over the cobblestoned streets. But getting the nod to serve in the driver's seat of her McLaughlin Buick ambulance had not been easy.

Her determination to do so, despite the odds, might have had something to do with being born, in 1895, the youngest of six children. When just a child, Grace moved with her family from Winnipeg to Vancouver, where she didn't seem content to spend her days biding her time in their comfortable home on Hornby Street. She was active, had an outgoing personality, and made lots of friends, but she clearly had designs on a career too; she studied typing and shorthand and taught youth at Sunday school. In a statement of her independence, Grace made quite the splash around town—while employed at a typewriter firm—when she bought her own Paige-Detroit automobile and wasn't the least bit fazed by having to repair the flats on her own.

If the mechanical realities of operating her own vehicle didn't toughen her view of life, however, the war soon did. By September 1915, Grace's brother Alex had been killed in Gallipoli and she complained in her diary, "Oh, this terrible war."[33] What might have been the catalyst in her life, however, occurred during an emergency in the streets of Vancouver. Confronted by a man in need of immediate first aid, Grace sensed that flagging down a cab or calling an ambulance wasn't good enough;

she drove him to a downtown hospital herself. Here, she suddenly sensed, was a way to contribute. "I'm going. I'm going to drive an ambulance," she announced to her mother.[34]

Grace immediately wrote to the War Office in Ottawa and to the British Red Cross to volunteer. Neither seemed particularly enthusiastic about her skill behind the wheel. Nonetheless, she inscribed in her diary, "I certainly hope for sufficient willpower and courage."[35] In time she managed to persuade officials at the Canadian Pacific Steamship line to offer her transatlantic passage. By August 1916 she had made the crossing and arrived on the doorstep of VAD headquarters at Devonshire House in London. A day earlier and she could have filled a vacancy available in France; instead, she had to settle for a temporary job handing out chits to troops on leave at the Canadian Army pay office.

Wartime London proved an adventure at every turn for the Canadian volunteer. MacPherson dined out at Lyons Corner House, attended vaudeville at the Palladium, danced at the Trocadero, and often travelled about in a friend's motorcycle sidecar. She still took repeated first-aid classes in anticipation of another VAD vacancy in France. But in her free time, she seemed the life of the party.

On one occasion, she recounted in her diary, she and a half-dozen of her chums had gone out to dinner and were joined by a handsome, apparently wealthy soldier from South Africa. "I'm going to get married tomorrow," he told MacPherson during the meal.[36]

"I wish you all the joy in the world," she responded.

However, the young soldier made repeated advances to MacPherson, kissing her hands in front of everyone and saying, "If I had met a little Canadian girl a couple of days ago, I would not be getting married tomorrow."

"Oh, but perhaps you *would* be getting married tomorrow, just the same," she retorted, and that brought hoots of laughter.

The young South African persisted, holding her hand and drawing her toward him while MacPherson's friends tried to help her escape, in a kind of tug-of-war at the door. "You have wonderful girls in Canada," he told her pals. "I simply can't get out of getting married tomorrow though. The girl threw over an artillery boy for me. And I've got to go through with it."

MacPherson wrote in her diary later that she'd saved her best retort to the last; she told the amorous South African that she'd just been posted to France. In fact, she had been thwarted in her every attempt to get there. But, undeterred, Grace MacPherson learned in the autumn of 1916 that Sir Sam Hughes was on his latest mission to Britain. She pressed for a private interview with the minister of militia and defence at his London headquarters, atop the Savoy Hotel. As she entered his enormous suite, apparently populated by "ten crossed swords and generals," she put her case to him.[37]

"I've come from Canada to drive ambulances," MacPherson announced.

The long-time military man, knighted in 1915 and clearly playing to the officers seated around him in the suite, began strutting around the room. "I'll stop any woman from going to France," he bellowed. "And I'll stop you!"

"I'm just impatient to go," she explained, "and I thought perhaps you could help me get there." She even pointed out that she'd heard Hughes's own daughter had been allowed to go over.

He repeated his position but suggested as a compromise that he would give her a letter that might help her get a driver's job in England.

"Well, Sir Sam, I am going to France and you are not going to stop me. And I can get there without your help," she said finally, and left the interview.

It's no surprise that the needs of the war undermined the wisest of plans and those most resistant to change. Conditions on the Western Front superseded Sam Hughes's bombast about women at the front when the War Office determined that the men in ambulance driver's seats could better serve the war effort closer to the front. And so the driving jobs—ferrying the wounded between hospitals on the coast of France—were reassigned to VAD women. On March 28, 1917, Grace MacPherson got her marching orders, joining twenty other women in a reinforcement draft of drivers for the convoys that would transport the wounded from the railroad station at Etaples to all of its military hospitals. Feeling the excitement of her wish come true, MacPherson dashed about London assembling her kit—boots, warm underwear, leather coat, and helmet—all of which she paid for herself. One of her male friends in London bought her a pair of goggles for good luck. And she was off to France.

"When I stepped off the ship at Boulogne and got into an ambulance with eight or ten other women," she said, "I felt I had been there all my life. It was so commonplace."[38]

Indeed, the nature of her routine reflected that. MacPherson noted that each day she had to clean and maintain two ambulances—each with space for four stretcher patients in the back and two more seated beside her in the cab. The toughest job when making repairs was fixing flats. All the tires had inner and outer tubes, and the driver had to jack up the vehicle, remove the blown tubes, patch them up, and then re-inflate the tubes by hand; at one point the women suggested taking up a collection to buy a mechanical pump, but their commandant suggested that was "sissy stuff."[39]

The job of the ambulance fleet—twenty-five vehicles per section, about 110 drivers in all—was to connect the area railroad stations with the network of hospitals; in Etaples there were approximately 50,000 beds among eight different military hospitals. As each hospital train arrived with coaches full of incoming wounded lying on rows of shelves, each ambulance would either ferry its wounded to the appropriate hospital or sometimes evacuate them right to a waiting hospital ship bound for "Blighty." VAD drivers worked twelve hours on followed by twelve hours off; often a convoy and an evacuation required three hours each and would fill a full shift. Everything changed when there was a major operation underway at the front, and drivers would have to work thirty-six or forty-eight hours without sleep. As compensation, MacPherson received four shillings a week for laundry and ten shillings to pay for food in the mess.

Lieutenant (it was an honorary rank) MacPherson arrived in France on April 7, 1917, just two days before the Canadian Corps' historic assault on Vimy Ridge. Late in the afternoon on the first day of the battle, Easter Monday, a call arrived in Etaples for the Red Cross to have as many as sixty-five ambulances at the station for incoming wounded.[40] The weather had closed in that day, with snow and slush on the roads. And with the entire Canadian Corps involved in the attack—forty regiments, and some 7,000 wounded over the four-day battle—the medical echelons at Vimy were swamped. Field ambulance crews simply bypassed clearing stations and carried their cases directly to the hospital rail cars for the non-stop trip to Etaples. Some even went straight to hospital ships for the cross-Channel trip to England.

"They were a very sorry looking bunch," MacPherson thought when she saw the first of the wounded from Vimy.[41] "We knew so many of them." And yet during this, her baptism of fire as an ambulance driver, she knew she couldn't let their medical conditions interfere with her responsibilities or meeting her schedule. If a soldier groaned from the back of the ambulance, she would immediately shout back, "You cut that out! Nobody's riding in my ambulance moaning like that!"

"Oh, I got a leg off," another might say.

"Look, I bashed my thumb," she'd respond, not allowing herself to think about a man with that severe a wound. She also hoped it might momentarily distract her patient's attention.

"You're a queer sort of bloke" might be the comeback.

And she'd reassure the man finally by saying, "You're going to get the best ride you ever had in your life."

She meant it. Without the advantage of lights at night and during blackouts, or well-maintained roads through winter conditions, ambulance drivers had to negotiate their way along darkened, often muddy or slippery routes at speeds no faster than a walking pace, five miles per hour along the nearly mile-long route to hospitals in Etaples. Despite the apparent snail's pace, however, most of the Vimy casualties arrived at the coastal hospitals within three hours of receiving their wounds on the Western Front. MacPherson's ambulance—RA660—

completed ten trips carrying Vimy wounded that night, many being evacuated to England straightaway. Following her first night's initiation into the ambulance service, transporting many of her countrymen, she commented, "I was very proud of my Canada [patch] on my shoulders."[42]

When Grace MacPherson found a few hours on her off-shift to sleep, she retired to the bell tents or Nissen huts set up as dormitories for most of the medical personnel in and around Etaples—doctors, orderlies, ambulance drivers, and nurses. She wasn't far from a host of other Canadians housed in the tent and hut cities adjacent to the hospital facilities. Like the ambulance drivers, most of the nursing sisters were dressed in blue, and with the addition of their white veils, they were nicknamed "bluebirds." The Canadian Army Nursing Service recruited over 3,000 nurses, more than half of whom were serving overseas.

Among the nursing sisters who arrived at No. 1 Canadian General Hospital about the same time that Grace MacPherson did was Nursing Sister Katherine Maud Macdonald. Nursing Sister Macdonald had graduated from nurse training at Victoria Hospital in London, Ontario, in April 1917, and she immediately enlisted with the Canadian Army Medical Corps. She took on responsibility willingly and ably; for the transatlantic trip, she was put in charge of a contingent of nineteen other nurses. "I have everything to look after," she wrote to her mother at home in Brantford, Ontario, "nineteen tickets, all their documents, baggage, [and] if they are sick. . . . One developed German measles, but she has just been inoculated."[43]

First in Eastbourne, England, where she served at No. 10

Canadian Stationary Hospital, and then when the facility was transported to Calais, France, the higher-ups in the nursing staff and the doctors found her an asset in surgery. She wrote that she regularly got the call to scrub up and contribute in the operating room, for which they "praised me up sky high."[44] In January 1918, they transferred her closer to the front, at No. 1 Canadian General Hospital in Etaples. The flow of letters home to her mother and sister, Florence, slowed to a trickle because the pace at the hospital consumed so many of her waking hours. When *Kaiserschlacht*, the German offensive, began on March 21, 1918, Macdonald wrote that suddenly the casualties were not getting first aid behind the lines at clearing stations, but immediately being sent by rail and ambulance to the hospitals in Etaples. The wounds she and the surgical staff faced grew more hideous and untreated on arrival, but despite feeling swamped by the tide of cases around her in the ward, Macdonald found a way to give individual solace.

"One man [had undergone] amputation of both legs above the knee," she wrote. "He has lost so much blood that . . . we had to send him to the O.R. again tonight. And when he came back he would not rest unless he had my hand. And there I sat, and thought every minute my back would break. He is a dear, but am so afraid he will go out."[45]

In the same letter and a subsequent note to her family, Macdonald noted that she had sought transfer back to No. 10 Canadian Stationary Hospital in Calais, but every time there was "another big push" at the front it seemed her request was delayed further. In fact, the reason for the delay was an administrative error; there were two Nursing Sister Macdonalds in the system, and transfer papers were sent to the wrong one.

On May 18, 1918, the hospital staff had discharged seventy-six patients, which meant that Grace MacPherson's ambulance crew had been busy transporting them back to the station en route to ports and ships bound for England. While No. 1 CGH still had over a thousand patients, one of the nursing sisters—not Katherine Macdonald—was transferred to another hospital. Still anticipating an imminent move back to Calais, Nursing Sister Macdonald decided to take a few moments to visit the cemetery adjacent to the hospital in Etaples. No doubt, even in the short time she'd served there, many patients whom she'd attended to were laid to rest there.

"They have millions buried," she wrote home, "some Canadians, lots of officers, and two VADs. The officers have graves to themselves, but the privates are two in a grave, each have a wooden cross at the head and all are fixed up nicely."[46]

The next day, Whit Sunday, the VAD ambulance convoy delivered eighty-two casualties from the train station to No. 1 Canadian General Hospital in Etaples. And that kept the surgical staff and nursing sisters busy most of the day. Medical teams managed to discharge forty-six patients, but even so, by Sunday night, No. 1 was still attending to a patient population of 1,156. With the casualties settled in the wards at the end of the day, the nursing sisters had time to attend a church service and an evening concert.[47] At 10:30 p.m. the moon had come up and the night air was still. But the calm was broken by the sound of aircraft approaching in formation, a squadron of them. Within seconds the hospital grounds erupted in explosions. Two waves of German bombers swooped in low enough to single out large structures or buildings clustered together.

Over the next two hours, the aircraft dropped 116 bombs.

"The raid was obviously planned to take place in relays," the No. 1 CGH war diary recounted. "A number of bombs, incendiary and high explosive, were dropped in the midst of the men's quarters. Fires were immediately started, which offered a splendid target for the second [wave] of the attack. The scene was immediately converted into a conflagration and charnel house of dead and wounded men. Bombs were also dropped on the Officers' and Sisters' quarters."[48]

While there were some bombproof shelters—either bunkers or sand-bagged huts—there was no warning, so no time for the nursing sisters to evacuate their quarters. One bomb fell directly on the hut housing Nursing Sisters Gladys Wake, Margaret Lowe, Barbara McKinnon, and Katherine Macdonald. The explosion caved in much of the building around them.

"We must move," one sister shouted in the smoke and dust.

"I am fainting," Macdonald called out.

Another sister and a recently arrived officer ran to Macdonald's assistance, but she collapsed almost immediately and died within a few minutes. The officer reported to Macdonald's fiancé that she had died "due to the severance of the femoral artery and concussion."[49] Eight patients were killed in the raid and another thirty-one wounded, while the No. 1 CGH medical staff sustained fifty-five killed and fifty-three wounded, including two nursing sisters—Gladys Wake and Margaret Lowe—who later died of their wounds. Nursing Sister Georgina Long, whose hut caved in during the blasts, said authorities had not heeded a warning they'd received.

"We had a meeting a month earlier, asking for tin hats to be served to the nurses," Long said to a reporter, "as word had gone 'round that Hun airmen dropped [leaflets] announcing their intention to bomb the hospitals. The authorities were considering the request when the raid happened."[50]

During the attack, British anti-aircraft gunners managed to shoot down one of the bombers. The German observer in the plane survived uninjured, while the pilot received shrapnel wounds; he was interrogated and, speaking perfect English, pointed out that "if the British choose to build their hospitals near railways, they must expect to get bombed."[51]

When she realized what was happening during the bombing, VAD driver Grace MacPherson raced around the barracks helping her comrades and their patients find cover. Then she jumped into her ambulance—which had by now been nick-named "Kangaroo"—and spent the rest of the night ferrying wounded from No. 1 Canadian General Hospital to other area hospitals unmolested by the attack. An officer wrote that "she was the first on the scene with her machine and she worked all night without quiver. . . . In the estimation of the officers here and of her own corps, Miss MacPherson is described as 'the bravest of them all.'"[52]

Nursing Sister Katherine Macdonald was interred with full military honours in the Etaples cemetery—with the "millions buried" that she had paid her respects to just a day earlier.*

---

* By the end of the Great War, 3,141 women had served in the Canadian Army Medical Corps; forty-six died as a result of enemy action or disease as they carried out their duties. While Canadian authorities campaigned for nursing sisters to receive the equivalent of officers' citations (e.g., the Military Cross), British authorities limited the honours to the Military Medal. In 1919 the *London Gazette* announced the awarding of the Military Medal to seven Canadian nursing sisters, the first Canadian women to win gallantry decorations.

CHAPTER SIX

"LIVES AFRESH TOGETHER"

I'M NOT QUITE SURE when the telltale photo first appeared. It had been tucked away in a suitcase in the basement of my parents' house in Toronto for many years. It was tightly rolled up—a cylinder of paper about a foot and a half long—and since the outside of the cylinder was the blank backside of a photo, it had gone pretty much overlooked inside this piece of Samsonite luggage. It was sister Kate who suddenly decided to take a closer look. And when she gingerly unrolled it, to a length of about five feet, she discovered it was one of those old-fashioned panoramic photographs. This stunningly clear black-and-white cyclograph,* taken in 1936, showed about 250 celebrants gathered for a summer picnic at North Beach Park in New York City. Most of the adults and kids were standing. The youngest were seated or held in their parents'

---

* A cyclograph was created inside a box camera with a spring-wound clock motor rotating film across the lens from one spool to another to create the wide-angle view.

arms. One or two had their hands in the air waving, although most—no doubt warned by the photographer—remained absolutely still in order not to blur the final image.

About halfway along the panorama, just to the left of a banner on a pole that identified these Greek picnickers as members of the Pan-Karabournian Society, two teenagers stood side by side. One of them, a girl, had a soft smile on a face warmed by a summertime tan. The other, a boy, was slightly taller, with hair tossed casually across his forehead; his complexion was a bit fairer, and he smiled more broadly. On closer examination, one could see that the girl had her hand almost imperceptibly resting on the boy's shoulder, as if to say "We are connected." That summer, Koula Kontozoglou was thirteen, while the boy whose shoulder she was touching would soon be fourteen. His name was Alexandros Barbaritis. That hand placed on that shoulder, if anybody had taken note of it, foretold a unique seventy-year relationship. Half of a Great Depression and a full world war later, in 1948, that couple would marry and become my parents— Kay and Alex Barris.

APRIL 3, 1945—KREFELD, GERMANY

BY THE TIME KOULA KONTOZOGLOU and Alexandros Barbaritis were teenagers in 1930s New York City, their families were already close. Both clans had been part of the city's vast blue-collar workforce—labouring in the food industry, stitching pelts in the fur coat business, and short-order cooking in restaurant kitchens to pay the rent, as well as feed and clothe seven children in total. And both families attended the same Greek Orthodox church, enjoyed friendly card games over Christmas and Easter, and attended functions such as the Karabournian Greek picnic each summer, often enough that Koula and Alexandros saw each other as children and adolescents regularly. Coincidentally, the two walked the same route to and from Haaren High School, near the Jackson Heights area of Queens. In fact, when Alex—after long neglecting to do so—decided to write Koula, it was their alma mater he reminded her about first.

"We have known each other so long, yet I never saw you very often after I finished school," Alex wrote to Koula in April 1945. "I remember many mornings when we met on our way to school at the El[evated train] station. Weren't those good old days—tell me, Koula, do you ever miss your high school days?"[1]

It was a leading question. Alex clearly did miss those days in class learning history, language, and literature. Like a lot of young Americans serving in the Second World War, Alex got as far as completing a high-school diploma, but that was it; the Barbaritis family hadn't had the wherewithal, and, as it turned out, neither did he have the time to go to college. Deprived of higher learning, trained for war, and rushed overseas to defeat the Nazis, Alex felt he'd missed out on a university experience. Indeed, in this letter from overseas, he told Koula that he'd "learned to appreciate things I once took for granted," including, he seemed to be saying between the lines, his friendship with her.

When Alex—his surname simplified when he went into the services from Barbaritis to Barris—sat down to compose this apparently long-overdue letter to Koula, a lot had changed in their worlds. Koula, who was now twenty-three and an honours graduate of stenography school, was working in retail helping her family make ends meet during the war. Meanwhile, Alex was a year older than her and, in the spring of 1945, had survived a couple of years in the army, including the bloodiest US engagement of the war, the Battle of the Bulge.

Now a veteran medical corpsman in the US Army, T/Sgt. Barris, along with the 94th Infantry Division in Patton's Third Army, had broken through the daunting German Westwall fortifications and forced the German armies defending the former Siegfried Line into full retreat. Finally, after three months of bitter winter weather and bitter close-contact fighting, his unit had gone into reserve. They'd been put on trucks, transported two hundred miles north to Krefeld, just outside the city of Düsseldorf, and given a few days' rest. Alex and the others in his war-weary unit had found time to wash in hot water, sleep between sheets in a billet, and clean their uniforms. He'd also found time to catch up on his correspondence, including this revealing letter to Koula.

"I've seen guys come and go—and they were in considerably worse shape in the latter act," Alex wrote to her. "I go on and on, and have high hopes of continuing to do so, my fingers are crossed."[2]

While Koula never considered Alex very romantic, she had a pretty good understanding of his comedic side. In an earlier letter she had poked at his sense of humour by kidding him about all the French women tempting him during the US Army's liberation of the Cherbourg peninsula, the Bocage in Normandy, and the city of Paris. Not surprisingly, Alex went for the bait.

"What's all this about French beauties?" he chided. "First of all, I'm in Germany, where women aren't any too beautiful. Furthermore, it's against the law to so much as look at them. . . . And if I may be allowed a word in my defense, I'll have you know I'm a good boy! (Ahem!)"

With just a bit more time on his hands, and a bit more hope in his heart that he might actually get out of this war alive, he opened up to his school-chum-turned-confidante about the future. He likely hadn't thought about such a thing in two years, but suddenly the prospect of sharing his hopes with someone he knew and trusted moved him to reveal more than usual. He described the pastimes of so many of his comrades now away from the battlefields—playing sports, writing, and reading. He was reading *The Great American Novel*, but for more than just Clyde Davis's take on a newspaperman in postwar America unable to find time to write that elusive manuscript. "The title fascinates me," he wrote Koula, "possibly because I have an ambition to be a writer someday. Of course, from where I sit, the chances of my becoming a writer are pretty slim, but I can dream can't I?"

His dreaming didn't end there. After seven pages of revealing his regrets about college, his perspective on the war, and some of his hopes and ambitions, he returned to Koula, asking her how she was doing, what she was doing, and if she had time to dream too. Finally, while not admitting exactly how he felt about her, he made her a pledge of sorts. "If you write again, and bring me up to date," Alex said, "I'll promise to answer and keep doing so whenever you write. Fair enough?"

...

JULY 12, 1917—BRAMSHOTT CAMP, ENGLAND

JUST LIKE T/SGT. ALEX BARRIS in front of Campholz Woods
during the battle in the Saar-Moselle Triangle in 1945, Capt.
Harold McGill, at Kemmel Trench on the Western Front,
served his medical unit on foot. In the winter of 1915 he
ensured that his 31st Battalion's wounded were quickly
carried by his stretcher-bearers to the regimental aid post,
about five hundred yards behind the front lines. There, in an
underground dugout, McGill and his two orderlies administered first aid and then passed their patients along, again
on stretchers, through a communication trench to dressing
stations farther back. Initially when McGill sent letters home
about his daily routine, he wrote guardedly about the front-
line fighting, the nature of battle wounds, and his treatment
of them. In a letter home in December 1915, for example,
he summed up his situation at the RAP, commenting that his
stretcher-bearers "are doing splendid work and not one of
them has had a scratch."[3]

In the spring of 1916, during the Battle of Sanctuary Wood
in Belgium, Canadian infantry regiments were defending the
southern sections of the Ypres salient near Hill 62. On June
16, while not revealing either his exact location or the units
involved in the fighting, Capt. McGill wrote a more detailed
letter than usual to an apparently understanding recipient. He
allowed that he'd witnessed "furious fighting at the front"
while barricaded in an abandoned mill (Menin Mill) employed
as a regimental aid post. He explained that the weather had
closed in with rain and cold temperatures, more like October than spring, as "the wounded came in soaked to the skin

and plastered with mud," most of them suffering from shell wounds "of terrible severity. . . . I have not yet counted up the number of wounded," the letter continued. "We started one evening at dusk, worked all that night, all the next day and until four o'clock in the morning of the following day."[4]

Only someone acquainted with the nature of attending to such life-threatening injuries, and the shock of that kind of trauma, might read this letter and understand what McGill had experienced trying to save lives behind the front lines at Sanctuary Wood. Only somebody he respected could McGill trust with the news that his cousin, another medical officer, had died in action with the 3rd Canadian Infantry Division. That he'd written this and similar letters to another person serving in the medical professions became clear as Capt. McGill brought his June 16 letter to a close. "I am enclosing you a rose which I picked in a garden among the ruins of a famous and historic city. . . . Sincerely, Harold W. McGill."

McGill had sent his letter to an acquaintance back in Calgary, a medical practitioner with whom he had worked when the city faced a typhoid epidemic before the war. That acquaintance was one Emma Mildred Griffis, a nursing sister on staff at Calgary General Hospital (CGH). And the rose he'd chosen to enclose, found in "the ruins of a famous and historic city"—Emma understood that to mean Ypres, still under siege by German forces that spring. Indeed, she would recognize "a garden among the ruins" as the former Cloth Hall, reduced to rubble by German guns firing from the heights beyond the salient. One detail McGill neglected to mention in the letter was that when picking the rose, he nearly bumped into the muzzle of a British field gun camouflaged in the Cloth Hall shrubbery. And why were the rose and the recipient so significant? Because the rose was a first romantic offering to Emma Griffis from a secret admirer. And the letter marked the start of a long-lasting and long-distance courtship that initially went in only one direction—from McGill to Griffis.

Though she had grown up in Canada, Emma Griffis was born in Kansas, in the United States. North of the border, as an adult, she had received her nurse training in Ontario and Alberta, joining the staff of Calgary General in 1910. Described by one historian as a vivacious young woman who enjoyed the attention of many admirers,[5] Emma clearly enjoyed life—a photo taken outside the CGH shows her perched playfully on the cornerstone of the entrance steps; she's wearing her hospital whites and a broad smile. Though Harold McGill had felt attracted to Griffis as they attended to Calgarians in the typhoid ward during the outbreak, she did not reciprocate, saying later, "I avoided him like the plague."[6]

Correspondence as regular, as rich with detail, and as honest as Capt. McGill's, however, left ever-deeper impressions on the home-front nurse. Griffis began to write in response and send packages to her former Calgary co-worker just as he was posted to the most challenging battlefields in the Great War. He wrote that he estimated his year at the front had made him a veteran, "thoroughly inured and accustomed to the signs of war." But the sounds, sights, and smells at the Battle of the Somme in the fall of 1916 outstripped anything in his experience, and "revolted and sickened me beyond my power of expression."[7]

On September 10, Capt. McGill led his medical team through the village of Albert to establish a regimental aid post close to

No. 3 Canadian Field Ambulance in a shallow gulley known euphemistically as "Sausage Valley," with the obliterated village of Pozières to their front. The captain noted in his journals that it seemed mortal enemies had fought back and forth across every inch of the valley. The expediency of advancing, digging in, and preparing for counterattack left no time for the new owners of the real estate to clean up the wreckage left by its previous occupants. The remains of unburied dead or bodies that shells had lifted back to the surface made any medical work nearby completely unsanitary, since any body parts on the surface of the battlefield soon displayed "a metallic lustre . . . clouds of loudly buzzing blue-bottle flies."[8] McGill's medics managed to acquire fly-tox pesticide to reduce the volume. But the whole environment left the inbound troops weary, disgusted, and unable to keep down any of their food rations. Barely dug in at the position after two days, Capt. McGill marvelled at the brutality and indifference of the scene. On a road into the valley, he wrote in his journal, he'd seen the remains of a man's arm, likely driven over and tossed about hundreds of times by the wheels of passing limbers; nobody had bothered to bury it or toss it off the road into a shell hole.

While the veteran medical officer didn't share that macabre anecdote with Nurse Griffis, in an October 1916 letter he did admit that he and his comrades, lately pushing German troops back to the east, were not about to rejoice, since their advance had sustained the loss of so many of their own officers and men, something he referred to as "the price of victory." In that same letter, though, Capt. McGill recounted one of the most difficult nights of his wartime experience. Fighting in mid-September along that section of the Somme battle line had depleted all ranks—casualty rates of 25 to 50 percent were commonplace—including members of his own medical unit. Of the nucleus of men with whom Harold McGill had enlisted in Canada, only one original stretcher-bearer remained. With him since mobilization in Calgary was a slight, wiry youth with blue eyes and red hair. Teddy Barnes was chief of the D Company first-aid men. McGill had often turned to Barnes and his experience to help new recruits learn the ropes. "I know that you have a number of green men," Barnes had told his captain, "and it may make it easier for you to have with you some of us that have had experience."[9]

Late in the afternoon of September 26, Barnes himself was brought in by other stretcher-bearers. "My stretcher bearer sergeant, the finest little fellow in the battalion," Capt. McGill wrote Emma Griffis, "had his leg torn off by a shell. . . . I saw him after he was hit. He bid me good bye saying he had tried to do his work and was sorry not to be able to carry on to the end."[10]

McGill recorded in his journal later that Barnes had lost a great deal of blood, that his face was deathly white, and that when he adjusted the tourniquet on his stump, Barnes seemed the coolest among those wounded men in the regimental aid post. The seasoned doctor hustled his friend to a field ambulance; if there was even the faintest chance the advanced dressing station could save Barnes, McGill would ensure that his closest aid man received immediate attention. Despite the severity of his wound, Barnes's gaze never left the face of his captain, his grip as strong as ever. And even as Barnes was carried away, he apologized to McGill for leaving him in the middle of the action. Sergeant Barnes died later that day. "It was not so much the loss of him as a stretcher bearer," McGill wrote finally to Griffis, "[but] the personal loss of a friend."[11]

Several weeks later, during a period when McGill's superiors had decided to give the long-serving captain special leave, he'd written Emma apologizing for what he called his blue letter about the price paid for military victories. He wrote that he felt ashamed for his apparent depression. He tried to show her that his spirits had been buoyed when he learned his friend Barnes had received a posthumous Military Medal, and that some of his previously wounded aid men had recovered enough to return to service, making the unit more like its old self again. Meantime, authorities confirmed that Capt. McGill would receive the Military Cross for conspicuous gallantry and devotion to duty during fighting at Courcelette. Nonetheless, in the same letter, he admitted that for at least some of the days during his special leave, he hadn't left the room at his hotel. Whether it was her growing affection for Capt. McGill or a growing concern for his health, not to mention her own sense of patriotism, in the new year Emma decided to enlist for overseas service.

On January 2, 1917, as she prepared for the cross-Canada train trip and her transatlantic passage from Halifax, she wrote McGill about his situation, his experiences, and (perhaps to provide some distraction from the war) mutual acquaintances. Though he hadn't seen her since his train left Calgary in May 1915, he had shared remarkable insights into life in the trenches. In his letters he had explained that conditions required that he sleep in his clothes, with orders never to remove his boots except to put on clean, dry socks.[12] He'd explained his responsibility for dispensing the tots of rum to the men—each ration measured out by his corporal "in a teapot" and given in the RAP dugout to bombers, snipers, signallers, machine-gunners, and wiremen.

Throughout two years of correspondence, McGill's writing had always remained businesslike—still signing off "Sincerely yours"—but when he received word in France that Nurse Griffis had arrived safely in the UK, McGill's tone changed. His greeting became "Dearest Emma" and signed off with "Yours with fondest love."[13] And they each—she serving at the Bramshott Military Hospital and he while billeted in northern France—began plotting to coordinate their subsequent leaves.

As if scripted, in late June 1917 Emma sprained her ankle and was briefly hospitalized, but then discharged July 7. Meanwhile, Harold had secured his leave beginning June 29, but he had to ride horseback from Houdain to the railhead at Aubigny for the train to Boulogne and the cross-Channel boat to Folkestone. By July 5 he'd reached Bramshott to meet Emma. There was tea, and commitments to meet friends for dinner and a dance; the couple did arrive, but fashionably late. Their leaves had coincided. They shared five days in London—where one day German bombs fell on the city—seeing shows, attending concerts, dining out at the Savoy Hotel, and, on the final day of Harold's leave, agreeing in secret to be married. With the die cast, at least between the two of them, Harold made his way back across the Channel to rejoin the 31st Battalion at Liévin on July 11; the next day he composed his first love letter to Emma.

While his correspondence referred to the battalion and being back at the front line, Capt. McGill had little else on his mind but his leave that "seemed almost too good to be true, especially when you . . . gave me the promise I so longed to receive. I was prepared to have that taxi drive around London until the petrol gave out or I knew my fate," he wrote her on July 12. "I hope we may be able to begin our lives afresh together."[14]

As much as their engagement lifted their spirits, the exigencies of the war made planning a marriage difficult. Emma worried for Harold's safety and suggested he seek a transfer to a Canadian military hospital in England; in correspondence, he rejected the idea because it would look as if he were abandoning his comrades. At the same time, demand for more and better hospital services upgraded Bramshott to No. 12 Canadian General Hospital, which meant that Emma and the nursing staff might be transferred to the Continent to take up casualty clearing duties; but Emma contracted influenza and was forced to take sick leave. Meanwhile, Capt. McGill left the 31st Battalion to lead the No. 5 Canadian Field Ambulance just a month before the Canadian Corps received orders to capture the village of Passchendaele, the last point of resistance by the enemy along the Ypres salient. The 5th established its advanced dressing station in the former Ypres prison. The ferocity of the battle tested each army's medical units to the core; McGill's ambulance aid men handled more than a thousand walking cases and seventy wounded German POWs in one sixteen-hour period.

After Passchendaele, Harold got leave and met Emma in London; they got their licence and were married on December 12. Their honeymoon seemed to pass in an instant, and by Christmas Day Harold was back where he was needed, on the Continent as an acting major. Emma, it seemed, was not needed; as a married woman she'd had to resign from the Canadian Army Medical Corps, and even when she attempted to reapply, it was apparent that the CAMC had plenty of qualified nurses arriving in England to choose from. Emma eventually took a position at Roehampton House, a convalescent hospital for soldiers with amputated limbs. The work paid nothing—she was on a spousal allowance from the CAMC—and proved strenuous without the benefit of healthy food.

Meanwhile, as the war ended, Harold's No. 5 Canadian Field Ambulance marched with Canadian troops—250 miles—through Belgium to the Rhine. Responsible for tending any sick or wounded on both sides of the war, McGill's medical team coped with inadequate rations, insufficient supplies, and enmity from German civilians. And Emma, waiting in England for Harold's release from occupation duties, reached a low ebb—she was pregnant, unwell, and without work; she even wondered whether Harold was sorry that he had married her.

Fittingly, the couple that had become acquainted by way of wartime correspondence, had supported each other through depression and doubt with their letters, had illustrated their commitment to military medicine with their prose, and had revealed their love for each other, ultimately resorted to written words when all seemed bleakest.

"I do not blame you in the slightest for being troubled with doubts," Harold wrote. "How did you ever come to accept me? You know I do not dance, [with] no social graces, and when it comes to music, I am simply *non est*. . . . I am afraid I am one of those that Shakespeare spoke of being fit for treasons, stratagems, and spoils. You must take me in hand early and see what you can do for me."[15]

The McGills sailed from Liverpool in May 1919 aboard RMS *Olympic* and returned home to Calgary by the end of the month. Despite a miscarriage while she was still in England, Emma eventually gave birth to two daughters. She remained connected to her profession through the Alberta Association of Registered Nurses and the local branch of the Overseas Nursing Sisters' Association.

Meanwhile, Harold returned to his civilian medical practice and eventually became a representative on the Alberta Council of the College of Physicians and Surgeons; he entered politics at the municipal, provincial, and federal levels, becoming Prime Minister R.B. Bennett's Deputy Superintendent-General of Indian Affairs.

Thanks to Emma, and ultimately the Glenbow Alberta Institute Archives, Harold McGill's remarkable correspondence about war and love—his letters to Emma—survived; then, thanks to the skilful editing of Marjorie Barron Norris, Capt. McGill's account of front-line medicine in the Great War took shape in her book *Medicine and Duty*.

Norris also published what she could about Nursing Sister Emma Griffis in *Sister Heroines*, but she was limited. As an ironic postscript to their story of love by correspondence in war, Harold did not save the letters Emma had sent him while overseas; he sensed some difficulty about holding on to them while on active service, and instead burned them after reading them.

...

JUNE 18, 1918—ST. PAUL'S ANGLICAN CHURCH, LONDON, ENGLAND

THE GREAT WAR was well into its third year when yet another couple, brought together by the war and in the service of the army medical corps, sealed their relationship. Indeed, just when the massive German springtime offensive was sputtering along the Western Front, and as an Allied counteroffensive was being launched in response, a small garden reception took place across the English Channel. Just outside London on June 18, 1918, Nursing Sister Louise Ann Spry quietly celebrated her marriage to Sgt. Frederick Charles Lailey, both serving with the Canadian Army Medical Corps. The two secretly exchanged vows at St. Paul's Anglican Church, at Kingston Hill, and slipped away for a short honeymoon.

That they made it to their wedding day, that they survived their duties in the military, that they even made it out of their childhoods makes the love story of Louise and Fred Lailey nearly miraculous. At any one of a hundred different turns in their lives, each might have chosen to turn back or give up. That neither of them did, that they managed to find each other amid the chaos of the Great War, and in spite of military protocol, suggests they were two of a kind.

Born one of three brothers and three sisters in England in 1892, Fred faced the breakup of his family when his parents died prematurely. The uncle who acquired Fred abused the boy, didn't allow him to attend school, and tasked him with chores most adults couldn't manage. At age ten he ran away to join another uncle and aunt, and to a more conducive upbringing; with them, Fred received some schooling and at home learned survival skills, including basic gardening, culinary arts, and sewing. Not tall or broad in stature, as a teenager Fred arrived on the wharf in Liverpool and approached a merchant navy captain, seeking work with his crew.

"You . . . applying for a position on my ship?" the captain bellowed.[16]

"I can work as your cabin boy." Fred said.

"Doing what?"

"Sir, your uniform is missing a button," Fred pointed out. "And your jacket has an open seam, not befitting a captain."

"What else can you do?"

"I can cook, make wine, and the ladies love my desserts," Fred said.

The captain noted Fred's impertinence but told him the ship left for Australia within days and to report to the cook. Thus began his short career at sea. Whenever work dried up on board the merchant ships, Fred found employment ashore in such faraway places as St. Petersburg, Russia, and Quebec City, Canada. By the spring of 1914 he'd become a crew member in the galley aboard a transatlantic passenger liner owned by Canadian Pacific Steamships and operating between Liverpool and Quebec. As their ship left port and plied the deep current of the St. Lawrence River on the morning of May 29, Fred was making bread with another young galley worker from Winnipeg.

"We were busy in the kitchen baking bread," he told his granddaughter years later. "Suddenly there was a very loud noise and the ship went way over on its side. My young friend said we should go to the lifeboats."

They were below decks, and Fred sensed that would take too much time. He yelled at his galley partner to pull a door on the upside of the kitchen from its hinges. They dashed through the opening and out on deck, where Fred told his friend to jump straight into the water. He couldn't believe it when his friend told him he couldn't swim; Fred threw the door overboard, jumped right after, and encouraged his friend to follow.

"I managed to pull him onto the door," Fred continued. "It was May, but the water was cold. We drifted down the river and were picked up by rescuers eleven hours later," two of only 465 who survived (1,012 died) in the worst maritime disaster in Canadian peacetime history—the sinking of the *Empress of Ireland*.

A year later, Fred had enlisted in the 20th Battalion of the Canadian Expeditionary Force serving on the Western Front in France and Belgium. Along the Ypres salient in 1916, the Germans attacked behind a cloud of mustard gas, and while Fred's unit held the line, he and many of his comrades were wounded and withdrawn for treatment back in England. During his convalescence at No. 16 Canadian General Hospital at Orpington, in Kent, hospital authorities learned that Sgt. Lailey had culinary skills. The Canadian Army Medical Corps quickly assigned him to lead the cooking staff in the officers' mess.

Louise Spry arrived at the same hospital facility several months later, but not before she'd followed an equally circuitous route. Originally from London, Ontario, she and her family moved to Toronto in 1899, when Louise was fifteen. With her good high-school grades, Louise applied to the Toronto General Hospital's

School of Nursing, but given the family's financial situation, she feared she might not be accepted, since she couldn't afford the required uniform. No matter, concluded her resourceful mother; almost overnight she'd refashioned the household living room curtains into a hand-sewn nurse's uniform. Louise graduated in 1910 and began her service at Toronto General.

Like Fred, Louise was not tall, and on some occasions when she assisted surgeons such as Dr. Herbie Bruce in the operating theatre, she needed to use a stool in order to reach the table. On one occasion, as Dr. Bruce prepared for a particularly tricky surgery, he looked around the operating room for Nurse Spry but couldn't find her.

"Get 'Squirt,'" the surgeon told the nursing supervisor. "I need her for this operation!"

The supervisor went to the nurses' residence, knocked on her door, and told Louise to come to the operating theatre quickly.

"Where were you?" Dr. Bruce asked when she appeared in the OR.

"It's my night off," Louise protested.

"I need you for this difficult case," he said. "Grab the stool."

After six years in the nursing service at TGH, and with the Great War raging overseas, Louise offered her services to the military just after Christmas in 1916. She volunteered for the Canadian Army Medical Corps, passed her medical exam and training requirements, and by the spring of the following year had crossed the Atlantic aboard a troopship and been assigned to a number of Canadian field hospitals in southern England. And that's where Nursing Sister Spry, on transit duties, met Sgt. Lailey, in charge of the twelve-man crew in the officers' mess at the same base hospital. The nurses ate their meals in Fred's officers' mess. But the CAMC officer in charge made it clear to medical servicemen that the nurses were not to be interfered with; in other words, as Fred put it, "Look but don't touch."

Neither protocol nor orders from the brass could keep the two apart, however, and their relationship flourished. A year later, probably because the nursing sisters and the medical corps NCOs knew how to short-circuit the system better than anybody, Louise and Fred managed to obtain simultaneous leaves. They met at St. Paul's Anglican Church, just southwest of London, and were married in that private ceremony.

Coincidentally, unofficial duty called before their marriage was hours old. Following their garden wedding reception, Mr. and Mrs. Lailey boarded a train en route to a honeymoon escape for the night. The train came off the rails and people on board were badly hurt, so the newlyweds jumped into action providing first aid to passengers. They found an army general among the injured, with blood streaming down his leg. Fred cut off the general's boots and Louise dressed the wound on his leg. Apparently the general grew suspicious and wondered why they weren't in uniform. Just in time, stretcher-bearers arrived and took the senior officer to the hospital before the newlyweds were exposed.

Regulations aganist married couples in active military service at or near the front were pretty clear. Louise was reassigned to serve back in Canada, but the crossing in October 1918 proved nearly fatal; she came down with typhoid fever and only round-the-clock attention from other nurses aboard the ocean liner saved her. She was also pregnant with twins. Back in Toronto, hospitalized with synovitis, Louise could barely provide for herself, much less the babies that were about to arrive. Mercifully, Fred received his honourable discharge and permission for transatlantic passage home just in time; he arrived back in Toronto eighteen days before Elma and Velma Lailey were born, on April 29, 1919.

SEPTEMBER 15, 1944—CORIANO RIDGE, GOTHIC LINE, ITALY

DESPITE THE ODDS against their survival, some friendships born in the Second World War—when medics were racing against time to save lives—outlived both the battles and the conflict itself. By the summer of 1944, the British, Americans, and Canadians had forced the Italian army to capitulate and had broken through German fall-back positions—the Hitler Line and the Caesar Line—and on to Rome, the first Axis capital city liberated in Europe.

Then, in August, Allied commanders had withdrawn three American and four French divisions for an amphibious landing on the south coast of France. That left the Canadian Corps with the prospect of assaulting the Gothic Line, the Germans' daunting defensive works that straddled the Italian peninsula north of the Via Flaminia, largely on their own. Preparing for the advance north, Canadian infantry and armoured corps— among them the 8th Princess Louise's (New Brunswick) Hussars—faced six rivers between them and their objective, the west-coast city of Rimini.

It wasn't just the waterways that lay in their path; dug-in heavy German armament, including their Tiger tanks, also posed a lethal threat. "We kept hitting [the Tiger]," explained one 8th Hussars commander in his Sherman tank, "but our 75 mm shells just bounced off."[17] Meanwhile, if the Tiger's 88 mm shells struck the Allies' Shermans, it was no contest.

By mid-September 1944, the 1st Canadian Infantry Division, including the Hussars, had advanced toward the Gothic Line and into the hills around the Italian town of Coriano, on the verge of breaking the Germans' Apennine Mountains barrier. In a month of day-in-day-out fighting, however, the division had suffered 2,511 casualties, including 626 killed in action.[18] And the campaign had not spared the rural towns and villages on or near the battlefields. Everywhere, civilians cowered in barns, sheds, and even haystacks, while perhaps the most vulnerable living creatures—the country's livestock—dashed away from explosions and crossfire, attempting to stay alive. L/Sgt. Gerald Kelly, a medic with the Hussars, dealt with the carnage, both military and civilian. "Dead cattle were lying upside down, bloated and swollen—killed by the shelling," he reported. "Houses were broken. It was pretty messy."[19]

For a regiment made up principally of volunteers from rural New Brunswick, the sight of decimated barnyards and livestock corpses hit especially hard. Moving through recently seized ground near Coriano that fall, some of the Hussars heard the shrieking of a distressed animal. In a farmyard recently raked by shelling and small-arms fire, they found a mare crumpled and lifeless on the ground. She'd likely been dead several days. Beside the mare, a foal not more than a few weeks old whinnied in a frantic search for nourishment and shelter from its mother. The first Canadian armoured troops on the scene, including medic Kelly, realized the filly had belly and leg wounds. They corralled the frightened animal and led it behind the lines to Tom Dalrymple, medical officer at the 8th Hussars' regimental aid post. Together the medics cleaned and disinfected the filly's wounds with surgical powder and then applied bandages to keep the flies away. "It was pretty hard to put a dressing on a horse's belly," Kelly said, "but we did drop a bandage around it to hold the dressing in place."

Not many members of the Second World War edition of the New Brunswick regiment realized it, but tending a horse within their ranks was actually quite fitting. During the American Revolutionary War, Col. John Saunders, a loyalist in Virginia, had organized a regiment of riflemen, grenadiers, artillerymen, and cavalrymen to fight for the Crown. In 1783, members of the Loyalist regiment left the colonies, landed in Saint John, settled in the Kennebecasis Valley, and called themselves a cavalry militia. By 1884 they'd become the 8th Princess Louise's New Brunswick Regiment of Cavalry, known after 1893 as the Hussars. Princess Louise's Hussars, named in honour of the fourth daughter* of Queen Victoria and Prince Albert, had fought in the South Africa War and the Great War and by late 1944 had earned a string of battle honours in the liberation of Italy. Now, nearly 170 years after their founding, the Hussars

---

* In her public life, Princess Louise, Duchess of Argyll (1848–1939), supported the arts, higher education, and feminist causes. In 1871 she married John, Marquess of Lorne, later appointed Governor General of Canada (1878–84). In her role as viceregal consort of Canada, she developed strong feelings for the country. During the North-West Resistance of 1885, she sent medical supplies and financial assistance to Thomas Roddick and his militia medical staff, with specific instructions for the aid to be administered to the wounded on both sides.

once again had a horse in their midst.

"It was up to the boys, the mechanics and fitters," medic Kelly said. "They handled the vehicles, trucks, and were essential, [but] they had a little more time than we did." So, in the days that followed, the mechanics, including Gordon Bickerton, attended to the filly, changing her dressings and keeping the young horse fed and watered. Kelly lost track of the regiment's equine patient for a while, but then suddenly there she was, perfectly comfortable in the company of the soldiers who'd attended to her. "And the boys had somehow made a banner to throw over the filly's back and it had 'Princess Louise' [inscribed] on it."

The banner seemed to signify that the filly had become the regiment's official mascot. That meant feed and accommodation—including the mobile variety—were required. For a mobile regiment such as the Hussars, transport didn't pose any difficult logistics, until the armoured group received orders to pack up their men and equipment to join the liberation of the Netherlands. Regulations strictly prohibited taking livestock out of Italy. No matter for the Princess Louise's Thad Stevens, who'd taken on the job of tending the regimental mascot. It simply meant improvising with the transport available. "The boys made up their minds they were going to take her to Holland, so they fixed up a truck," Stevens said. "They put the machine-gun boxes up the sides, and in the middle . . . was the [makeshift stall] for the filly and a sergeant."[20]

Every time the regiment moved, Princess Louise moved with it inside her modified three-ton machine-gun truck, across France, Belgium, and Holland. But when the war finally ended, the regiment and its acquired mascot had to wait their turn coming home. As medic Kelly put it, "A good part of Canada was over there fighting, and there weren't enough ships to bring everybody home,"[21] so the filly, now a yearling, eventually crossed the Atlantic aboard the Dutch liner *Leerdam*. In New York, Trooper E.A. Jackson met Princess Louise and travelled with her to Montreal, then on to Saint John, New Brunswick, for a reception at the train station. With an honour guard and a band to greet her, Princess Louise received a hero's welcome in front of a brigadier, the mayor, enthusiastic city residents, and many of the 8th Hussars veterans who'd help to save her in Italy.

During the reception, Princess Louise received all the decorations awarded any other deployed member of the 8th New Brunswick Hussars: the 1939–1945 Star, Italy Star, France and Germany Star, Volunteer Service Medal, and (acknowledging her shrapnel gashes) three wound stripes. There was, however, one outstanding piece of red tape that needed attention before her immigration was complete. The *Kings County Record* offers excerpts from an interview allegedly given by the horse at the county courthouse, where she informed the reporter, "We had to go to Hampton for a formal welcome [including] the presentation of my naturalization papers," changing her citizenship from Italian to Canadian.[22] The certificate, dated March 27, 1946, read in part: "Princess Louise is hereby made and proclaimed a citizen of the great Dominion of Canada and a free woman of the Village of Hampton, and, as such, is entitled to roam at will over hill and vale and to devour . . . that which she so pleaseth . . . whether carefully tended garden or the bursting warehouses of Henry Sharp's Feed Store."[23]

Such proclamations of immunity came in handy. After the war, Field Marshal Bernard Montgomery came to Canada for the annual Remembrance Day observance in Fredericton; he had actually met the 8th Hussars' equine mascot with her regiment in Europe. During proceedings in New Brunswick, the former field marshal joined Governor General Harold Alexander and Lady Margaret Alexander for an inspection of the guard. As the dignitaries passed Princess Louise, she nonchalantly reached out, snatched, and devoured the flowers Lady Alexander was to receive. The regiment's favourite horse became so comfortable with her caregivers, including Hussars veteran Gordon Bickerton, and so blasé about participating in lengthy ceremonies on the parade ground, that she would often fall asleep standing up. On occasion, Bickerton recalled, he had to tug on her ear and scold her, "Princess Louise, wake up!"[24]

Princess Louise had three foals—Princess Louise II and sons Prince and Hussar—and died in her thirtieth year; she was buried in 1973 on park grounds next to the cenotaph in Hampton, New Brunswick.

War brought out the worst in its combatants, and sometimes the best. Somehow, in a race to kill or be killed, for the medics, mechanics, and others serving with Princess Louise's Hussars, pitching in to save the life of an innocent animal on a battlefield in the middle of Italy introduced some sanity. Perhaps it was a practical distraction. Maybe it allowed them a moment to feel some emotion in a place where there was little time or space for it. And as they attended this creature's simpler needs, it's possible it reminded them of home. "Yes," medic Gerard Kelly agreed, the whole enterprise had given the Canadians some hope, "even though we had to steal a horse to do it."

...

DECEMBER 24, 1944—BASTOGNE, BELGIUM

IN THE FEW DAYS leading up to Christmas 1944, nothing in the lives of two experienced medical people coping with circumstances inside the Belgian city of Bastogne felt like peace on earth, goodwill toward men. Earlier that fall, since the Allied breakout from Normandy, the 2nd Canadian Infantry Division had cut off the Fifteenth German Army in the Beveland peninsula and the Second British Army had liberated the Belgian cities of Tournai, Brussels, and Antwerp, while the US First and Third Armies had liberated Mons, Namur, Liège, and the Ardennes. In the middle of it all, the recently liberated city of Bastogne, at the hub of seven key crossroads in the Ardennes, was returning to normal. And with Christmas coming, the city's farmers' markets got busy again. GIs with the US 28th Keystone Division—their numbers badly depleted by the recent Battle of the Hürtgen Forest—had settled in for a bit of rest and relief. So some of the city's cobblestone streets, which dated from 634 AD, sprang back to life with civilian as well as military traffic. Downtown shops even displayed holiday decorations.

A week before Christmas, Augusta Chiwy, a twenty-three-year-old registered nurse (RN) originally from the Belgian Congo and employed for about a year at St. Elisabeth Hospital near Brussels, had received an invitation from her father to join him, Augusta's brother, and her aunt at home in Bastogne for the holidays. On December 16 she'd gathered some belongings, dressed herself in the warmest clothes she had, including her nurse's gabardine coat and woollen scarf, and made her way from Brussels by train, truck, Jeep, and bus—she'd even found a discarded bicycle with a flat tire to pedal part of the way—arriving after dark at her home on rue des Écoles in downtown Bastogne. After dinner and time to catch up with her family, Augusta retired to bed. A calm before the coming storm.

That same week, a medical officer from Vermont serving in the Alsace-Lorraine region with the US 10th Armored Division got a new assignment. Instead of dealing with cases of trench foot and venereal disease and preparing the battle-wounded for transit to evacuation hospitals behind the lines, Capt. Jack Prior was dispatched to the US 20th Armored Infantry Battalion (AIB). At age twenty-seven, Prior had previously graduated from a Reserve Officers' Training Corps program at university, completed an internship in New York, been inducted into the US Army, and shipped overseas in 1944.

Just ten days before Christmas, his new orders gave him command of a medical unit comprising a dentist and thirty stretcher-bearers and first-aid men. His transportation equipment included a handful of half-track ambulances and two Jeeps. The excitement of his new posting nearly overshadowed unwelcome news from home; his fiancée, Marion Golden, had decided to call off their engagement. But there was little time to worry about a "Dear John" letter. Almost immediately following his redeployment, Capt. Prior's medical detachment joined the 20th AIB; they told him it was an administrative march toward Luxembourg. In plain English, it seemed like an exercise. "Working in a safe climate, free of artillery, and small-arms fire," Prior wrote later, "I was ill-prepared for the baptism that was to follow."[25]

The day RN Augusta Chiwy arrived home for Christmas and Capt. Jack Prior's medical group rumbled through Luxembourg on an admin march, 1,600 German artillery pieces opened up a ninety-minute barrage along eighty miles of Allied positions across the River Our. Allied strategists dismissed the barrage as a feint, reacting to American advances at Metz and Aachen; Allied commanders seemed preoccupied, as well, with their next offensive moves into Germany, not defensive ones. Meanwhile, shrouding the entire Saarland front, overcast skies and heavy snow descended on the region, bringing with them reduced aerial reconnaissance and cover on both sides.

The barrage was not a feint at all. Adolf Hitler's breakout plan, *Unternehmen Wacht am Rhein* ("Operation Watch on the Rhine"), sent more than 400,000 German troops, spearheaded by 1,400 tanks and 2,600 artillery pieces, across the River Our headlong into the Ardennes. Their objective: to push the Allied beachhead at Antwerp back into the North Sea. In their path, just twenty-five miles to the west: sleepy Bastogne.

Rested, but on Sunday morning somewhat restless from hearing the crumping sound of artillery off to the east, Augusta Chiwy decided to travel out of Bastogne, partly to seek food for her family but also to visit her brother Charles, who was lodging with friends near Noville. The weather closed in. At just four foot eight in height, she tried pedalling her father's bicycle, but cycling through the snow eventually made no sense, so she paused at the Catholic church in the village. Ultimately she abandoned her journey to seek out her brother, returned to the church, rapped on the door, and was welcomed by the parish priest, Father Louis Delvaux.* He offered her shelter overnight; the next morning he gave her food for her family and sent her back down the road to Bastogne.

By the time Chiwy re-entered the city walls, the place was alive with motion. Tractors, cars, trucks, and carts overflowing with people were on the move out of town. Word of approaching German troops had panicked Bastogne's population. By December 18 nearly two-thirds of the city's 9,000 residents were fleeing south. The remainder gathered what food and warm clothing they could and descended into communal underground shelters beneath schools and churches.

Henri Chiwy, Augusta's Belgian-born father, a veterinarian, had volunteered to work in the communal shelter under the Sisters of Notre Dame school. When Augusta didn't find her father at home, she began searching the communal cellars, initially at the seminary on the edge of town. Two nuns stopped her at the entrance; since she wasn't known to the nuns, and because she was black, the pair looked her up and down and refused her entry. Eventually Augusta found her father beneath Notre Dame. The school had a bakery and, thanks to Henri Chiwy's contacts with the farm community, some meat and other produce to sustain those hiding there. Unwelcome at the seminary, Augusta's nursing abilities proved a godsend at Notre Dame; wrapped in an overcoat and her nurse's gabardine, she moved among the civilians—paying special attention to the children—offering whatever assistance she could. At night she scurried to the family home on rue des Écoles for a

---

* When forward units of the German offensive entered Noville, Gestapo agents converged on Father Delvaux's church, accusing him of harbouring a radio transmitter in the steeple and supporting resistance fighters; on December 21, the agents executed the priest and seven civilians.

few hours' sleep in the basement. "The only safe places in town were the cellars," she said, recalling how it felt to watch the city empty. "I really thought the Germans were going to walk up the main street any minute."[26]

With a clearer understanding of German intentions, Allied commanders were on the move too. Eisenhower met his generals at Verdun. Shortly thereafter, Gen. Patton's Third Army turned away from its push to the River Rhine and rushed north into the flank of the German breakout. Included in the redirection, Capt. Prior's medical detachment raced to Noville (along the same route Augusta Chiwy had travelled in search of her brother the day before) to protect one of the three main roads into and out of Bastogne. Codenamed "Team Desobry," for its commanding officer Maj. William Desobry, the force of fifteen medium tanks, five light tanks, a company of infantry troops, a platoon of tank destroyers, and some mechanized cavalry with half-tracks and Jeeps quickly set up defensive positions around Noville.

At the same time, Capt. Prior scoped out a location for a regimental aid post. "My Aid Station was located in a pub . . . best for our purposes since the large drinking area accommodated many litter patients," Prior wrote. "Within two hours of our arrival the little town had turned into a shooting gallery."[27]

The large drinking area suddenly became a hazard. Machinegun and tank fire quickly reduced the pub's front picture window to shards of glass, forcing Prior's aid men to crawl across the floor to avoid being hit as they treated a growing number of casualties. Though they didn't know the strength of the enemy (a full division of German tanks), Team Desobry was ordered to stand fast at Noville; but by midday on December 19, defensive positions were deteriorating perilously, Desobry himself was among the wounded, and the depleted force received orders to withdraw south to Bastogne. Prior and his medical detachment had ten minutes to evacuate themselves and their twenty patients. With no ambulances and no litters, Prior considered staying behind and surrendering himself and the twenty wounded to the Germans.

But just as the prospects for saving anybody left behind seemed darkest, one of Prior's medics dashed outside to flag down the departing tank squadron. Seconds later, members of the tank crews charged into the aid station, ripped down every available door, strapped Prior's patients to the doors, and tied the makeshift litters to their vehicles. All the wounded, now attended by medical corpsmen, were on the move. The column of tanks and Jeeps took three hours to retreat the four miles to Bastogne; every time the column slowed or stopped because of enemy shelling or small-arms fire, the medical corpsmen dove for cover until the firing stopped; they had no choice but to leave the wounded strapped to the vehicles. When an American tank was hit nearby, the wounded began calling for help.

"Before I could [move,] one of my litter bearers and the bravest man I have ever known, Pvt. Bernard Morrissey of Providence, Rhode Island, got up and said, 'I'll go, Doc,'" Prior said later. "Another litter bearer, Pvt. Ignacious Vaznon from Chicago, volunteered to go with him."[28]

The two medics dashed forward, joined by a Jeep driver, and the three saved the wounded strapped to the tank and even lowered each other into the tank to save the wounded crew inside. They retrieved all the casualties and brought them to safety. Prior called Morrissey "the man with a thousand lives."

"Every one of us was inspired by their bravery," Prior continued. "We forgot fear and set up an aid station around that jeep, treating the wounded who were brought to us. All the time snipers were potting at us . . ."[29]

Also involved in the firefight on the road from Noville to Bastogne that day were paratroops of the 101st Airborne Division, hastily summoned from a rest area and dispatched to assist in the pullback. It was only later that those who'd fought at the Noville outpost northeast of Bastogne learned that they had halted the entire Panzer Division that day. Outnumbered ten to one, the defenders had knocked out thirty-one enemy tanks in two days. That night, the newly arrived 101st established its battle headquarters at the Heintz Barracks in the city.

"I have never learned who to predict will be a hero," Prior wrote. "I'd still be in that ditch on the Bastogne road, if not for the arrival of the Airborne."[30] On rue de Vivier, just off a main street in Bastogne, Capt. Prior's medics moved into a vacant garage to function as an aid station. It was soon overflowing with patients, but as temperatures dropped and snow accumulated, Prior could provide little or no heat to keep the facility warm. A lot of his cases involved trench foot, frostbite, or hypothermia. Meanwhile, his fellow military officer (a dentist), Capt. Irving Naftulin, had found a three-storey private house. Prior and Naftulin and their corpsmen transferred more than a hundred patients to the new location. Records show that the medical detachment staff worked twenty-four hours a day; they recounted the difficulties of keeping plasma from freezing and medical supplies from running out. In particular, the aid station's supply of hydrogen peroxide to prevent GAS (Group

A streptococcal) or gangrene infection was critically low—a serious concern in cases where extremity wounds required irrigating. Worse still, there were as many as thirty patients with head, chest, and abdominal wounds facing "certain slow death since there was no chance of surgical procedures. We had no surgical talent among us," Prior wrote. "There was not so much as a can of ether or a scalpel to be had in the city."

Capt. Naftulin, already successful at finding a new hospital location, began beating the bushes for professional assistance. One contact led Naftulin and Prior to Place du Carré and the haberdashery shop of Gustave Lemaire, whose daughter Renée was a nurse. She in turn directed Capt. Prior to rue des Écoles and Henri Chiwy's residence. Augusta and her aunt heard him knocking and answered timidly.

"*Parlez-vous anglais?*" Jack asked.

"Not too well," Augusta said.

The well-educated medical officer admitted that his command of French was about the same. Nevertheless, RN Chiwy invited him out of the cold and into the basement, where she and her aunt were waiting out the latest bombardments. Somehow Capt. Prior managed to explain to Augusta that a block or two away, young American soldiers lay wounded and dying in a makeshift hospital. He had very little medicine and not enough qualified medical assistance.

Augusta asked Jack why the Americans and Germans were fighting in Belgium. In his broken French, he tried to paint her the larger picture, explaining that Allied forces were fighting elsewhere in the world, too, not just in Belgium. Presently Augusta's father, Henri, returned home from his duties at Notre Dame. When Capt. Prior's request was restated, Henri explained that it was up to Augusta to decide.[31]

"You would be safer with the US Army," Henri told his daughter. And he was about to ask the young American if he could give assurance for his daughter's safety when Augusta pulled on her overcoat. "Yes," she said to her father and the captain, later noting that she thought "the whole debacle would be over faster if I was busy doing something useful."[32]

Three days before Christmas and Bastogne looked like a ghost town. Any civilians remaining in the city were hiding underground. The American military units still on site— what was left of the 28th (Keystone) Infantry Division, the 10th Armored Division, and companies of the newly arrived 101st Airborne Division—dug in at strategic points to defend against two groups of the 47th Panzer Division, commanded by Gen. Heinrich Freiherr von Lüttwitz. By noon on December 21, the Panzers had severed all seven roads leading into Bastogne; the city was virtually encircled. But rather than deploy all its panzer resources against Bastogne, the main German force kept moving westward with operation *Wacht am Rhein*, leaving one regiment to assist the 26th Volksgrenadier Division, which was ordered to capture Bastogne.

Thus began a steady bombardment of downtown Bastogne, augmented by infantry assaults and (when the skies were clear) Luftwaffe air raids. Inside the city perimeter, the defenders— outnumbered five to one—assembled three artillery battalions, each with twelve howitzers, and forty light and medium tanks to operate as a mobile fire brigade, rushing to points where enemy incursions occurred. At the end of a daylong siege, on December 22, the Germans issued an ultimatum:

"There is only one possibility to save the encircled U.S.A.

troops from total annihilation," wrote Gen. von Lüttwitz. "That is the honourable surrender of the encircled town. In order to think it over a term of two hours will be granted beginning with the presentation of this note."

To which US Brig. Gen. Anthony McAuliffe responded: "NUTS!"

Bastogne seemed too attractive a prize for the Germans to pass up, too valuable an asset for the Americans to lose.

Capt. Jack Prior hardly had to direct Augusta Chiwy to his three-storey impromptu hospital on rue de Neufchâteau. She could smell its inhabitants and the environment in which Prior and his medical staff were working even before she entered it. Among the strongest odours was the sulpha. Most of the first-aid kits American soldiers carried included sulpha (or sulphanilamide) powder, which GIs were taught to sprinkle liberally into wounds to prevent infection. The putrid smell of gangrene infection and the hydrogen peroxide treatment was present among some of the wounded. There was the smell of wax candles too, since the city was without electricity or gaslight. A sweeter, less offensive aroma in the aid station was that of cognac; the nurses used it to disinfect their hands and, in small doses, as an alternative to morphine syrettes for patients in severe pain. Soon after his two Belgian volunteer nurses arrived, Capt. Prior recognized how best to employ their skills.

"Renée shrank away from the fresh, gory trauma," Prior noted, so he directed her to attend the litter patients, sponging their faces, feeding them, and distributing what medicine they had; she would circulate among the more severely wounded, spoon-feeding them cognac to alleviate pain when there was no morphine. Meanwhile, "Augusta" always was in the thick of the splinting, dressing, and hemorrhage control."[33]

Not long after she started to attend to the wounded at Capt. Prior's aid station, RN Chiwy showed her capabilities in an emergency; when a GI's neck laceration suddenly gushed blood, she helped Prior to stem the bleeding and suture the wound. Another time, GAS infection had shown itself in a wounded GI's lower leg and hand, both shattered by shell fire. The captain concluded that both limbs had to be amputated or the gangrene would kill his patient; so, with equipment more reminiscent of 1864 than 1944—a serrated-edge army knife and cognac anesthetic—medical officer and nurse prepared the man for the impromptu surgery. Jack administered the brandy and readied his primitive tools while Augusta assembled her sutures and bandages for post-op. With the man somewhat subdued by the brandy, Augusta held down the GI's leg as Jack sawed into it above the infection. The patient soon lost consciousness with the pain and shock; that enabled Jack to repeat the process on his hand, and Augusta to irrigate, stitch, and bandage the stumps. "Nice work, Augusta," Capt. Prior said to his assistant, "although if we don't get some disinfectant soon, he'll die anyway."[34]

To help her blend into the surroundings—and certainly to provide her with more suitable clothing, given the cold and the daily grind at the aid station—Jack gave Augusta some army fatigues. He marvelled at the emotional stamina of both nurses in the unit, but especially the diminutive Augusta. No matter the level of stress, she proved herself capable and resilient under the weight of responsibility. Equally capable but more at ease in conversation with the wounded than treating them in emergencies, Renée was always smiling, trying to cheer her patients.

As Christmas approached, she brought a tree from her father's store to decorate and brighten up the aid station. On December 23, the fog and snow cleared enough that US Army Air Force transports could drop much needed provisions—food, ammunition, blankets, and medical supplies. Even the parachutes were repurposed as bedding in the aid station, although Nurse Lemaire had raced out to retrieve a chute to use one day, she hoped, in a wedding dress. But someone had scooped up all the silk, and Renée returned empty-handed.

December 24 brought very little cheer Capt. Prior's way. Litter-bearers had delivered an officer with a severe chest wound. The lieutenant had served with Combat Command B of the 9th Armored, one of the so-called fire-brigade regiments, each day dashing to the latest attempted German incursion into the city. After working on this patient, knowing his chances of survival without more sophisticated surgical attention were nearly non-existent, Prior took a break inside the building next to his three-storey hospital. It was 8:30 in the evening.

"I've got to write a letter to that lieutenant's wife," Prior told one of his corpsmen.

"It's Christmas Eve," the corpsman interrupted. "We should open a bottle of Champagne."

There were far too few bottles of medicine available during the siege in Bastogne, but certainly sufficient supplies of wine and spirits around the city, and Prior's corpsman thought it appropriate to share it with his CO at that moment. That pause in the adjacent building to open the Champagne bottle, fill their cups, and toast Christmas Eve likely saved their lives. In the night there was the sound of approaching aircraft. As the two Americans raised their cups, the blacked-out room where they were standing suddenly lit up as bright as a welder's torch. It was a magnesium flare, dropped by a German bomber to illuminate the area—a precursor to something worse. Within seconds, a five-hundred-pound bomb[35] exploded on the hospital building and blew both men to the floor where they had been standing.

"I ran outside," Prior wrote later, "to discover that the three-story apartment serving as my hospital was a flaming pile of debris about six feet high."[36]

Following the reflex that was part of their training and the routine of their existence under siege, those members of Capt. Prior's medical crew not inside the aid station raced to the pile of burning timbers. The aid men began flinging debris aside. Others fought the flames caused by the magnesium flares and the explosives. In his rush to the inferno, Prior also called out to Augusta. When the bomb landed, she was working in the kitchen on the main floor of the aid station, and the blast had blown her right through the wall and windows of the hospital to the outside. Prior found her dazed, with minor cuts, and covered in dirt from the debris, but otherwise uninjured.

Meantime, another of the Luftwaffe bomber crews had spotted the sudden concentration of people out in the open around the burning building and made a strafing run of machine-gun fire across the scene. The rescuers threw themselves under vehicles parked in front of the hospital.

Capt. Naftulin, the acting medical superintendent at the time, took charge of the attempts to rescue wounded from the hospital cellar. Seven patients were trapped in the basement debris. Naftulin heard them shouting for help.

"Sgt. Kenneth Souder, an engineer from Michigan, found

a tiny hole at the rear of the basement," Naftulin reported. "While the rest of us fought the fire, he tied a rope around himself and went in and got out two of the wounded men before he was overcome himself. Another engineer named Riordan got out four more, and Corp. Bernard Morrissey got out the last man."[37]

Bill Kerby, a member of the 20th Armored Infantry Battalion, joined the rescue effort as well. Rumours had circulated that German paratroops dressed in white jumpsuits had parachuted into that quarter of the city, and Kerby had posted guards adjacent to the hospital. But when the bomb exploded, he raced into the wrecked hospital to bring out wounded as well. On one of his rescue trips, his path crossed that of Nurse Renée Lemaire, who was also retrieving any patients still alive. With her latest rescued patient safely away from the burning aid station, Kerby said he saw Renée disappear back into the building to search for others. That was the last time she was seen alive.[38]

Five of the aid station's medics had died in the raid, and thirty GIs already wounded were killed. When Capt. Prior managed to recover Renée Lemaire's body from the rubble, he notified her family. Though it was always the toughest of his responsibilities, he attempted to put into words the nature of her service. He recalled that she had first come to the aid station just days before, when it faced the impossible task of attending to 150 patients. He wrote that Renée had "accepted the herculean task" of working without adequate rest or food, cheerfully changing dressings, feeding patients, dispensing medications, and making all in her care as comfortable as possible. He noted that her very presence was "an inspiration to those whose morale had declined from prolonged suffering."[39] After a description of her death under fire, Prior officially recommended to the divisional surgeon of the 10th Armored Division a posthumous citation for Nurse Lemaire. Then he paid a personal visit to her family. "I brought her remains to her parents, encased in the white parachute [silk] she so dearly wanted," Jack wrote later. As far as he knew, no citation was ever officially considered.

With his hospital gone, Capt. Jack Prior, along with his dental officer Capt. Naftulin and surviving corpsmen, relocated to the Heintz Barracks. The former Riding Hall had become a military hospital for the 101st Airborne and other wounded. Jack quickly asked Augusta if she would come to the barracks and help. She answered his plea and appeared at the barracks soon after in the army uniform and Red Cross arm band he'd procured for her days previously. But, like Jack, Augusta hadn't shaken off the trauma of Christmas Eve. "The first day, I didn't say anything," she recalled. "I just helped. Otherwise, I just waited, saying nothing [until] they told me to do this or that."[40]

As traumatic as coping with such primitive circumstances was for nurses such as Augusta, sometimes the insensitivity and prejudice of those around her in the makeshift hospital proved most devastating of all. Despite their severe wounds and helpless condition, some of the GIs on the aid station litters balked at the prospect of receiving treatment from an African nurse. Augusta Chiwy knew instinctively which patients didn't want a black woman to touch them.[41] Indeed, US Army regulations stipulated that black medical personnel could not treat white soldiers. Even in 1943, the US Army Nurse

Corps had accepted only 160 black nurses into its ranks. Segregation and discrimination had made them a rarity. In the Heintz Barracks, however, when one wounded soldier from the southern United States protested Augusta's presence—his language loaded with racist epithets—Capt. Prior made clear the rules on *his* ward. "Either Augusta treats you," he said, "or you die. Your call!"[42]

Once again, the young American captain and his nursing assistant were thrown into endless hours of triage and treatment by the seat of their pants. Despite the risk, the US Army managed to fly in a bona fide surgeon aboard a small spotter aircraft. However, somewhere between Army HQ and the Heintz Barracks, the assessment that the Bastogne aid station had six hundred surgical patients was misinterpreted as sixty patients; the incoming surgeon had only a basic instrument kit with him, and a few cans of ether. The frustration and fatigue grew. One night, Capt. Prior escorted Augusta home. He'd gone without sleep too long and was exhausted. All they had to rest on were mattresses in the cellar, but Augusta and her father led him to a divan in the family dining room, tucked him under a feather quilt her grandmother had made, and, when he'd closed his eyes, left him to sleep in peace.

The day after Christmas, news filtered through that Gen. Patton's Third Army was close to breaking through the German encirclement of Bastogne. As well, the army managed to fly in a medical surgeon; he too faced the daunting task of triaging critical internal wounds versus extremity wounds severely infected with gangrene. Meantime, the medical officer in charge of the barracks had managed to rig up a shower for his personnel. Capt. Prior made sure that his faithful volunteer nurse was among the first to enjoy the cold-water amenity.

Late on the afternoon of December 26, 1944, an American army officer entered the Riding Hall where Capt. Prior's medics were busy with attending to hundreds of patients. The intruder managed to get everybody's attention long enough to announce that tanks from the 4th Armored Division of Patton's Third Army had broken through the encirclement and help was on its way. Even if she couldn't quite understand what a breakthrough meant, Augusta Chiwy recognized from the jubilation in the place that things were going to change. Medical supplies would soon arrive. Lives could soon be saved because ambulances would carry the wounded to clearing stations and military hospitals beyond the city. US Army surgeons, anesthetists, nurses, and orderlies would shortly arrive and relieve the beleaguered medical aid men at the barracks. The siege of Bastogne would end. And inevitably, Augusta recognized, Jack's superiors would order him to new postings far from Bastogne.

The beginning of the end of the Battle of the Bulge occurred on December 27, when Patton's Third Army re-established ground communications with the 101st Airborne in Bastogne so that ambulances could travel unmolested out of the city, delivering wounded to the rear. During the week-long siege in and around Bastogne over Christmas 1944, the 10th Armored Division's Combat Command B group had suffered five hundred casualties, while the 101st Airborne Division had sustained over 2,000 casualties—killed, wounded, sick, and injured or missing. Many hundreds of those wounded and sick passed through the aid station at the Heintz Barracks, where Capt. Jack Prior and Nurse Augusta Chiwy had treated them. By the middle of January, Bastogne had once again been liberated, the barracks had emptied, and the last units of the 10th Armored had packed up to resume the advance against the enemy into Germany's Rhineland region.

On the last day Capt. Jack Prior was stationed at the Heintz Barracks, Henri Chiwy visited him and asked the American officer what plans he had for his daughter. Uncertain as to what Augusta's father meant, Jack offered his gratitude to the family for its assistance during the siege, but in particular to Augusta for her voluntary service at his aid stations. Henri explained that he wanted his daughter to stay with the US Army medical units, meaning that Jack was to take her with him. The man expected Jack to continue protecting her, and had in that sense "willed" her to him. Jack could no longer promise him that.

In the Riding Hall, Jack and Augusta spent an awkward few minutes, first as he tried to interpret her father's demands and then to say goodbye. As much as he cared for her, he was still a soldier; he couldn't take her along. He hugged her to express what his words could not.

"Give me your address," she said finally. "I'll be your *marraine de guerre*."

Jack couldn't understand Augusta's being "willed" to him by Henry Chiwy, or her offer to be his confidante, a moral support via correspondence. He would never forget her will to work in the face of overt racism or her devotion to the wounded. When Capt. Prior left Bastogne, RN Chiwy wrote to him right away. Fifteen days later she received her letter back, *Deceased* stamped on the envelope. The US War Office, censoring the mail, routinely dissuaded what it considered GIs' European girlfriends or mistresses from pursuing American soldiers.[43] Believing that her dear friend had been killed, Augusta tore up the letter and burned it. "I cried when Jack left Bastogne," she told documentarian Martin King in 2013. "It broke my heart, but I knew he had to go."[44]

After two years' overseas service, Capt. Jack Prior returned home to the United States. Along with his honourable discharge, he received the Silver Star, the Bronze Star, the Legion of Merit, and the Belgian Croix de Guerre among his service awards. He worked in pathology at Syracuse University, and then as a professor at the Upstate Medical Center. He maintained reserve status in the 376th Combat Support Reserve Hospital, retiring with the rank of colonel in 1977. He married Elizabeth Troy in 1948 and they had six children. Each December, his family would listen to Jack as he told his version of "The Night Before Christmas," in which two courageous nurses and a staff of medics attempted to save soldiers' and civilians' lives while under siege at Bastogne.

Jack and Augusta reunited in 1994. That December, veterans travelled from the United States to Bastogne to pay homage to their fallen comrades and to the civilians killed in the siege fifty years earlier. At the museum, the retired pathologist and retired nurse embraced while conversing with the help of a translator. As the entourage revisited the spot where a plaque commemorates Prior's three-storey aid station, Jack recalled that at Christmas 1944, his medical staff had no training as nurses.

He praised Renée Lemaire and Augusta Chiwy as his "angels of mercy" for volunteering to help him care for the wounded. He paused before leaving, looking around the street one last time. "I wonder if my grandchildren will ever remember the sacrifices that we made in this small town, years ago," he said to his son Jeffery Prior.[45]

Jack Prior died in 2007, Augusta Chiwy in 2011.

IN JANUARY 1945, shortly after Capt. Jack Prior loaded the last members of his medical unit aboard trucks to follow the 10th Armored Division into its next clash with the Germans, deeper in the Rhineland, he dashed off a quick note to his mother back in the United States. "Dear Ma. I guess they gave us write-up," he wrote, alluding to the siege he and his comrades had endured over Christmas. But just in case she was in the dark about their little corner of the war, he added, "I was one of those sweating it out in Bastogne. Don't believe those who say they caught us asleep, 'cause when the whole story is out you will know they didn't."[46]

My father offered much the same sentiment in his letter to his confidante Koula Kontozoglou when he wrote to her from Germany in April 1945. Like Jack Prior, T/Sgt. Alex Barris figured Koula had no idea where he was or what he was doing. "I suppose [they've] told you some of the exploits of the 94th Division," he wrote her. "[But] most accounts of war I've ever read are horribly distorted, and aimed more at selling [war] bonds than giving truthful news."[47]

Both Capt. Prior and my father didn't believe that anybody

who wasn't on the ground in Bastogne or along the Siegfried Switch Line could possibly have understood what they had experienced in this prolonged Battle of the Bulge. Worse, they feared nobody would recognize their actions as anything other than a skirmish on the way to eventual victory in Europe. They couldn't have been more wrong. Across the Channel and around the world, the Battle of the Bulge had military leaders and war correspondents singing their praises.

"Youth and courage were the deciding factors in the battle of the Belgian Bulge," an Associated Press war correspondent wrote at the time. "It took youthful stamina to stand the biting frosts, winds and cold . . . when relief was impossible and soldiers had to fight on with no help in sight."[48]

"Undoubtedly the greatest American battle of the War," British prime minister Winston Churchill concluded on January 18, 1945. "[The Battle of the Bulge] will, I believe, be regarded as an ever-famous American victory."[49]

And despite his earlier disdain for elements of his own army, Gen. George Patton claimed the Third Army had "moved further and faster and engaged more divisions in less time than any other army in the history of the United States, possibly in the history of the world."[50]

CHAPTER SEVEN

BLOOD OF THE ENEMY

I
N ALL THE STORIES my father chose to tell me about his war, I don't think he ever talked about being situated at the business end of a gun. In none of the photos I found in his files, years later, did I see him either holding or even close to a weapon. I don't know if my father was a conscientious objector, but I do know that he never allowed a weapon, not so much as a BB gun, into our household when I was growing up. I didn't much care for guns either, but at some point I asked him if his loathing of weapons had influenced his decision to become a medic. He told me that the vagaries of the army put him in the medical corps; in other words, on the day he joined up, the army was low on medics, so without regard for either his educational background or his civilian experience, the US Army chose to make him a medic.

My father's medical corps buddy, Tony Mellaci, told me he was allowed a .22 at his house for shooting squirrels that raided the garden or rats at the local dump. But Mellaci said that during advanced training at Camp McCain, Mississippi, all medics received live-fire training,[1] crawling on their bellies while live bullets whizzed above their heads and shells exploded around them; instructors told them it would help them get accustomed to the sights and sounds of combat. That probably sealed the deal for my father. He admitted, as well, that he never felt the "killer instinct" that appeared to be a basic requirement for becoming an arms-bearing soldier.[2]

As mentioned earlier, both my father and S/Sgt. Mellaci, his comrade in the 319th Medical Battalion, understood what the Geneva Convention said. Or at least they had a working knowledge of the basics. Going back to the nineteenth century, one article stipulated that hospital orderlies, medics, nurses, or stretcher-bearers who were collecting, transporting, or treating the wounded and sick "shall be respected and protected." In other words, shooting a medic was considered a war crime. Equally vital in a war zone, the convention stated that a wounded combatant had the right to be collected and to receive care; once a soldier became a casualty, he became neutral, a non-combatant, and a patient of medics on either side of a war zone.

Another article spelled out rules for medics when captured, saying that as POWs medics were expected to perform medical functions only as the need arose. The convention also stated that if a medic were armed and chose to use a weapon offensively, that medic would forfeit the convention's general immunity. The risk, as my father described it, was calculating whether everybody on the battlefield had read the fine print. During their service in the battle of the Saar-Moselle Triangle and beyond, medics in the line of fire couldn't always rely on an enemy's abiding by the rules.

...

MARCH 1945—LAMPADEN RIDGE, GERMANY

WHETHER OR NOT MEDICS could rely on immunity in the battlefield didn't seem to preoccupy the minds of too many medics during the Battle of the Bulge. It was all they could do to manage the relentless flow of wounded in and out of their aid stations. Few regimental war diaries noted the toll that such day-in, day-out triage and lifesaving first aid took on medics, in addition to worries—conscious or subconscious—about whether the enemy might ignore the red cross on their sleeves or helmets and open fire. However, one GI's personal journal did reflect on the physical and psychological pounding that US medics endured that winter of 1945. During the latter stages of the 94th Infantry Division's push through the Saar-Moselle Triangle, William Foley kept track of his experiences by sketching on paper.

At age eighteen, Bill Foley went from US Army volunteer to hurriedly trained rifleman, to transatlantic passenger on a troopship, to front-line combat soldier in G Company, 2nd Battalion, 302nd Infantry Regiment, with the 94th Infantry Division of Patton's Third Army. In barely a year, Foley's career path led him from life in small-town New Jersey to infantry replacement in the middle of the Battle of the Bulge. In March 1945, that assignment found him up Lampaden Ridge, nearly surrounded by the German 6th SS Mountain Division.

To prevent fear getting the better of him—while withstanding artillery barrages, dodging mines and booby traps, crawling through no man's land to snatch prisoners, and seeing comrades cut down in battle—Foley had rediscovered a childhood pastime, pencil drawing. In his pack he always carried the US Army-issue V-mail form* and a pencil, but instead of jotting down notes to send home to his family, he would draw. The habit was both a response to what he witnessed and a means of coping. "From somewhere in me, a surge of self-esteem welled up higher than the lift I gained from proving I could, so far, take infantry combat," he wrote. "I had arrived at the point where I could call myself an artist."[3]

In early March, in the town of Hentern, his platoon had dug foxholes around a building where their battalion medic, Fred Buckner, had set up an aid station in the basement. Waiting his turn for medical attention for a mild chest wound he'd sustained days earlier, Foley watched Buckner attend to a German prisoner with a broken arm. The sixteen-year-old POW couldn't stop crying as the American medic set and splinted his arm; meanwhile, members of Foley's squad shared rations with the captured soldier. That's when Foley noticed how poorly their medic Buckner appeared to be coping. "This Louisiana boy with the beautifully chiseled facial features could not control his eye tic and badly shaking hands," Foley wrote. "His black hair was graying over his ears and his voice was anything but steady."[4]

Everything was different about life in the front lines. Foley noted how some of the rules and regulations had become pretty lax as well. Nobody could get or keep clean. In place of regulation army long johns, Foley admitted he'd resorted

---

* A V-mail form consisted of a light sheet of letter paper, about seven by nine inches, on which the sender wrote correspondence in pencil. Once read and cleared by censors, the note was photographed and transported to the United States as a quarter-sized negative on microfilm. Once in the US, the negative was printed and sent on to its designated recipient as traditional mail.

to a couple of pairs of long-unwashed green flannel pyjamas. Then one day a Jeep rolled up and men Foley described as "shockingly clean, pink-faced officers" entered the command post and started ordering people around.

"Everyone fall out for a short-arm inspection!" a sergeant called out.[5]

This inspection for cleanliness required GIs to drop their pants and to roll back their foreskins so medics could check for venereal disease.

"This hadn't happened since before D-Day," Foley noted. "And how long had it been since anyone had even seen a girl, much less gotten close to one?"

Nevertheless, Foley and the rest of his platoon lined up for the embarrassing inspection.

"Pull 'em out and roll 'em back," the officer demanded. The sight of such unclean members provoked sharp intakes of breath among the reviewing officers and then sharp reactions. "Get out! Next! Move on, soldier. Next!" When half a dozen of the soldiers being examined failed to pass muster, one of the reviewing officers marched out and tore a strip off Foley's commanding officer. As absurd as the order seemed—with no such facilities nearby—he demanded the GIs get baths daily.

Foley remembered a platoon mate saying that not even their own officers understood what front-line troops were up against. The scene left such a deep impression on Foley that he later made a sketch of it. Within a few days, the cleanliness protocol was forgotten when the battle for Lampaden Ridge took a turn for the worse. The building in which their medic had previously treated the wounded had become consumed by the combat. And medic Buckner had finally cracked. Foley recalled the man crouched on the stairs to the basement, holding his head and shaking badly. There was little refuge for medics in such situations, least of all the immunity of an article in the Geneva Convention. Instances throughout the winter had proven that.

On January 16, 1945, when the 376th Infantry Regiment advanced headlong into a snow-covered minefield at Monkey Wrench Woods (as described in chapter 3), medical corpsman Bill Cleary rushed forward to assist members of F Company wounded by exploding land mines. Despite the red cross on his helmet, German snipers shot him dead.[6] Three days later, during the 302nd Infantry Regiment attacks near Nennig, medic John Riskey moved through the battlefield attending to wounded from C Company; administering first aid in the open, Riskey had his heavy jacket shredded by enemy fire and barely managed to save himself and his patients.[7] Nevertheless, a number of situations during the battle for the Saar-Moselle Triangle forced both sides to trust that the Geneva Convention articles would be respected.

In February, the US 376th advanced north of Sinz into another wooded area, called Bannholz. The GIs encountered heavy return fire from artillery, tanks, and mortars concealed in the woods. They tried desperately to hold on to the section of Bannholz they'd entered, and then struggled to evacuate wounded out of the line; two medical aid men had been cut down in the attempt. This brought Lt. James McCullough of the US Medical Administrative Corps (MAC) into the battle zone. He drove a jeep into Sinz and then walked to within three hundred yards of the German tanks camouflaged at the south end of the woods. He waved his helmet, plainly showing the Red Cross insignia.[8]

Eventually a German officer emerged from the woods and waved McCullough forward. In broken English, the panzer commander negotiated a deal with the MAC lieutenant. The panzers would maintain a ceasefire over the area as long as the US medics evacuated both American and German wounded from Bannholz at the same time. Lt. McCullough agreed to the compromise and moved into the woods, where he immediately heard calls of "Hey, Doc!" The voices drew fire from enemy gunners who were unaware of the truce. Flying tree fragments exacerbated the wounds on both sides, but McCullough had soon taken care of the GIs and at least five German walking wounded. Eventually they all emerged from the woods, but before any of the wounded reached the safety of their home lines, both American artillery and German guns brought down more fire on the evacuation convoy. Thankfully, no further casualties resulted. The intermittent ceasefire and brokered evacuation had saved a few lives.

For GIs and medical corpsmen reversing the Bulge in the winter campaign of 1945, the Germans' interpretation of the articles of the Geneva Convention would always present uncertainty and risk. As volunteers and draftees, they would always have to ask themselves if the immunity of long-ago rules of engagement applied on the ground in all-out war on the German front. Inevitably, they would regularly be forced to make snap decisions about respecting the immunity of medical personnel and the rights of casualties, whether comrade or foe.

For Raiden Winfield Dellinger, an officer in the 319th Medical Battalion on that German frontier, it wasn't so much the

Geneva Convention that governed his actions as the Hippo-
cratic Oath. Dellinger had come by his respect for the sick or
injured quite naturally. His father had been his role model.
Dr. Arthur Dellinger had received his medical degree in 1916,
done post-graduate work in Chicago and New York, and then
come home to Rome, Georgia, to run a practice for over thirty
years. Raiden pursued a related path, completing his degree in
1938 and his internships in New York and Florida, and then
returning home to conduct hospital surgery. But when the war
came, he needed to meet his military draft obligations.

In 1940 he joined the US Army Medical Corps, serving as a
first lieutenant at Fort Ethan Allen, Vermont, as an orthopedic
and surgical specialist, all the while keeping an eye on the war
and "brushing up on my French in the event I have to use it."[9]
But he finished his required year of active service, got married,
and secured employment at a hospital in Florida, expecting to
now focus on his career. Five months later, the Japanese attacked
Pearl Harbor and everything changed.

On December 9, 1941, the medical corps called for his return
to active duty, and by March 1942, at age twenty-eight, he was
a major serving with the medical detachment of the 301st Infantry Regiment of the 94th Infantry Division, en route overseas.

As it was for most of the 94th during its posting to western France in 1944, containing the two German armies at St.
Nazaire and Lorient proved a relatively uneventful deployment.
Maj. Dellinger and his friend, Capt. Jovell, enjoyed their relatively leisurely front-line service in their Brittany bungalow.
They acquired a dog mascot (for a pack of cigarettes) and, at
least in Dellinger's case, enjoyed the comfort of sleeping at night
in "blue silk pajamas," as he wrote his parents. "Jovell kids

me about them, but I find them convenient. Probably the only soldier in France with them!"[10]

Once the 94th hurriedly joined the American counteroffensive into the Saar-Moselle Triangle, sending letters home to his parents and his wife, Ruth, became a lower priority for Maj. Dellinger. And the correspondence from them reflected their fears for his safety. In February 1945, Ruth wrote her husband that the news "seemed to shorten the European war a lot, but I'm not laying any bets."[11] It turned out that as a CO in the medical battalion, Maj. Dellinger had indeed been quite busy. In the 209 combat days that the 94th Infantry Division had served in the European theatre, it sustained a total of 5,884 battle casualties—1,087 killed, 4,684 wounded, and 113 missing. Another 5,028 were put out of action because of trench foot, frostbite, or illness.[12]

Dellinger had served right in the middle of all that, often first into the fray—directing traffic at aid posts, attending to casualties directly, and when necessary dropping everything to deal with surgical life-and-death situations, even as bullets flew around his impromptu operating theatre. He never boasted about such actions, and even when credit was due—he was awarded a Bronze Star medal—he dismissed it as fulfilling his commitment to his country. During its push across the Saar-Moselle Triangle, the 94th had also taken 26,638 Germans prisoner—seven of them captured by Maj. Dellinger.

"My driver, Capt. Jovell, and I were driving down a road when . . . a [German] lieutenant, a sergeant and five men . . . stepped out and stopped the jeep and surrendered," he wrote to his parents. "For a minute, there was some question of who was surrendering to who, but when we asked them, were they surrendering, the answer was 'Ja.'"[13]

It's unlikely that group of German prisoners of war realized how fortunate they were to have surrendered to Raiden Dellinger—an experienced medical officer and a resident of both big cities and small towns in the United States. The major coolly loaded all seven of the Germans aboard his Jeep and brought them in for processing and medical attention. It wasn't so much a matter of respecting the Geneva Convention. For Raiden Dellinger, it was a reflex of experience and wisdom—and a belief that the welfare of those in his care, no matter what their military affiliation, was paramount.

JANUARY 1942— BANGKOK-TO-MOULMEIN RAILWAY, BURMA

EVEN MEDICS WHO EXPERIENCED combat medicine under fire might not agree on whether they felt as if they were targets or not. During the Second World War, news outlets among Allied nations that were prone to propagandize such things chose to vilify German soldiers when they printed the story of Pte. Louis Potts. An American corpsman with the 26th Infantry Division—and clearly wearing his Red Cross helmet and arm bands—Potts dodged sniper fire on Christmas Day 1944, when he entered no man's land to attend to a wounded GI. Moving to a second casualty, Potts was struck in the forehead by a sniper's bullet.[14] Similarly, news reports on the German side played up the violation of medic immunity with the story of a German

Jeep racing through the village of Vierville, France, on D-Day Plus Two. The vehicle carried two wounded men on stretchers lashed to the seats. At first no one responded, because the Jeep was flying a large Red Cross flag. Eventually, however, the Jeep was stopped, the medic shot (allegedly for carrying a pistol), and the two casualties left to die at the roadside.[15]

During the Battle of the Bulge that began in mid-December 1944, doctors and nurses at the US 77th Evacuation Hospital learned quickly that red crosses on or near their sites meant nothing to an enemy bent on driving perceived invaders from its fatherland. At Verviers, east of Liège, the 77th established a casualty clearing centre for American wounded. As per echelon protocol, doctors and nurses decided then and there how they would attend to incoming casualties. In some cases the medical staff could dress relatively minor wounds and send troops back to front-line duty. In other cases they might tag casualties and send them to a hospital in Liège. At the height of the German offensive, hundreds of American casualties went through the casualty centre, and the triage area took direct hits from German artillery and then strafing runs from Luftwaffe fighter aircraft. More than twenty nurses became additional casualties.[16]

Arguably, atrocities against medics, surgeons, and nurses occurred most often where the fighting raged between deeply philosophical opposites. A volunteer in the Republican Army during the Spanish Civil War recalled a nursing sister caught in the crossfire between those fighting for the restoration of the monarchy and democratic rule, and the Nationalists intent on replacing the monarchy and its communist sympathizers with a fascist state. The Republican rifleman recalled that the war had hardened him and his comrades in the Mackenzie-

Papineau Battalion from Canada and the Abraham Lincoln Brigade from the United States. When a wounded German parachutist fell into Republican hands, the casualty lay on a stretcher unattended until Nursing Sister Carrie approached the injured man and offered him a cigarette. "It wasn't because we had forgotten the code of the medical corps," the rifleman wrote, "but because still fresh in our minds was the work of the German flyers that morning."[17]

Earlier in the day, he had recorded the entire Republican brigade retreating. Nurses and patients fleeing in ambulances. Equipment tossed willy-nilly into trucks. He remembered that the casualty clearing station had to be evacuated and that the roads were crowded with refugees—old men, women, children—all of them lugging their meagre possessions. The road was free of combat troops, but suddenly Nationalist fighter aircraft filled the sky and swooped down, machine guns blazing. In their wake, the Canadian reported, women, children, nurses, patients, and old men lay dead or dying. He wrote that he saw a mother with her slain baby in her arms, cradling it "as if her life's strength could close those gaping wounds, close those staring eyes or shut the stilled mouth."[18]

Few could be blamed for the intense hatred directed at the enemy paratrooper in their midst that afternoon; only their esprit de corps, he wrote, kept them from killing this man lying on a stretcher in front of them. He surmised that Nursing Sister Carrie had simply felt her duty more than others, or that her sense of Christian forgiveness had taken care of this wounded man where others wouldn't.

"In two days came her reward," the rifleman wrote. "A new raid. A new attack on the helpless and unarmed. Nurse Carrie carried another wounded man into a little depression just large enough for one. Her body helped to protect him. Nothing protected her. Machine gun bullets ripped off the top of her head. Death came to this fine woman. Thus, Fascism repays her debts."[19]

In spite of this Republican soldier's general condemnation of Nazi-indoctrinated troops in the Spanish Civil War, a post–Second World War survey of medics' accounts from northwestern Europe claimed that German violations of the Geneva Convention were uncommon. The report showed that, despite some instances of aid men wearing Red Cross insignia being shot, such killings were rare. Generally, US medics serving in France, Belgium, and Germany responded by wearing arm bands on both sleeves and by keeping the red cross in its white square plainly visible on their helmets. Medics genuinely hoped their German enemies would respect such insignia if clearly visible. The survey also indicated, however, that all bets were off in the Pacific War, where Allied medics wearing red crosses became special targets of the Japanese. In response, medics often removed their arm bands and erased any helmet insignia completely, preferring to be invisible; some even dyed their white bandages green to disappear into the jungle even further.[20]

The apparent disregard for the convention that confirmed the immunity of medical staff is perhaps clearest in the Japanese Imperial Army siege of Hong Kong, which began eight hours after the attack on Pearl Harbor, December 7, 1941. From the middle of the month until Christmas, virtually all 14,000 Allied troops were overrun by the Japanese invading force of more than 50,000. An estimated 10,000 Hong Kong civilians were executed, and more than 1,500 Allied troops died in the slaughter. As each area of the island fell under Japanese control, so too did all medical facilities, including an advanced dressing station in the Wong Nai Chung Gap, a strategic passage between north and south Hong Kong. T.R. Cunningham, a sergeant in the Royal Army Medical Corps, documented events at his ADS beginning on December 18, when he recorded that the aid station housed an RAMC officer, a lance corporal, two privates, and a driver, as well as himself and ten St. John Ambulance personnel. The Japanese surrounded their position early the following morning.

"At daybreak we heard [Japanese soldiers] on the roof trying to force their ventilators open, but they were unsuccessful," Sgt. Cunningham wrote. "After a series of explosions, we were able to see the St. Johns [sic] bearers with the Indian constable come out of their shelters and surrender. Although the bearers were full dressed, complete with Red Cross brassards, the Japanese killed everyone."[21]

Similar atrocities befell many of those defending the British colony—whether the Middlesex Regiment, the Royal Rifles of Canada, the Winnipeg Grenadiers, or the Hong Kong volunteer defence corps—as well as patients and their caregivers at hospitals and aid stations across the island. At the Wong Nai Chung Gap, the ADS personnel spent a horrific night as Japanese forces sprayed their station with machine-gun fire or tried to break down the doors. Some inside suggested that the staff and casualties surrender, while others, fearing for the fate of the wounded, reminded the rest of their obligation to attend to them no matter what. Eventually Capt. B.D. Barclay improvised a Red Cross flag with a note attached saying that those in the ADS were unarmed. But when he pushed the flag through a crack in the building wall, the Japanese opened fire again.

"We heard a large body [of Japanese troops] assemble round the A.D.S.," Cunningham continued. "So, we all came out and surrendered. We were then beaten, securely tied and our Red Cross brassards torn off. We were brought before a few officers [and] after interrogation we were again beaten."[22]

The casualty numbers in the fall of Singapore were six times worse than Hong Kong's. During seventy days of siege, nearly 9,000 British, Indian, and Australian troops lost their lives, and nearly 85,000 became prisoners of war (in addition to 50,000 already captured during the fighting down the Malay Peninsula). Among the casualties in what Prime Minister Winston Churchill described as "the worst disaster and largest capitulation"[23] in British military history was a forty-two-year-old Romanian-born physician. His story would outlive even the mightiest of wartime empires. During the battle for Malaya, Jacob Markowitz served as a surgical officer at No. 5 Casualty Clearing Station, an Indian medical unit. Operating and retreating southward for days on end, Markowitz and his staff attended to casualties day and night for a month, until his medical team, like the British Army, ended up with its back to the sea.

"In this war, Dunkirk is . . . the outstanding example of an orderly retreat, followed by an evacuation by a fleet," he explained later. "No such luck eventuated in Singapore Island . . . . As one Tommy put it, 'When we ran out of earth, and had no place to retreat, we surrendered.'"[24] Right away, Markowitz reported, his anesthetist had been killed and his sergeant dresser in the surgical team was missing, presumably killed.

As the Japanese conquerors continued their orgy of killing in Southeast Asia into 1942, Capt. Jacob Markowitz began an almost subterranean campaign to save as many around him as he could. After the capture of so many POWs, the Japanese essentially starved their prisoners for the next six months in Malaya. Markowitz recorded in his illegal diary that he'd lost twenty-eight pounds by summertime. He'd also witnessed the first outbreaks of disease—beriberi (paralysis followed by dropsy) and pellagra (sore tongue, loose bowels), and at least a thousand cases of dysentery (diarrhea with blood). Then, according to Markowitz's notes, the Japanese moved thousands of the POWs farther inland with a promise of better working conditions and improved food. They delivered neither.

Instead, the Japanese transported about 50,000 British and Australian prisoners of war into the jungles of what was then Malaya, Siam, and Burma to build the Bangkok-to-Moulmein Railway. Pierre Boulle called his epic novel based on this POW story *The Bridge over the River Kwai*, and Columbia Pictures spent a then unprecedented $3 million filming the movie adaptation. To the 55,000 POWs and several hundred thousand South Asians forced to build the original, however, it was known as "the Death Railway," and it cost more than 200,000 lives. "[In] the first year alone," Capt. Markowitz later told newspaper reporters, "15,000 whites and 150,000 coolies died there. For every tie that was laid a native died; for every rail, a British Tommy."[25]

Markowitz quickly discovered that the Japanese attitude in the POW camps was that the sick and injured were a nuisance and if they died it was the doctor's fault. His job was to prevent workers from dying. In the Chungkai camp, at the Siam end of the railway, he attended to 9,000 patients, most suffering from tropical ulcers that bared the leg bones from the knee to the ankle. Markowitz would attempt to scrape out the stinking pulp of necrotic flesh with a sharpened spoon, but all too often gangrene would win out, and there would be no alternative but amputation.[26] The Canadian doctor and his staff of four junior medical officers performed more than a thousand amputations with a hacksaw borrowed from the camp carpenter.[27] They were allowed no medical instruments. The only anesthetic available was Novocain, injected at the base of the spine. He employed broken bottles as funnels for blood transfusions, and as he transfused a patient his orderlies kept the blood from coagulating by whipping it with a stick. Markowitz and his team administered 3,800 transfusions this way and, despite some severe reactions, recorded no deaths due to transfusion.

Just when the RAMC doctors sensed things could get no worse, there was an outbreak of cholera. "The Japanese who were terrified of this illness, supplied large quantities of cholera vaccine," Markowitz wrote. "Medical officers inoculated 7,000 troops in twenty-four hours. . . . We had 152 cases of whom 60 died."[28]

Markowitz proved as meticulous a note-taker as he was a surgeon. The Canadian Press reported later that he recorded the comings and goings of patients every day, and then each evening he slipped his notes into a corked bottle and hid the container under the shroud of a corpse. After the war his notes were unearthed, published, and heralded in the *Journal of the Royal Army Medical Corps*.

Capt. Markowitz's route to the Death Railway was a circuitous one, but as it turned out, few medical men were better qualified for the primitive conditions he faced. Born in Romania in 1901, Markowitz came to Canada as an infant. His post-secondary studies led him routinely through the University of Toronto, graduating with his MD in 1923 and his PhD three years later. He moved to the University of Glasgow as an assistant professor in physiology, and then to the University of Minnesota to complete a degree in a medical practice that was off the beaten path, something called "experimental surgery."

At the Mayo Clinic in 1932, he pursued investigative medical procedures and focused his attention on blood science, becoming the first surgeon to successfully transplant the heart of one warm-blooded animal—a dog—to another. And though he took his unique surgical techniques quite seriously, even he was amused by good-natured jokes that called him "the dog surgeon." Markowitz lectured, travelled, wrote, and published his revolutionary concepts, although he had to pay $3,500 for the cost of printing the manuscript himself. His book, *Experimental Surgery*, sold 25,000 copies.

In 1940 Dr. Markowitz offered his medical services to the Canadian Army, but recruiters wouldn't accept him because he didn't have naturalization papers.[29] So he sailed for England and enlisted in the Royal Army Medical Corps. He arrived at his wartime posting in Singapore seven days before the Japanese invaded the Malay Peninsula.

"Now occurred . . . the fulfillment of all my background," he wrote in his curriculum vitae. "As a POW of the Japanese, I found my training of great use."[30]

More than once Capt. Markowitz noted that the primitive hospital conditions seemed more like "an environment resembling the days of Moses." Markowitz and his surgical team often operated out in the open, where fresher, cleaner air might circulate and where the light was brightest; but with the out-of-doors would also come dust and hundreds of flies to be "flicked off when they settled."[31] Of particular note, the medical officer they called "Marko" recorded treatment for an Australian soldier who underwent an amputation at the hip. Though the medical team had anesthetized the man with a spinal injection of percaine, Markowitz claimed the patient was saved on the operating table by a technique recorded in the Old Testament. Twenty minutes into the operation, the patient stopped breathing. The operating team applied artificial respiration, but since the man's chest had collapsed into the expiratory position, trying to compress his lungs proved futile.

"Luckily there happened to be a piece of rubber tubing nearby, which we put in his mouth," Markowitz wrote. "He was given artificial respiration by the method used by Elijah the Tishbite when he resuscitated the widow's child. The patient's lips and nostrils were compressed and air was blown into his chest about twenty times a minute."

A few whiffs of air later, the man's heart began beating again. After forty minutes of artificial respiration, the man could breathe on his own. Markowitz then commenced the amputation. The operation was successful. The wound healed, the patient survived, and Markowitz even recorded the soldier's first remarks upon learning about the artificial respiration: "I'm glad you guys don't eat onions," the Australian had said. "I don't like onions."

Initially their Japanese jailers did not allow any living quarters for Capt. Markowitz's medical staff, so they slept in open ditches until they could lash together pillars and posts with coconut bark and cover their camp area with thatched roofing. Since the Japanese did not allow them to carry matches, the POWs maintained a perpetual fire. They dug freshwater wells by hand. Their rations consisted of rice and little else, although the medical team soon tried supplementing the prisoners' diets with indigenous grass. To keep up his own strength, Markowitz drank an occasional sip of beer that was brewed from rice, with a rotten banana added to provide some yeast. In spite of their weakened physical state, Capt. Markowitz and his team worked up to eighteen and twenty hours a day for weeks at a time. "We lived under conditions such as might have existed 3,500 years ago," he later told Canadian newspaper reporters.

The Japanese permitted no news from the outside world into either the railway construction camps or the jungle hospital. Sometime late in the summer of 1945, Markowitz was informed that he and his men were no longer prisoners of war. But none of the Japanese bothered to tell the POWs that Japan had surrendered (on August 15) until a squadron of Allied Dakota transport aircraft parachuted in supplies and a rescue party. Markowitz was finally repatriated to Canada in January 1946.

A decade later, the story gained international fame with the production and release of Columbia Pictures' blockbuster movie *The Bridge on the River Kwai*. The movie grossed $33 million at the box office in 1958, had everybody whistling the "Colonel Bogey March," and swept the Academy Awards. But amid all the hoopla, there was little or no mention of the unassuming doctor from Toronto who'd kept thousands of prisoners alive in the jungles of Siam, where their Japanese captors abused Allied POWs as forced labour building the railway bridge.

Dr. Jacob Markowitz got no mention in the movie credits,* even though he received postwar accolades from King George and the British Army.

"[During his] service in prisoner-of-war camps in Siam," read his citation for Member of the Most Excellent Order of the British Empire, "using the most primitive and improvised apparatus, Capt. Markowitz has shown skill and ability of an outstanding degree."[32]

JUNE 7, 1944—ABBAYE D'ARDENNE, FRANCE

THE TREATMENT OF PRISONERS OF WAR on both sides during the first days of the Normandy invasion became the basis of both war diaries and court testimony. On D-Day, more than 15,000 Canadian troops landed in the Juno Beach sector. Among the 9th Brigade soldiers landing in front of Bernières-sur-Mer, Pte. Hollis McKeil and his North Nova Scotia Highlanders all carried collapsible bicycles; they had trained to race inland from beachheads secured by the first wave to capture

---

* On Academy Awards night in March 1958, Columbia Pictures' *The Bridge on the River Kwai* made nearly a clean sweep of the major categories, winning seven Oscars (for best picture, best actor, best director, best screenplay, best cinematography, best editing, and best musical score). In accepting his Oscar, director David Lean remarked at the podium, "When we were sweating in the jungle for so long, I never dreamed that the bridge would bring us to Hollywood." As he sweated out the real war in that Siamese jungle from 1942 to 1945, Dr. Jacob Markowitz no doubt never considered winning anything but his freedom. As it was, the pioneer of experimental surgery was able to enjoy that freedom for only a few years. He suffered a severe coronary in 1962 and died a few years later. His memoirs make no mention of ever viewing the wartime movie drama set just outside his hospital window on the Death Railway.

the villages of Buron and Authie and the airfield at Carpiquet. While the Canadians penetrated German defences deeper than any other Allied units that day, neither the North Novas nor their armoured units, the Sherbrooke Fusiliers, reached the planned objectives. Miraculously, Pte. McKeil and members of his platoon had made it ashore without a scratch. The next day, June 7, would be altogether different.

After a false start at dawn, McKeil and his platoon mates hopped aboard the Sherman tanks of the 27th Armoured Regiment (the Sherbrooke Fusiliers), which carried them straight south on the road to Buron, Authie, and, ultimately, the airport at Carpiquet. The advance moved swiftly—knocking out enemy guns, capturing prisoners, and gobbling up German-occupied territory—until about midday. Suddenly the Canadian column of infantry and tanks came under fire from positions on their exposed left flank. Despite their quick dismount from the tanks, McKeil and his 12th Platoon sustained casualties, McKeil himself being hit with shrapnel in the chest and ankle. He and another wounded Highlander received medical assistance from a stretcher-bearer but were then left behind to be evacuated later.

Although no one knew it at the time, the entire 9th Brigade advance was under surveillance by Col. Kurt Meyer, commander of the 25th SS Panzer Grenadiers, a regiment whose rank and file consisted of *Hitlerjugend*, German youth (no more than eighteen years old) highly indoctrinated with Nazi ideology.[33] From a steeple at the Abbaye d'Ardenne, about a mile to the east, Meyer directed his artillery, tank, and infantry counterattack so effectively that the entire 9th Brigade advance stalled and fell back, leaving some—including wounded North

Nova Scotia Highlander Hollis McKeil—behind in an open grain field.

The day's losses were heavy on both sides. The four companies of North Novas engaged in the battle had sustained 242 casualties—eighty-four fatal, and 128 becoming prisoners. The Sherbrooke Fusiliers had lost twenty-one tanks, with seven more damaged, and suffered sixty casualties, including twenty-six deaths. The 25th Panzers now had scores of Canadian POWs crowded within the walls of the Abbaye. Among those Sherbrooke tankmen wounded and held captive at the monastery was Hubert Thistle, a twenty-year-old wireless radio operator from St. John's, Newfoundland. Manoeuvring a Sherman Firefly tank under fire, he and his crew had fought until their tank burst into flames; the crew barely managed to abandon the vehicle before its fuel ignited and exploded and Tpr. Thistle fell into enemy hands. "These young SS captured us and took our watches, cigarettes," Thistle said. "And they took us to Abbaye d'Ardenne."[34]

Thistle's captors were members of the 12th SS Panzer Division under the command of Col. Meyer but, as Thistle soon learned, they had also been given carte blanche with their prisoners—wounded or otherwise. En route to the monastery, several of the Hitler Youth troops drew their weapons, shot individual captives on the spot, and in some cases tossed the bodies of the murdered men onto the roadways, where German vehicles pulverized their remains beyond recognition. At the Abbaye, SS officers confiscated the tags and pay books of surviving POWs and interrogated them for strategic information. Then they demanded volunteers, and North Novas and Sherbrookes were dragged away.

"They took us into this barn, five of us, and lined us up. We were next," Thistle said. "They had a sniper in front of us ready to go. We shook hands, you know, like it was the end . . . when in came some high-ranking [German] officer and stopped him. Just a split second and another five of us would have been among the dead."[35]

That night, the *Hitlerjugend* executed six of Tpr. Thistle's comrades in the Sherbrooke Fusiliers, as well as five North Nova Scotia Highlanders. The next day, June 8, the SS troops killed eight more Novas, including the wounded Pte. Hollis McKeil, who was shot in the back of the head.* When the killing spree ended, the surviving prisoners were transported to POW camps.

In the same battle sector as the Canadian 9th Brigade advance south of Juno Beach on June 7 and 8, 1944, members of the Royal Canadian Army Medical Corps struggled to get a toehold for their wounded. Near the town of Basly, about four miles inland from the beaches, S/Sgt. Henry Duffield had managed to find suitable natural shelter and set up a field hospital. Duffield had always known ways to improvise. When the skilled soccer player immigrated to Canada in the 1920s, the sanatorium in Prince Albert, Saskatchewan, took him on as a medical orderly so he could play for the institution's city soccer squad. Later, in British Columbia, he parlayed his position as an orderly into first-aid medic jobs with lumber com-

* In July 1944, Roland and Francine Vico and the rest of their farming family returned to their living quarters at the Abbaye. Despite several visits and searches by members of the Canadian War Crimes Investigation Unit, it was the accidental unearthing of bodies in Mme. Vico's flower garden that revealed evidence of the murders. In the spring of 1945, investigators excavated the gardens and recovered eighteen bodies. An autopsy revealed that, in addition to his chest and ankle shrapnel wounds, Hollis McKeil had received fatal bullet wounds to the head.

panies on the Pacific Coast. In 1940, with medic work on his resumé, Duffield was allowed to enlist in the Royal Canadian Army Medical Corps, first administering No. 11 Canadian General Hospital in England, and then running field hospitals as the invasion began.

Despite the relatively successful landings at the two British and one Canadian D-Day beaches, German counterattacks had left the actual front-line configuration, an east-west line about four miles inland, in flux. For S/Sgt. Duffield, however, the challenge of a growing number of wounded—both Canadians and Germans—required the immediate attention of first-aid medics and surgeons. There was no time to deliberate about whether or where to erect a marquee tent for the field hospital. Nevertheless, the decision to set up shop near Basly suddenly triggered an extraordinary encounter.

On June 8, as Col. Kurt Meyer was riding a motorcycle from his 25th Panzer headquarters at the Abbaye to several German battalion positions along the front line, more than once he was driven to ground by incoming artillery shells. During one barrage, shrapnel struck his motorcycle and Meyer was forced to abandon it beside the road. Momentarily on foot and with several SS troops accompanying him, Meyer came across a field position covered in canvas, and he raced inside. "In comes [Col.] Meyer with his SS guys, all with Schmeissers drawn," Henry Duffield told his son Ray.[36]

At that stage of the Normandy campaign, S/Sgt. Duffield wore a 9 mm pistol on his belt. But the sudden realization that his field hospital had been invaded by the commanding officer of a panzer division left Duffield frozen on his feet. The field hospital housed scores of wounded men on cots, including

Canadian and German casualties. Meyer broke the momentary pause, Ray Duffield said, and strode right up to several of the wounded, unarmed but clearly wearing German uniforms as well as bandage dressings and splints.

"Are you being treated the same as the Canadian wounded?" Meyer said in German to one of the German casualties on a cot. Duffield spoke the language, so he understood the question immediately. The next moments seemed eternal.

"Yes," came the response.

Just as quickly as the incident had begun, it ended. Meyer turned, motioned those SS troops with him to leave, and without another word, they all disappeared through the canvas door.

More than a year later, as the German armies retreated across the River Meuse, local partisans discovered Kurt Meyer hiding in a barn and turned him over to American authorities. In December 1945, he was put on trial for war crimes in the German town of Aurich. Among the indictments was the murder of Canadian POWs at Abbaye d'Ardenne.

In a postwar memoir, as a retort to the accusations, Kurt Meyer recounted at least one action committed by Allied troops that he said violated the Geneva Convention. He wrote that on June 9, D-Day Plus Three, he'd found a group of German troops—from the 21st Panzers and 12th SS Panzers—south of the village of Rots in Normandy. Their bodies were lying beside the road "all shot through the head"; the colonel reported the killings back to his corps headquarters. Meyer further contended that the scene inside Abbaye d'Ardenne was quite the opposite of the account reconstructed by the Canadian War Crimes Investigation Unit.

"In the monastery orchard our wounded comrades are being tended, the young grenadiers are lying side by side cheering each other up," Meyer wrote on June 7, 1944. "Canadian [POWs] lie next to German soldiers. The doctors and medical orderlies make no distinction between the uniforms, there is nothing separating the soldiers anymore. The only issue at stake here is the lives of human beings."[37]

Despite his plea of not guilty, Meyer was found responsible for the deaths, but not guilty of directly ordering the killings. In his final statement before sentencing, he defended the record of his military unit and the innocence of his soldiers. In his diary he complained about the difficulty of transporting wounded away from the front lines during those early days in Normandy. He noted that Allied fighter-bombers routinely attacked ambulances and that German regimental doctors cited aircraft strafing and bombing of medical companies that were clearly marked with white paint and red crosses to distinguish them from military vehicles. "The red cross no longer offers any protection," he wrote.

In 1946, Kurt Meyer began his imprisonment at Dorchester Penitentiary in New Brunswick; he petitioned for clemency in 1950, was transferred from Canada to a military prison in Werl, West Germany, in 1951, won his release for good behaviour in 1954, and died in Westphalia in 1961.

Henry Duffield's momentary confrontation with the former panzer commander would prove to be his closest shave during his overseas service in the Second World War. The veteran medic rose in rank to warrant officer in postwar regular service, in part by maintaining a tough but fair attitude when dealing with people. And how did his son Jim describe his father's demeanour at home?

"Stubborn," he said without hesitating. "He was a take-no-prisoners kind of guy."[38]

Chapter Eight

MEDICS, MYTHS, AND MARTYRDOM

As A SOLDIER, my father was more a pragmatist than a patriot, more a realist than a romantic. His view of the military and war was more Ernest Hemingway, who saw war as a crime, than it was Douglas MacArthur, who said it required the will to win. His sensibilities were more Franklin D. Roosevelt, who called war a contagion, than Winston Churchill, who said success in war came only to those who deserved it. But perhaps the perspective of war my father espoused most was that of comedic writer Larry Gelbart: "A war is like when it rains in New York and everybody crowds into doorways. . . . And they all get chummy together. Perfect strangers. The only difference, of course, is that in a war it's also raining on the other side of the street and the people who are chummy over there are trying to kill the people who are over here who are chums."[1]

In particular, I'm sure my father, a born and raised New Yorker, could quickly draw that picture in his head. More than that, Alex Barris—who spent a lot of his time before, during, and after the war writing newspaper and magazine stories—eventually saw the parallel between his aspirations and those of Larry Gelbart, the scripting genius behind the 1970s hit TV series *M*A*S*H*. Like my father, Gelbart wrote as much as he could during the Second World War; the difference was that T/Sgt. Barris wrote stories, some serious, others satirical, for his medical battalion, while Pfc. Gelbart wrote variety scripts for show-business stars on radio.

When he turned eighteen in 1944, Gelbart received his draft notice and was shunted from one training camp to another until the army spotted the young Californian's writing ability and arranged to have him posted to the Armed Forces Radio Service in Hollywood; he wrote a kind of radio request show (often staged in front of a theatre audience) for American service personnel longing to finish the war and get home. Among other things, he and the producers of the popular show *Command Performance* arranged for the radio broadcast of Ann Miller tap dancing in military boots, Lana Turner frying a steak amid armed guards at centre stage, Errol Flynn taking a shower, and Bing Crosby mixing a bourbon and soda for Bob Hope. Larry Gelbart's war meant he was stationed in Hollywood, able to live at home and hobnob with a who's who of show business.

By comparison, at that stage of the war, Pvt. Barris was living in a drafty barracks hut at Camp Phillips, Kansas, a long way from his mom's home cooking. And yet he applied all his creative juices to the extracurricular task of editing the *Weekly Dose*, the newsletter of the 319th Medical Battalion. He led a staff of four, including himself, scouring the training facility for printable tips, tales, and gossip. In the March 6, 1943, edition, for example, he composed an editorial extending sympathy to all the battalion ambulance and truck drivers, suggesting they fly their imaginary flags at half-staff because "Henrietta" and her companions were no more. Apparently the powers that be at Camp Phillips had decided that assigning feminine names to their vehicles in honour of their girlfriends back home was inappropriate; instead, the corpsmen-in-training had to choose medical names.

"Slowly but surely they're taking all the sentiment out of the army," Editor-in-chief Barris wrote. "Pretty soon they'll have us using medical names for the litters and, who knows, some day we may hear of Sgt. Sulphadiazine, Cpl. Capillary, and Pvt. Pneumonia!"[2]

In his own small way, my father was scratching an itch he'd always had: to write as a reporter, a feature writer, and a columnist. Eventually all those forms of professional writing would become Alex's livelihood when he returned to the United States and ultimately moved to Canada in pursuit of work as a peacetime journalist. I think it's fair to say that the wit and satire my father regularly stitched into his newspaper columns for the *Globe and Mail* and the *Toronto Telegram* in the 1950s and '60s had a strong connection to some of the tongue-in-cheek writing he'd generated at the helm of Camp Phillips's *Weekly Dose* in 1943.

For his daily newspaper column in Canada, "The Barris Beat," my father chased leads, contacts, and original stories in show business. Not surprisingly, when CBS Television premiered *M*A*S*H*, a show about wartime medics, my father took notice. Not only was the writing on *M*A*S*H* razor sharp and funny, its context and message resonated with my father's memories of army life as well as his views on war and peace. It wasn't long before my father became a regular viewer of the show and a dedicated fan of its head writer, Larry Gelbart.

*M*A*S*H* originated as a novel by Richard Hooker, the pen name of Dr. H. Richard Hornberger, a graduate of Cornell University Medical School who served as a doctor with the 8055th Mobile Army Surgical Hospital (MASH) during the Korean War. Like Hornberger's novel, the movie released in 1970 reflected the experiences of a MASH unit coping with the rhythm of life and death behind the lines in the Korean War. Eventually producers approached Larry Gelbart to adapt the successful movie for television. The sitcom enjoyed great ratings and lasted eleven seasons (251 episodes). Throughout its run, from 1972 to 1983, Gelbart instinctively sensed that the show had to present characters and situations that were respectful of the Korean War veterans' experience as well as the experiences of those still serving in Vietnam.

He wrote the initial TV episode in two days, but once CBS decided to produce a full season, Gelbart spent countless hours interviewing military surgeons, nurses, patients, helicopter pilots, and orderlies to maintain the show's authenticity. From those conversations, word for word, came the poignant image captured in one *M*A*S*H* script by the chaplain character, Father John Mulcahy: "When the doctors cut into a patient—and it gets very cold here, you know—steam rises from the body, and the doctor will warm himself over the open wound. Could anyone look on that and not be changed?"[3]

Former army corpsman Barris never missed an episode of

former Pfc. Gelbart's take on military medical personnel at work and play in a war zone.

MARCH 25, 1945—KREFELD, GERMANY

NONE OF THE FORMER *Weekly Dose* staff members was on editorial duty for most of the Saar-Moselle campaign in the winter of 1945. All of its reporters and editors were otherwise occupied, performing the medical duties they'd been trained to carry out. That doesn't mean there were no stories to document; on the contrary, by March 1945 most corpsmen of the 319th Medical Battalion had far more experiences fresh in their memories than any four-page newsletter could accommodate.

And in addition to the personal stories, there were the regimental ones. Trier, the crown of the Saar-Moselle Triangle, fell that first week of March. And with that, the race to the River Rhine had begun, with the 94th Infantry Division, to which the 319th was attached, chasing German troops eastward. In the middle of the month, just as the division was about to break through the enemy's front lines along the rolling, wooded terrain of the Schwarzwälder Hochwald, Gen. Eisenhower visited Gen. Patton's Third Army headquarters and agreed to allocate the 12th Armored Division in support of the 94th's advance. On March 14, 15, and 16, the division captured 344, 341, and then 700 German soldiers, respectively; after that, an average of as many as 3,000 troops surrendered per day. With limited space available in the forested areas, the roads grew congested with infantry and tanks racing eastward and POWs going in the opposite direction.

"In the last weeks of the war," T/Sgt. Barris wrote, "I remember the mad race across Germany in pursuit of a tattered, thoroughly demoralized Nazi force no longer interested in fighting, only surviving."[4]

Indeed, the only thing that appeared to matter, according to the grapevine that informed my father and others, was Patton's single-minded focus on crossing the Rhine before anybody else. In particular, he was anxious to best his nemesis Field Marshal Bernard Montgomery and the 21st Army Group, whose Operation Plunder planned to make the crossing on March 23. The 94th was ordered forward at double speed to get Patton there first. Between March 12 and 24, Patton's so-called Ghost Corps advanced over a hundred miles, taking objectives in more than two hundred villages and towns. In the course of the rush eastward, the 94th captured more than 13,400 German troops. The division was then allowed to backtrack by rail and truck through Luxembourg, over the former battlefields of the Battle of the Bulge, and north to Krefeld, just across the river from Düsseldorf, to await its final orders of the war.

On March 25, as the GIs of the 94th settled into rest areas at Krefeld, they cleaned, overhauled, repaired, or replaced vehicles, weapons, equipment, and clothing. For the first time in two months the daily routine orders slowed to a leisurely pace as command posts attempted to catch up on overdue clerical work. Among the missives came one from Gen. Patton, who finally acknowledged "the splendid work your Division has accomplished during its tour of duty with us."[5]

At the time, S/Sgt. Tony Mellaci remembered, many of the

medical units that the Saar-Moselle campaign had scattered across the front for weeks were temporarily reunited in the rest area. And as the corpsmen settled in, the regimental bureaucracy posted a number of citations, promotions, and awards to be presented. One caught Mellaci's eye.

"Hey, Al Barris is getting the Bronze Star," he announced to his buddies in the 319th motor pool.[6] And he recounted the unit assembling for the presentation by Capt. Laurence J. Sykora. Mellaci said it was the first such award given to a member of B Company of the medical battalion, and that my father seemed embarrassed at being in the spotlight for retrieving the four litter-bearers from Campholz Woods back on February 12. Nevertheless, the events of that night were read aloud as the award was presented.

"Tech-4 Barris has repeatedly expressed initiative and foresight in discharge of his duties as liaison Sgt.," the citation said. "His total disregard for personal safety and his continual service to his organization over and above the call of his particular duties are in keeping with the highest of army traditions."[7]

It was S/Sgt. Mellaci's turn several weeks later, when the appropriate paperwork was processed and he too was awarded the Bronze Star for his meritorious service across the Saar-Moselle Triangle. Such recognition was hardly the stuff of feature films, books, or even news copy. But for those around him, T/Sgt. Barris sensed, this was welcome recognition—despite Gen. Patton's earlier accusations of their malingering—that the corpsmen, litter-bearers, and ambulance drivers of the 319th Medical Battalion had committed themselves to a greater cause that winter of 1945.

...

OCTOBER 12, 1915—BRUSSELS, BELGIUM

IT HAD BEEN THREE MONTHS since the armies of Kaiser Wilhelm II marched into Belgium. Ahead of them, in August 1914, the Belgian government went into exile while King Albert I and what was left of the Belgian army joined Allied troops as they fought while withdrawing westward. Behind the lines of German occupation, inside occupied Brussels, the Belgian capital, Germany assigned senior military officers to rule the country. They in turn deported Belgians to become forced labour at German military installations and munitions plants, while making concessions to radical groups in an attempt to placate the Flemish population. Nevertheless, an active Belgian resistance sabotaged German military sites, operated an underground press, and regularly ferried Allied troops trapped inside occupied Belgium to Holland. Amid deteriorating economic conditions and the struggle for power in occupied Brussels, one service continued to operate with relative immunity under the auspices of the Red Cross—*L'École Belge d'Infirmières Diplômées*, the Berkendael Medical Institute.

One afternoon in November 1914, two wounded British soldiers in disguise arrived at the institute, located on rue de la Culture, seeking assistance. The nursing sister who had run the school of nursing since 1907 welcomed the men as patients. Matron Edith Louisa Cavell operated the facility on the principle that all wounded soldiers—friend or foe—had to be treated alike. Indeed, despite her British origins, Cavell directed emergency services at the institute and at relief stations elsewhere to tend German casualties, an order that almost overwhelmed the nursing staff; that summer and fall the nurses slept fully clothed on their beds, ready to attend to the flood of wounded. But by accepting the two disguised British troops, Matron Cavell knew that the city's German administrators might consider her humanitarian efforts as "aiding and abetting the enemy."

Cavell was no innocent. Born in 1865 at Swardeston, in Norfolk, as a vicar's daughter, Edith attended a school for girls and for a short time served as governess for a family in Brussels in the 1890s. She received her nurse's training at the London Hospital, where her "self-sufficient manner" was not encouraged or appreciated.[8] Rescued from what might have become a lifetime of short-term nursing positions in Britain, in 1907 she was approached by a Belgian doctor to supervise a school for nursing in Brussels. Her hospital grew to become a thriving facility with more than two dozen fully trained nurses. As matron of the hospital, Cavell, at age forty-two, had overnight become a senior figure in Belgian nursing circles.[9] Not only did she have full authority over nursing instruction at the school in Brussels, but she had also befriended Antoine Depage, founder and chair of the Belgian Red Cross.

When the Great War began, Cavell was looking after her mother at home in England, but she quickly returned to her duties, preparing the nursing school for the realities of tending the onslaught of war-wounded in occupied Belgium. By 1915 her associate Depage, also the personal physician of King Albert, was in exile, and his wife, Marie Depage, had travelled to America seeking funds for the Belgian Red Cross. Returning to Europe in May 1915 aboard *Lusitania*, Marie Depage drowned in the German torpedoing of the ship. Meanwhile, Cavell's work continued in Brussels, attending to both German

wounded and what the French called "*les enfants perdus*"—
Allied soldiers who'd become isolated in German-occupied
territory.

Matron Cavell did not stop there. For the first two British
soldiers in disguise and others who would follow, she sought
out safe houses and an underground network to secretly lead
the men to neutral Holland. Before long she had concealed
about twenty British soldiers in an attic, provided them with
false papers manufactured by Prince Reginald de Croy at his
chateau near Mons, and arranged for the disguised men to
receive money and guided passage to the Dutch frontier. The
underground railroad brought together Belgian aristocracy,
church leaders, and even the British Secret Service.[10] Cavell
kept as tight a rein on her "casualties" as possible, warning
them not to travel in groups, to abide by nighttime curfews,
and to be mindful that German officers were billeted close by.

However, one night a group of Allied troops awaiting transit to Holland got drunk, began fighting, and were overheard
singing "It's a Long Way to Tipperary."[11] When a postcard
later arrived from two British soldiers thanking Cavell for their
safe return to England, the German authorities closed in. They
arrested Cavell on August 3, 1915, charged her with harbouring Allied soldiers, and held her in St. Gilles prison to await
trial for treason, even though she was not a German national.

During ten weeks of imprisonment, Cavell presented three
depositions to German authorities. She admitted that she had
conveyed as many as sixty British and fifteen French soldiers,
in addition to about a hundred Belgian civilians of military age,
to the Dutch frontier.* She admitted to housing many of them

---

* In her 2010 book *Edith Cavell: Nurse, Martyr, Heroine*, author Diana Souhami
indicated that the number of Allied soldiers Cavell assisted was more like 1,500.

at her hospital and to receipt of correspondence thanking her for their safe passage. The German penal code made "conducting soldiers of the enemy" a crime, but not necessarily a capital offence. Further, by using her medical immunity under the Geneva Convention as a protection to harbour and transport a belligerent, the German tribunal claimed, she had fallen outside any protection the convention might have afforded her. The tribunal found her guilty and sentenced her to execution.

In her final two weeks in custody, her German jailers kept her in solitary confinement. Announcement of the verdict sparked a diplomatic response from Brand Whitlock, the US minister to Belgium, and the Spanish minister, the Marqués de Villalobar, requested that the death penalty be commuted. The British Foreign Office claimed it was "powerless" to intervene. But Hugh S. Gibson, the secretary of state for the United States, which was not then involved in the war, spoke out. "We remind [the German civil governor] of the burning of Louvain and the sinking of the *Lusitania*," Gibson wrote, and "that this murder would rank with those two affairs and would stir all civilized countries with horror and disgust."[12]

"[We] would rather see Miss Cavell shot," German Lt. Col. Count Franz von Harrach responded, "than have harm come to . . . the humblest German soldiers, and [our] only regret was that [we] had not three of four English old women to shoot."[13]

Of thirty-five prisoners accused of related crimes, only Cavell and Belgian patriot Philippe Baucq were condemned to death. Matron Edith Cavell's final hours illustrated her resolve and foretold her stature in history and mythology. Beyond answering the questions put to her in the tribunal—offering no more than 130 words in her own defence—she made no further attempt to refute the German claims. The night before her execution, Reverend Stirling Gahan, an Anglican chaplain, was allowed to pray with her. Apparently without being prompted, the guard at her cell commented to the chaplain that Cavell was a fine woman, illustrating by stiffening his back. Gahan made notes of his final conversation with Cavell. "Patriotism is not enough," she told him. "I must have no hatred nor bitterness to anyone."

The chaplain spoke quietly with her for an hour, during which she acknowledged that she had seen so much death during her time as a nurse that the idea didn't frighten her. Finally, knowing that the execution was scheduled for dawn, Reverend Gahan suggested he had better leave. "You will want to rest," he said. "Yes," she said. "I have to be up at five."[14]

On October 12, 1915, sixteen riflemen in two firing squads carried out the sentence—eight shooting and killing Cavell, the other eight, Baucq. Immediately following the gunfire, Belgian women took away and quickly buried the remains next to St. Gilles prison. Cavell's body was exhumed at the end of the war and returned to England, and on May 19, 1919, in a Westminster Abbey filled to capacity, King George V led a memorial service. A special train transported Cavell's body to Norwich Cathedral; the shaft of the wooden cross erected over her Belgian grave was later delivered for display at Swardeston Church, where her father, Frederick Cavell, had served as rector for forty-five years. It would become a mecca for those paying their respects to the fallen nurse. But long before the church displayed the wooden cross, the Edith Cavell story had transformed her from British patriot to international martyr.

Indeed, even before the Great War was over, the Edith Cavell mythology grew daily. Journalists, poets, cartoonists, painters, musicians, and moviemakers all helped—in either fact or fiction—with the creation and enhancement of the Edith Cavell myth. The *American Journal of Nursing* printed the hearsay that Cavell had fainted and fallen because she'd refused to wear a blindfold at the execution, and that a German officer then shot her dead with his pistol. This account of a woman, a nurse, a patriot facing a heroic death undoubtedly ramped up American support for war against Germany. By April 6, 1917, both the House and the Senate had passed President Woodrow Wilson's declaration of war.

While they had seemed oddly resigned to the German death sentence, following Cavell's execution, British officials turned to Wellington House, the British War Propaganda Bureau, to characterize the nurse matron as an innocent victim of a ruthless enemy. Nurses from the home front to the Western Front looked to the Edith Cavell execution for motivation and inspiration. Agnes Warner was typical. As the matron of Ambulance Mobile No. 1 attending to the wounded of the French army, she regularly warned her nursing-sister staff to be ready for difficulties such as dealing with gas masks and pounding air raids. And she drew the sisters' attention to posters showing the torpedo sinking of the hospital ship *Llandovery Castle*, which had drowned fourteen nurses in 1918, and the execution of Edith Cavell as a denunciation of "German barbarism."[15]

War bond posters appeared with Cavell in her nursing uniform shown prominently. Postcards circulated widely showing renderings of the firing squad and/or the German officer shooting a defiant nurse, with captions reading "the assassination of Edith Cavell" or "Miss Edith Cavell cowardly murdered." Overnight, Edith Cavell became the most celebrated British casualty of the war. Recruitment campaigns across Britain adopted the catch phrase "Remember Edith Cavell," and enlistment doubled from 5,000 to 10,000 for eight consecutive weeks.[16]

Elsewhere, the Edith Cavell martyrdom story emerged in every conceivable form. The senior doctor representing the Brussels administration, Gottfried Benn, who had witnessed the execution, later published *Wie Miss Cavell erschossen wurde* or *How Miss Cavell Was Shot*, to acclaim. Within three months of Cavell's death, motion picture producers had already capitalized on the drama of her life story; *The Martyrdom of Nurse Cavell* was released in January 1916 by Australian silent film directors Jack Gavin and Charles Post Mason. And on October 27, 1918, less than two weeks before the Great War ended, American movie producer John G. Adolfi cast Julia Arthur in another silent picture, *The Woman the Germans Shot*. Not to be outdone, playwrights C.S. Forester and C.E. Bechhofer Roberts wrote a three-act play called *Nurse Cavell*, produced on stage in 1933. British movie director Herbert Wilcox shot two versions of the story—a black-and-white silent with Sybil Thorndike in 1928, and a black-and-white feature film, *Nurse Edith Cavell*, in 1939.

In one poignant scene in the movie, actress Anna Neagle as Matron Cavell attends to a British soldier, preparing him to follow a guide and escape to Holland.

"Don't you ever want to go back home? Not be here among all these foreigners?" he asks her.

"There's only one human race, my dear," the matron says.

"What would they do if they found out you'd got me here?" he asks. "I'd be all right if you'd hand me over to them, now that I'm all right again."

"Do you think I've nursed you back to life just to have you shot?"

The movie follows her arrest, trial, and conviction. It ends with her march to execution and Neagle's voice offering her final thoughts to Reverend Gahan: "I have no fear nor shrinking. I have seen death so often it is no longer strange or fearful to me."

The sound of the firing-squad rifles flashes ahead to Westminster Abbey and her memorial service over a crescendo of the hymn "Abide with Me" and a final image of Edith Cavell offering her benediction: "Patriotism is not enough. I must have no hatred nor bitterness to anyone."[17]

In a case of art imitating life, the film was released to American movie houses on September 1, 1939, the very day Hitler's armies invaded Poland.

SEPTEMBER 1951—YELLOW SEA, OFF THE COAST OF NORTH KOREA

WHEN AUDIENCES ATTENDED either the play *Nurse Cavell* in 1933 or the movie *Nurse Edith Cavell* in 1939, they readily understood that behind the acting and Hollywood embellishment was the story of an actual nursing sister martyred in the Great War. In 1960, however, when Universal Pictures released *The Great Imposter*, the line between fact and fiction was blurred at best. The story of a navy doctor in the Korean War being found out seemed awfully far-fetched to be real. But it, too, was based on a true story.

During its second tour in late September 1951, the Canadian naval destroyer HMCS *Cayuga* supported units of the South Korean marines who were conducting raids along the west coast of North Korea from the Yellow Sea. One such raid left about a dozen South Korean troops wounded, including one with a bullet lodged in his lung.

On the after-canopy deck aboard *Cayuga*, Royal Canadian Navy (RCN) surgeon Lt. Joseph C. Cyr did a quick triage of the South Korean wounded and requested an operating area be readied for the soldier with the punctured lung. Capt. James Plomer offered his cabin. According to the ship's supply officer, Bill Davis, Dr. Cyr—with a gunnery officer acting as his assistant and an ordnance officer as his anesthetist—"opened up the [Korean] marine's chest, took out a bullet, held it up, and said it had been a quarter of an inch away from his heart. He sewed the man up and proceeded to deal with all the other wounded on deck."[18]

Later, Lt. Davis joked about his ordinary shipmates Fred Little and Frank Boyle being asked to serve as surgical assistant and anesthetist, respectively, during Cyr's expertly conducted bullet extraction. "It felt like just another event on board ship," Davis said. "Anyway, our public relations officer wrote up a piece for publication about Joe Cyr, that he had taken a bullet from next to this guy's heart, that he had attended all the wounded, and on another occasion had even removed the captain's abscessed tooth."[19]

When the real Dr. Joseph C. Cyr informed the Royal Canadian Mounted Police of the coincidence, the extraordinary tale of Ferdinand Waldo Demara Jr. came to light. And his life's story as a repeat impersonator did indeed read like a Hollywood script.

Born in Lawrence, Massachusetts, in 1921, Fred grew up with plenty of exposure to fantasy; his father, Fred Sr., ran a chain of private movie theatres in the region, but he lost everything in the Depression. At sixteen young Fred ran away from home and joined a Trappist monastery in Rhode Island. With only a high-school education, he served as a teacher and guardian at a home for boys, but then, on impulse, in 1941 stole the home's car and dashed off to join the US Army. Not enamoured of basic training in Biloxi, Mississippi, he took on his first false identity, choosing to go AWOL as Anthony Ingolia.

His family back in Lawrence eventually convinced Demara to stop masquerading and turn himself in. But, at the last minute, he changed his mind and joined the US Navy under his own name. He chose to be trained as a medic, but when his grades fell short, Demara stole the identity of a doctor to support his application for a commission. Despite service on the North Atlantic aboard USS *Ellis*, his qualifications for advancement in military medicine fell short. That's when he decided to fake his death, leaving a pile of clothes and a suicide note at the end of a pier and disappearing into the night.[20]

Becoming Dr. Robert Linton French next, Demara offered bogus services as a former naval officer with credentials as a psychologist, a science teacher, and eventually a doctor of medicine at a Benedictine abbey college near Seattle, Washington. But eventually those false qualifications were challenged in court and led to a charge of desertion from the navy and a jail sentence.

Following eighteen months in prison, Demara resurfaced in Canada, at Grand Falls, New Brunswick, where he met and assisted Dr. Joseph Cyr, a physician with aspirations to work in the United States. Demara borrowed Dr. Cyr's credentials and attempted to use them to convince another college of his medical and administrative skills. When he was turned down, he stole another vehicle, drove to a Royal Canadian Navy recruiting centre in Saint John, New Brunswick, and—with those borrowed certificates—enlisted for service as Dr. Joseph C. Cyr.

"The only [real] medical background I had was that which I had obtained as a hospital corpsman in the United States Navy," Demara explained later. And yet he managed to convince medical personnel at the RCN headquarters that he could lecture and lead seminars on internal medicine. He sensed that his delivery was credible enough, since the doctors in the sessions "were avid note-takers."

In 1951 Canada's tribal-class destroyers began rotation through tours of duty in the Korean War. On board HMCS *Cayuga*, the personable and readily convincing Dr. Cyr got on well with the captain and appeared perfectly at ease performing routine procedures in the ship's sick bay, as well as emergency surgery such as removing the bullet from the Korean soldier's internal organs.

On October 24, 1951, a month after the famous lung surgery, *Cayuga* received a message informing the captain he had an impostor aboard. When Capt. Plomer confronted his ship's now celebrated doctor with the information, Demara produced Joseph Cyr's notarized birth certificate and his physician's sheepskin and then retreated to his cabin. Unmasked and accused of impersonating the Canadian physician, Fred Demara took an overdose of barbiturates and slashed his wrists. He was given first aid at sea, transferred ashore, shipped home to Canada, and discharged from the navy.

The real Dr. Cyr did not press charges because Demara hadn't harmed any of his so-called patients. One of his former *Cayuga* shipmates, Gil Hutton, claimed that a number of Canadian Navy officers offered Demara funds to pay for a real medical education. Ultimately, Fred Demara was deported to the United States, where he became a hospital chaplain and where, in 1960, Hollywood released its version of his story, with Tony Curtis in the role of *The Great Imposter*.

FEBRUARY 1952—SEOUL, SOUTH KOREA

IT'S THE MIDDLE OF THE KOREAN WAR. The fictional 4077th Mobile Army Surgical Hospital, made famous by the 1970s and '80s hit television series *M*A*S*H*, faces an unexpected, unknown enemy. Col. Sherman T. Potter (Harry Morgan) has called a meeting of his senior staff—Frank Burns (Larry Linville), Margaret Houlihan (Loretta Swit), B.J. Hunnicutt (Mike Farrell), and Hawkeye Pierce (Alan Alda)—to compare notes about an inexplicable fever that's infecting both patients and staff in the camp. Potter acknowledges that everybody has worked tirelessly around the clock attending to those with the rapidly spreading fever, but that the trend will continue until they learn the source of the sickness and its cure.

"Any news from the lab in Seoul?" somebody asks.

"Father Mulcahy's down there now on R and R," Potter reports.

"Rest and resurrection?" Hawkeye wisecracks. But the real problem the MASH staff faces is attempting to deal with a disease that for them has no name, doesn't respond to antibiotics, and is spreading like wildfire. Potter offers what little information he's gathered, that the fever might be caused by rat-borne mites and fleas. He asks if anybody has noticed more rats around the camp.

"Just the couple that's been building a family room in my shaving kit," one of his staff quips.

A few scenes later, in this twelfth episode of season four of the TV sitcom M*A*S*H, Father Francis John Patrick Mulcahy (William Christopher) returns with the lab analysis from Seoul. He reports a history he's uncovered that both Japanese and Russian soldiers suffered from much the same symptoms during the Sino-Soviet war in northern Manchuria in the 1930s. "[Its] name is hemorrhagic fever," Mulcahy says. "The doctors then were just as perplexed as you are now."

"Great," a MASH staffer says. "We know what to call it, only we don't know how to cure it."

"There isn't a cure," the padre says. "The only treatment is common-sense medicine."

The TV MASH, as its creator Larry Gelbart appropriately commented, was better remembered than the costly war that inspired it. In his memoir *Laughing Matters*, Gelbart wrote that his adaptation of Richard Hornberger's original book was principally a sitcom, obviously going for the laughs. But it was equally ready to sacrifice laughter for a greater message, or, as he put it, "to give the audience either a laugh or a lump in the throat." He also referred to the show's realism as life imitating art. And for at least one of its viewers, truer words could not have been uttered.

Don Flieger, a service corps corporal in the Canadian Army during the real Korean War, recalled the round-the-clock life of what was called "moving control" at Kimpo Airfield, near Seoul. In 1951, as the war moved toward a stalemate at the thirty-eighth parallel to the north, Flieger and his supply and service crew of twenty men scrambled onto the tarmac dozens of times each day to service the flying transports, mostly from the Royal Australian Air Force. The Dakota aircraft would barely have rolled to a stop when Flieger's crew converged to off-load its food, medical supplies, weapons, ammunition, beer, and cigarettes destined to head north toward the front lines. Then, if required, the moving-control crew would load casualties heading for hospitals in Japan or, occasionally, when loading for US destinations, coffins of war-dead bound for home.

"Seeing all these coffins going back was a pretty graphic way to remind you of the life and death of the war," Flieger said. "But I was never close to the battle. You could just hear it in the distance."[21]

In what some called a bombproof job, Flieger continued the repetitive routine of off-loading and loading, day and night, for the better part of eight months. During rare moments of down time, Flieger and his comrades amused themselves with an odd form of target practice. Armed with flashlights and 9 mm pistols, the men sat at the edge of Kimpo Airfield in the dark tracking down and shooting rats, some as large as house cats, Flieger remembered. Rat hunting was both a distraction and a way to contain an exploding rat population around the supplies, which were sometimes stored on the airfield. But one February morning he awoke in his tent to discover redness on his ankles and wrists, the only skin on his body exposed at night.

"It started out as a rash and then the rash turned into blisters," Flieger said. "Some were pinhead size, some the size of a fingernail. . . . Then the blisters broke and started to bleed. . . . I didn't know whether I had leprosy or what. I was just terrified."

Uninformed and unable to diagnose his ailment, but wise enough to seek help, Kimpo Airfield staff raced Cpl. Flieger to the 8055th MASH in Seoul. By that time he had a body temperature of 104 degrees. The MASH doctors were not familiar with hemorrhagic fever, and tried penicillin. After several days, when Flieger's condition hadn't changed, they shipped him to the military hospital in Kure, Japan, where an American doctor recognized the symptoms and reacted with the only antidote he knew. "He told me that all the tests indicated I had hemorrhagic fever," Flieger said, "and the only possible cure [was] massive blood transfusions."

What the American doctor didn't tell his patient was that the mortality rate was as high as 80 percent. Hospital medical staff transfused Flieger right away. He remembered that the procedure required seven or eight bags of blood, all introduced into his system in less than three hours. Four days later they flew him to the island of Midway and from there to Hawaii, where they transfused his system yet again, and again at a military base in San Francisco; he received another transfusion in Tacoma, Washington, and another in Chicago.

"It took me a month to get home to Saint John, New Brunswick," he said. "I had eight complete transfusions. I was one of the few survivors."

Had the MASH staff in Korea, the American doctor in Japan, and the military medical staffs in North America not responded with as much "common-sense medicine" as fictional character Father John Mulcahy recommended in that episode of *M*A*S*H*, real-life patient Don Flieger might never have made it home alive—nor, as it turned out, back to Korea for a second tour of duty when he regained his health.

CHAPTER NINE

"ABOVE AND BEYOND"

A TTEMPTING TO PLACE EVENTS in time at the Barris household when I was growing up usually came down to a couple of descriptives. "Before the war . . ." meant when my folks lived in New York City, when their parents and they as youngsters coped with the Depression in the 1930s, or as a generally understood synonym for when times were tough. Similarly, my mother and father often used "after the war . . ." to distinguish the point in their lives when peace returned, when they got married in the late 1940s, or when they eventually found the means to begin careers, have a family, buy a bungalow, and get on with their lives. While the war in Europe technically ended with the official capitulation of the German armies on May 8, 1945, my father often admitted that he could never really remember VE-Day. He was certainly there. He and his medical unit had taken over a bombed-out apartment building a couple of blocks from the River Rhine in Düsseldorf. There was no furniture in their quarters, just a bare floor on which they set their sleeping bags, half a dozen men to a room.

More memorable for this war-weary medic were the events of April 13, 1945. The day began, he recalled, when a member of his medical battalion entered the apartment room, where they were just waking up. "The president is dead," he said reverently, and then moved on to another room to spread the news. My father remembered the stunned silence that followed. "I remember we spoke in soft voices of Roosevelt's death, almost as though he were laid out in the next room," he wrote. "It felt as if we had lost someone close to us, almost a member of our immediate family."[1]

My father had idolized the man since he was a boy in the 1930s. He had just turned ten in 1932 when Franklin D. Roosevelt was first elected. In 1940, when he ran for his unprecedented third term, Dad had been too young to vote. But in 1944, when FDR ran for the fourth time, Alex, like all overseas American troops, received a ballot, and he voted for the president's re-election. With word of FDR's death, my father recalled, even those men in his company who had expressed disapproval of Roosevelt's policies were sensitive enough to the gloom of the day to avoid any provocative outbursts of joy at his death. Much of the preoccupation of that day and those that followed was wondering what FDR's death meantin terms of the war, in terms of their future. "Nobody among us knew much about this Harry Truman, the recently elected vice-president, who was now in command of everything, including us," my father wrote.[2]

For my father, life "after the war" began in Düsseldorf in

that empty apartment block remembering his beloved president. Then, as the city got used to US occupation troops running things, the installed provisional authorities began registering the non-military population, revitalizing civilian administration, restoring railway operations inside the city, reopening banks, and attempting to distribute food and medical supplies to those in greatest need, those in the formerly industrialized but still densely populated downtown. The 94th Division arranged for truck convoys to retrieve hundreds of tons of onions, potatoes, sugar beets, and rhubarb.

My father found it particularly difficult to watch children scrounging for food, many just outside their army kitchen, rummaging through garbage cans and picking out scraps they could take home. He noted that a few of the less timid and more enterprising German children tagged along as a soldier made his way to the garbage cans. The child would offer to wash the GI's mess gear, and if successful in his quest would find a bit of food left for him near the cans. In turn, some of the medics might pile on a bit more food than they could eat in order to leave decent portions for the children. The ritual allowed rules to be observed on both sides—nobody was begging, just receiving recompense for work completed.

My father recalled a skinny teenager the medics named Charley, who had a constant craving for cigarettes. When he cleaned my father's mess kit, he would ask for a cigarette in return rather than food. Alex generally obliged. Then, for some reason, the ration of cigarettes for the US occupation troops failed to arrive, and he had to refuse Charley's request.

"You have none?" he said with surprise.

"No, Charley. I really haven't."

"Here," he said, and took out a rusty metal cigarette case. "Have from mine."[3] He had half a dozen in the case.

US Army generals realized the GIs needed more than just a regular supply of Camel cigarettes to occupy idle hands. In Düsseldorf they liberated breweries and took over the Park Hotel to operate as an officers' mess; the sign outside read "The First American Red Cross Club East of the Rhine, courtesy of the 94th Infantry Division." Meanwhile, they arranged for 120 English-speaking women from Venlo, Holland, to be guests at dinner-dances at the Rheinterrasse for the men of the 302nd Infantry. By June the 94th had staged softball, swimming, and track and field competitions, the latter at Adolf Hitler Sportplatz, home of the athletic trial competitions for the Fuhrer's 1936 Olympics. They even reactivated a horse-racing facility just outside Düsseldorf, dubbed it "Truman Park," and on June 6, 1945, staged a full card of racing that featured the sixty thoroughbreds housed at the track, while a GI band played "My Old Kentucky Home."[4]

Meantime, my father had acquired his most precious wartime souvenir. The day before T/Sgt. Barris's 319th Medical Battalion packed up and left Düsseldorf, the teenager the medics had befriended while hanging around the garbage cans behind their living quarters suddenly appeared. This time Charley had something other than cigarettes to hock—a working portable typewriter that another potential American buyer had declined because it was a German machine and the keyboard was "different." Alex paid Charley exactly what the boy was asking—a full carton of American cigarettes—and in that moment Dad acquired a significant tool in what would become his first meaningful career "after the war." He was soon typing stories as a reporter for the 94th Division's weekly newspaper, *The Attack*.

JULY 4, 1945—VODŇANY, CZECHOSLOVAKIA

IT WAS JUST ABOUT THE LEAST LIKELY PLACE to stage a national American holiday. Nevertheless, on US Independence Day, hundreds of American troops marched through the downtown streets of Pilsen, near the western frontier of Sudetenland, in a victory parade. It was no coincidence that the celebration took place in that part of Czechoslovakia, the first land conceded by European allies in 1938 to placate Adolf Hitler. Most of the Czech civilians who lined the streets eight and ten deep along the parade route had waited nearly six years for this moment. In place of Nazi swastika flags overhead, they watched the national flags of Czechoslovakia, the United States, and the Soviet Union unfurled amid great pomp and ceremony. They listened to brass bands playing US military marches, and they applauded the passing columns of GIs as their conquering heroes.

T/Sgt. Barris did his bit to contribute to the festivities that July 4th. From his earliest days in the US Army my father had demonstrated his love of popular music and, in particular, of performing it. In the winter of 1943, while in training at Camp Phillips, Kansas, he had organized a vocal quartet from among his medic comrades; Jim McConnel, from New York City, sang bass; E.D. Eutzer, from South Bend, Indiana, and Walter Weeks, from Peru, Indiana, provided the tenor harmonies; and my father filled in all the baritone parts. They'd entertained during basic training and aboard the *Queen Elizabeth* Atlantic crossing in 1944, and while it wasn't quite part of his job as a medic, my father hoped he could reunite the group to perform for troops and civilians in newly liberated western Czechoslovakia.

"McConnel had been wounded—so much for the Geneva Convention's rules protecting medics," he wrote. "So, we got a replacement for the quartet and worked up a version of Cole Porter's 'Don't Fence Me In,' with original lyrics."[5]

The song choice was highly appropriate. The Czechs loved every aspect of their restored freedom. And when the 94th Infantry Division and its medical support unit arrived at a quickly designated command post in the city of Vodňany, "it felt like an explosion."[6] As American Jeeps and trucks motored into the downtown, radio stations that had been shut down by the Nazis for four years began blaring the Czech national anthem through speakers into the streets. The main square filled with people screaming deliriously. They showered the Americans with flowers and mobbed the soldiers in their vehicles while the children looked for treats in return. Everybody just wanted to touch the GIs, shake their hands, embrace them.

One teenager, Jaroslava Svatkova, had gone to great lengths for the celebration. "We waited so long for this," she said. "I had nothing fancy to wear. My mom made me a red skirt right out of a German flag. I wore it with a white blouse and felt so pretty."[7]

A young Czech boy, Vladimir Krizek, couldn't believe his eyes. He watched his parents carrying platters of drinks and traditional Czech pastries to the Americans as they arrived. He and the other boys surrounded the Sherman tanks, trucks, and Jeeps and looked for handouts. And the GIs obliged with plenty of chocolate and treats that Vladimir had never seen before. "For the first time we saw chewing gum," he said. "They gave us some, but we had no idea what to do with it. Almost every American soldier was chewing. . . . It took a bit for us to figure out how to chew it."[8]

The Krizek family—two adults and three sons—had run a lumber mill before the war. In Vodňany they owned a modest home. When members of the 94th Infantry Division and the 319th Medical Battalion arrived in the town, the Krizeks offered to billet two Americans, including T/Sgt. Alex Barris. Initially communication posed a bit of a problem, but eventually the Americans acquired an English-German dictionary to explain themselves, while the Krizeks referred to their German-Czech dictionary to speak the proper responses. As the two American billets settled in, their US Army superiors marvelled at how effectively Czech civil and military groups had purged their country of Nazi officials, authorities, and sympathizers. Army diarists reported that the liberated Czechs wrought vengeance upon the enemy so thoroughly and rapidly that they were essentially doing the work of military intelligence in the zone. The division diarists went so far as to describe the Czech civilian population as "one vast counter-intelligence agency, imbued with an intense hatred for things German."[9]

Vladimir Krizek, the family's eldest son, had served in the Czech underground and offered the American billets insight into life under Nazi fascism. When Hitler's troops entered Sudetenland, Vladimir said, everything changed. Singing the Czech anthem was forbidden. German bosses assumed leadership and control of Czech auto and steel factories. All men over the age of sixteen were scooped up as forced labour. Czech currency lost its value. In September 1941, when Reinhard Heydrich became governor of the Protectorate of Bohemia, all Jewish property was confiscated and Jewish families transported to concentration camps. The German regime seized all privately owned radio receivers, replaced Czech signs with German ones, and made German the official language in school and on the street. In one odd statement of control, the Germans removed all the historic bells in Vodňany and melted them down; however, in a daring move, Mayor Thomas Holat managed to hide one town bell—nicknamed "Mark"—before the Germans could seize it.*

In the spring of 1945, Vladimir Krizek could sense that the Germans were on the run. He witnessed many German civilians who'd occupied Sudetenland during the war fleeing west. Whether on foot, in horse-drawn carts, or in motor cars, they carried away as many belongings as they could. Emboldened Czechs spat on them or beat them up with sticks (or whatever was handy) as they streamed away. But towns such as Vodňany had a greater problem on their hands than simply squaring accounts with the Nazis. Their community infrastructure had disintegrated: no food distribution, no functioning schools, and, worst of all, few means for delivering medical care and no medical supplies to treat the sick and wounded. That's why the Krizek family welcomed the medics of the 319th so readily.

Medical officers with the 94th and medical corpsmen,

---

* "Mark" would remain hidden for the duration of the German occupation but was reinstalled at Vodňany city hall in time to ring in the liberation of Czechoslovakia on May 8, 1945.

including my father, spent the summer transforming a former school into a general hospital, treating first the local population and eventually survivors of nearby concentration camps. They installed 115 sickbeds in the school and then 100 beds in a second building; eventually they began treating the civilian population for tuberculosis, lice, and malnutrition. For some of the American medics, this vital service was beyond their experience; organizing hospital schedules, getting nearby restaurants to cook food for five sittings a day, and treating communicable disease among civilians were a long way from the daily routine orders of front-line warfare. Mind you, if nobody was shooting at them and if they could sleep in a bed with clean sheets, US medics welcomed the trade-off.

Meanwhile, for civilian Vladimir Krizek, having an American medic living with his family brought unexpected benefits. T/Sgt. Barris invited him along to watch the Americans play baseball and volleyball in the city square. The young Czech also got in to see US Army dances, with local girls in their best dresses and the Americans in their pressed uniforms. T/Sgt. Barris appreciated the Krizeks' hospitality and gave back whenever he could. "The medic gave me a flag and an army sweater, and I never wanted to take it off," Krizek said. "We were all high on the feeling of freedom."[10]

Family meant a lot to the occupying soldiers too. Members of my father's medical unit had not seen their families since leaving the United States. Alex regularly wrote to his mother, his sister, and his older brother Angelo, who was stationed in Heidelberg, Germany, at the end of the war. Formerly part of the US Army 67th Antiaircraft Artillery, during the occupation Angelo became an MP directing traffic, keeping the peace, and making a few dollars tailoring on the side. "There was an empty high school with a sewing machine," Angelo explained, "so I started stitching army patches and stripes onto guys' jackets. I made a fortune at three bucks a stripe."[11]

In July, Angelo managed to get a three-day pass and decided to use it to find his kid brother. He learned from the US mobile records unit that the 94th Infantry Division had been posted to Czechoslovakia. So, at five o'clock in the morning, Angelo started hitchhiking the five hundred miles from Heidelberg to western Czechoslovakia. Miraculously, by eight o'clock that night he'd found his way to the 94th's headquarters in Pilsen and was reunited with Alex the next day. "We laughed and got together with some of the people there and had a great reunion," Angelo said. "And I kidded him about not having the service points I did."

Any GI with eighty-five service points—a point for every month in the army, a point for every month overseas, and five points for every battle star—was automatically entitled to an honourable discharge. Angelo had eighty-six points. Alex had less than was required to get out of the service. "So, he'd have to go back to the States and train and go to Japan," Angelo said. Of course, within a month the US had dropped atomic bombs on two Japanese cities and ended the war in the Pacific.

Meanwhile, the 94th Division—including the 319th Medical Battalion—had spread itself out across a newly consolidated Czechoslovakian Occupation Zone. About 10,800 American troops had taken on the job of reorganizing services and reinstalling Czech authority in about 3,600 square miles of occupied territory, as well as protecting ninety so-called security targets and manning twenty-two roadblocks along

190 miles of the Russian-American Control Line. The high-stakes security work belonged to other members of the 94th.

Meantime, T/Sgt. Barris had approached *The Attack*, the division's daily newspaper, and enrolled in journalism classes to prepare him for future reporting assignments with the paper and, he hoped, a crack at the real thing one day at the *New York Times* when he got home. Not long after he'd begun journalism instruction, in September my father was faced with a three-day hiatus in classes. And suddenly the world beyond the high-security roadblocks beckoned. Just seventy-five miles away sat Prague, a Czech city my father had always yearned to see. So tantalizingly close. The problem was that Prague lay in the Russian-occupied zone and was therefore out of bounds for American troops.

No matter, decided medic Barris and three of his GI pals. The four Americans decided to go AWOL—or, in their words, to do an exploratory expedition by crossing legitimately at a roadblock, dashing across the frontier, and entering the prohibited confines of Soviet-controlled Prague. First they hopped on a wood-burning truck crossing the border, but they were turned back by Russian guards. Next—with two of the four having aborted the mission—my father and one remaining fellow traveller snuck aboard a civilian train bound for Prague. The following morning they managed to skirt more guards and enter the city limits.

"To the best of my knowledge," Barris wrote, "except for a small U.S. government contingent in Prague, we were the first Americans, the [city] had seen since the war. They certainly treated us wonderfully."[12]

Three days and three raucous nights later, the AWOL pair

boarded the return train, using their classroom mock press passes to convince guards they had the authority to be travelling inside the Soviet zone. Back across the Russian-American Control Line, they hitchhiked the last few miles and just managed to get back to the American military installation in Vodňany before roll call. That Monday morning, Barris and company returned to *The Attack* journalism class, just in time for the lecturing junior officer to announce he had exciting news: "We're working on a plan to allow you to visit Prague!" he said.

It would be another few months before the 94th Division completed its occupation service and made its way to the French port of Marseilles and a waiting Liberty troopship bound for New York. Meantime, the purpose of his summer-long mission to Czechoslovakia had become abundantly clear. My father's medical battalion and infantry division comrades weren't in Vodňany so much to help the Czechs as they were there to prevent the Russians from moving any farther west. "The Cold War had unofficially already started," T/Sgt. Barris wrote.

SPRING 1951—SOUTH OF THE THIRTY-EIGHTH PARALLEL, SOUTH KOREA

T/SGT. BARRIS MAY HAVE CONSIDERED the Cold War a kind of international charade of force between former allies, the United States and the Soviet Union, in faraway Sudetenland. It's also possible that when he returned home to New York, my father might have read the topical essays of Eric Arthur Blair (a.k.a. George Orwell), including one from 1945 in which he described the emerging nuclear stalemate as "two monstrous super-states, each possessed of a weapon by which millions of people can be wiped out in a few seconds."[13]

But Frank Cullen, a Canadian medical officer stationed south of the thirty-eighth parallel on the Korean Peninsula several years later, would not have used any of the naive euphemisms of the day—"police action," or "Cold War conflict"—to describe his circumstances. He considered the Korean War a dirty shooting war. "We all carried a Browning pistol," Cullen said. "I think it was the first time medical officers were allowed to carry arms . . . to protect yourself and to protect your patients."[14]

In the spring of 1951, Canadian units of the Canadian Army Special Force, among sixteen member countries of the United Nations supporting the Republic of Korea forces, were on the move north toward the thirty-eighth parallel. On June 25 the previous year, the UN Security Council had told the Democratic People's Republic of Korea (North Korea) it had illegally invaded and occupied the territory of South Korea, and a state of war existed. As a signatory to the UN peace charter, Canada had deployed Royal Canadian Air Force (RCAF) No. 426 Thunderbird Squadron to provide transport back and forth across the Pacific Ocean; three Royal Canadian Navy tribal-class destroyers to join a sea blockade of North Korea; and troops of the Royal Canadian Regiment (RCR), Princess Patricia's Canadian Light Infantry (PPCLI), and the Royal 22nd Regiment (the Van Doos) on the ground in South Korea. Before the early spring of 1951, none of the Canadians had faced North Korean or Communist Chinese forces in combat.

Then, from April 22 to 25, although nearly surrounded in the Kap'yong valley, the PPCLI halted a Communist Chinese army advance on Seoul, South Korea's capital city; their action earned the US Presidential Distinguished Unit Citation but had cost the regiment thirty-one killed, fifty-nine wounded, and three captured. On May 30, 1951, the RCR advanced through positions held by the Van Doos to meet Chinese troops invading from the Chorwon Plain; they clashed at Chail-li, where six Canadians were killed and fifty-four wounded.

Right behind the fighting forces, in what were called rear echelons but were, in fact, very much within the range of enemy artillery and mortar fire, members of two Canadian units worked to provide supplies and medical support. The Mobile Laundry and Bath Unit (MLBU) provided soldiers with an assembly-line arrangement of showers, washtubs, and clothes dryers that allowed a continuous stream of troops to enter the showers at one end and emerge from the other with a clean change of clothes in less than thirty minutes. Right beside them, and taking full advantage of the cleaning services, the Royal Canadian Army Medical Corps set up its casualty clearing stations (the Canadian equivalent of the US mobile army surgical hospitals) to attend to Canadian wounded. Both the MLBU and the RCAMC units always positioned themselves close enough to the line of fire to be of greatest value to their fighting comrades.

On May 28, 1951, as the MLBU set up its cleaning apparatus at a stream near the brigade's centre line, a Chinese Communist army patrol stumbled into the location and, finding itself outnumbered by the MLBU staff, was quickly captured. Apprehending enemy troops was not considered part of the MLBU or medical officers' job descriptions. But all that changed in the first armed defence of the UN peace charter.

In the summer of 1950, Frank Cullen had been interning at Toronto Western Hospital, working eighteen-hour days and making sixty dollars a month. He was already an air force veteran; he'd flown Baltimore aircraft with the RAF's 117 Squadron in the Mediterranean during the Second World War. Despite the rush among infantry to join the Special Force for Korea, the army was short of doctors. Cullen suddenly became a prime candidate for Korea. By the spring of 1951, his superiors in the 3rd Battalion of the Van Doos had posted him as the medical officer in charge of a section of the No. 25 Field Ambulance, attending to Canadian wounded in a regimental aid post amid the dust and heat near the thirty-eighth parallel. Conditions in Korea seemed more like those in North Africa, which he'd experienced in Egypt during the Second World War.

"Nothing was ever really sterile there," Cullen said. "Rats ate your soap, chewed your toothbrush, and the only way to discourage them was not to organize your medical equipment on open tables, the way you're supposed to." Instead, Cullen insisted on keeping surgical tools and dressings in metal panniers to be opened by his staff only when actually administering first aid. Making matters worse was that the battle lines were always in flux. That meant Capt. Cullen was constantly setting up and then breaking camp. "I remember at Chorwon . . . we set up this big bloody tent, got ready for the wounded . . . then nothing happened. Then we're told we're moving again," he said. "I think we set up and moved five times in one day."[15]

Cullen's RAP was the first point of contact behind the front lines—the place stretcher-bearers carried wounded for immediate first aid. Often working at night, Cullen packed shrapnel injuries, introduced intravenous lines, applied tourniquets, or set splints by the light of a Coleman lantern; sometimes he wore a headband with a lamp attached, directing the light at the patient and his wounds. From Cullen's RAP, a litter Jeep carried wounded to the casualty clearing station, where another medical officer could remove dressings, do minor surgery, and stabilize those patients in shock. Beyond the CCS, the wounded went farther back in four-stretcher box ambulances to the bigger advanced dressing station, where they could be tended until stable enough to move by helicopter to a sixty-to-seventy-bed mobile army surgical hospital or flown all the way to a hospital in Japan. Generally Cullen attended to Canadians, but during his second night on duty, stretcher-bearers arrived with five Turkish officers whose Jeep had run over a land mine; Cullen's RAP treated and moved them on. "Prepared for anything" seemed to be the motto of the medical corps.

Like Frank Cullen, Keith Besley left an internship in Toronto, at St. Michael's Hospital, to serve in Korea. Besley also had Second World War experience, flying Spitfires in support of the British 8th Army in North Africa. In 1951, as a medical officer in Korea, Capt. Besley was immediately sent forward to establish the casualty clearing station behind the Van Doos' front lines. Just like Cullen, Besley too had to grapple with the mobility of the war. On one occasion he found a dry riverbed where he and his medical team set up their CCS for the night. They had just settled down to catch some shut-eye in anticipation of the night's work ahead, when a British mortar platoon moved in beside them and began firing at nearby Chinese Army positions. Before long the Communist artillery had zeroed in on the riverbed location and began returning fire. Besley's medical station was forced to make a hasty retreat.

Sometimes, however, encounters with enemy soldiers couldn't be avoided. At six o'clock one morning that spring, Capt. Besley was up doing his daily ablutions. He'd placed a mirror on a tree to shave when he sensed he was being watched. He turned and found himself facing a Chinese soldier armed with a rifle. The man began chattering at him, suddenly dropped his gun, and threw his hands in the air. Interrogators soon arrived to take away "the first prisoner of war captured by the RCAMC!"[16]

Capturing Chinese troops was not among Capt. Besley's responsibilities. But after the morning shaving incident, the medical officer made a habit of carrying his assigned Browning pistol. As the fighting drew the Chinese Communists from the north and UN Command forces from the south closer together across the thirty-eighth parallel, incidents involving medics increased. Before the stalemate in the middle of the peninsula in 1951, Besley routinely found as many as ten armed guards surrounding him whenever he entered an operating room at his casualty clearing station to work on a patient. The guards became more commonplace, even travelling with ambulances behind the lines.

"The Chinese began attacking our box ambulances," Besley said. "They would stop them on the way down the road. In one instance, one stopped the ambulance and killed the driver. But the guards nearby immediately killed him.

"Yes, the idea of medical officers carrying pistols was foreign to us. And I shot fifty rounds a day and became a very,

very accurate pistol man," Besley concluded. "In order to protect myself."[17]

JANUARY 1968—CAM RANH BAY, SOUTH VIETNAM

IN THE SPRING OF 2016, Norm Malayney made a visit to a reunion he chooses to attend regularly—it's staged every two years—bringing together men with whom he served in Vietnam. Most of the vets served in the US Army, a few in the US Navy or Marines, and, like Malayney, some in the US Air Force. At the 2016 gathering, one of Malayney's fellow Air Force vets, Cal Schuler—who was well past retirement age but still practised emergency ward medicine—addressed the reunion of the Canadian Vietnam Veterans Association. He reflected on some of his own experiences from his service as a medical officer overseas, and acknowledged some of the others who'd served with him in the 483rd US Air Force Hospital at the Cam Ranh Bay Air Base in the Republic of Vietnam. At one point in his talk, he paused to offer an observation that perhaps startled some of his fellow vets. "Norm Malayney had the worst job in the Air Force," Schuler said. "I knew that unit. I had guys I served with there. They didn't want to come back the next day. They wanted a transfer out of there . . ."[18]

The former medical corpsman at Cam Ranh Bay Air Base wouldn't disagree with Schuler's assessment. When Norman Malayney arrived there in April 1967—carrying his Air Force–issue summer and winter uniforms, combat boots (as well as oxford shoes), hospital duty uniform, raincoat, toiletries, towels, washcloths, and other baggage (not exceeding sixty pounds)—the United States had officially been at war in Vietnam for three years, since the Gulf of Tonkin Resolution.* America had by that time committed nearly half a million troops to the conflict, and in 1967 alone it had sustained more than 11,000 men killed in action. But Airman 3rd Class Malayney had no airborne duties flying fighter jets, or ground duties maintaining aircraft engines or air frames. Malayney reflected on his year-long tour of duty at Cam Ranh Bay as a hospital medic—working twelve hours on and twelve hours off—as gruelling, exhausting, eye-opening, in many ways rewarding, and, as he put it, "one of the two greatest experiences of my life."

Malayney served in 483rd USAF Hospital, the second-largest military facility in South Vietnam, with 485 beds for general surgery, chest surgery, neurosurgery, orthopedics, urology, ophthalmology, and dental surgery and a 200-bed-capacity casualty staging unit (CSU). Each month, Cam Ranh Bay Air Base handled approximately 8,000 aircraft takeoffs and landings, 40,000 tons of cargo, and no fewer than 130,000 passengers.[19] Cam Ranh Bay served as one of three aerial delivery and mobility bases—the other two were at Saigon and Da Nang—supporting the US war effort in Vietnam. Located 175 miles northeast of Saigon, the South Vietnamese capital, Cam Ranh Bay was home to the 12th Tactical Fighter Wing of the USAF and was about as

---

* Passed by US Congress on August 7, 1964, the Gulf of Tonkin Resolution allowed President Lyndon Johnson to take any measures he believed necessary to retaliate against an aggressor and to promote the maintenance of international peace and security in Southeast Asia.

close to the action as a non-combat medic could wish to be. It was Malayney's wartime address for a year.

Twice during Malayney's tour at Cam Ranh Bay, US Air Force jets crashed on takeoff. The first explosion of a Phantom killed the pilot and left the second airman aboard with burns to 80 percent of his body. The second accident occurred when the jet fighter failed to clear a barrier and tore the aircraft's fuel tank and two missiles away from the fuselage; the resulting fire killed the two aircrew and then cooked and launched one of the plane's missiles, which penetrated the jet's fuselage and struck one of the air base rescuers, a fireman, severing his arm.

Following such crashes, a siren blared a steady three-minute blast, for "Condition Yellow," calling all personnel—surgeons, nurses, medics, and orderlies—to report to their emergency duty stations. In the missile-exploding incident, within minutes a flight surgeon on the base had raced to the scene and attended to the injured fireman, applying a tourniquet to what remained of the man's arm, while medics from Malayney's CSU loaded him into a field ambulance bound for the base hospital for emergency surgery and further treatment. But even under regular circumstances, Malayney and his fellow corpsmen had their hands full.

"Every day, first thing, a [Lockheed Starlifter] C-141 arrived," Malayney said. Any patients requiring more than thirty days' attention were carried aboard the transport jet, which was equipped with four tiers of stretchers. "Our job was to load the wounded between 6:30 and 7 a.m.,"[20] when the C-141 took off for military hospitals in Japan. But that was just the start of an Air Force CSU medic's day.

Once medics had cleared the ward of outbound patients, they then had to treat the 120 beds in the ward. First they stripped the beds of their linen and blankets to be washed for reuse. Mattresses were cleaned and turned, the bed frames—from springs to bed rails—were washed down, and the floors were scrubbed with a special iodine cleanser. With the cleaning complete, the medics placed fresh sheets of paper on top of the mattresses, the full length of each bed.

Around noon or 12:30, when the corpsmen had finished disinfecting the ward, the first of the day's new wounded began arriving aboard transport aircraft. Doctors converged on stretchers coming off the transport and conducted triage, while medical corpsmen like Malayney took patients' vital signs, recorded findings on placards, and then added ranks and serial numbers before attaching the placards to wardroom beds. Their patients were US Army or Marine Corps troops, but it was sometimes difficult to tell; many of the wounded arrived with red (high-iron-content) soil caked all over their battledress and wounds. During the washing phase of treatment, the medics often covered a soldier's open wounds to prevent infection. But Malayney recalled one doctor triaging a soldier whose leg wound was covered in the ferrous soil. "Put him in the shower," the doctor told Malayney. "It couldn't get more contaminated than it is right now."

Managing under the circumstances came naturally to Norman Malayney, via his bloodlines. Both sides of his family traced their peasant roots to Bukovina, Ukraine, in the Carpathian Mountains, during the nineteenth century. When they immigrated to western Canada in 1902, they gave farming a try on rock-strewn prairie land in southern Manitoba that was more suited to raising sheep than growing grain; by the 1930s they had abandoned farming and moved to Winnipeg for better work opportunities and to ensure that their children got educations.

Norman's father managed to find high-paying work after the Second World War building military installations on the Distant Early Warning (DEW) Line in the Arctic; he'd go north for a year, come back for thirty days, and then return north; but he died prematurely in 1956, leaving Norman's mother as the sole wage-earner in the family. By the 1960s Norman had matriculated, tried auto mechanics, and finally found work with a TV sales and repair shop on Sargent Street in Winnipeg. "There was no future in TV servicing," Malayney said. "So I figured I'd go to the US, get a green card, join the Air Force, and get training in electronics."

As a registered alien—unable to acquire security clearance or US citizenship until he'd been a resident for four years—Malayney had no choice but to go where the USAF sent him; they posted him to San Antonio, Texas, for basic training as a medical corpsman. At Lackland Air Force Base, recruit Malayney worked in the orthopedic and urology ward, where for the first time he encountered army and marine troops who'd been wounded in Vietnam, men with burn wounds, head injuries, or limb amputations. Then, in the spring of 1967, with US deployments at their highest level since the beginning of the war, casualty rates just as high, and those on a previous deployment coming to the end of their tours, the 26th Casualty Station Unit at Cam Ranh Bay Air Force Base

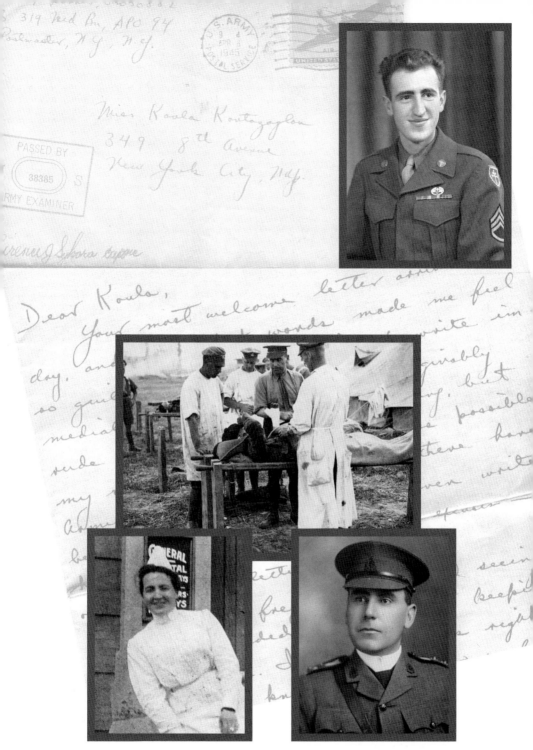

Relationships spawned by circumstances of war: In 1945, army medic Alex Barris (TOP RIGHT) composed this letter to his school-chum-turned-confidante Koula; he offered insights, shared secrets, and hoped they could one day get back together. In contrast, medical officer Harold McGill (MIDDLE, IN DARK UNIFORM, AND BOTTOM RIGHT) corresponded regularly throughout the Great War with Nursing Sister Emma Griffis (BOTTOM LEFT); eventually that connection by mail blossomed into a commitment of love, marriage, and a return to civilian life together.

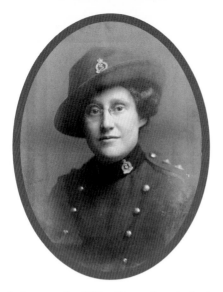
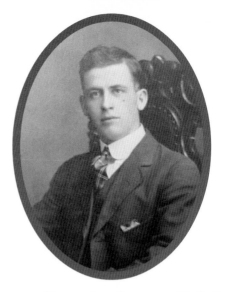

Regulations at the UK military hospital where they served in the Canadian Army Medical Corps restricted staff cook Fred Lailey (TOP RIGHT) from fraternizing with Nursing Sister Louise Spry (TOP LEFT). As Fred put it, he was told, "Look but don't touch." But the couple proved that love has a way, and secretly married just outside London on June 18, 1918.

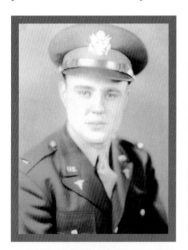

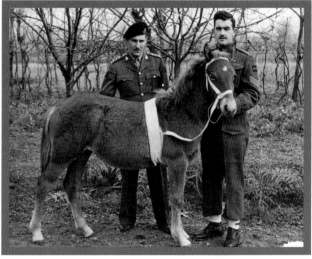

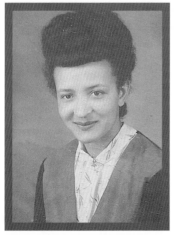

When the 8th Princess Louise's (New Brunswick) Hussars found a foal (ABOVE) wounded in the crossfire of a battle-field near Coriano, Italy, their regimental medics attended her shrapnel wounds with salves and a belly bandage. It was the beginning of a unique relationship; christened "Princess Louise," the horse mascot travelled with the Hussars all the way to VE-Day and home to Canada.

At Christmas in 1944 in Bastogne, Belgium, American medical officer Jack Prior (MIDDLE LEFT) and Congolese-born nurse Augusta Chiwy (BOTTOM LEFT) were thrown together as the Battle of the Bulge raged around them; their struggle to save lives and to survive themselves brought this unlikely pair of heroes together in a nearly doomed city.

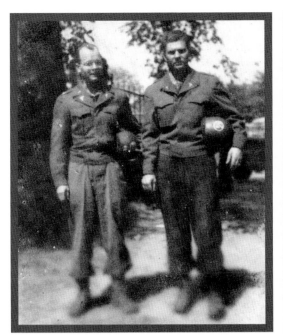 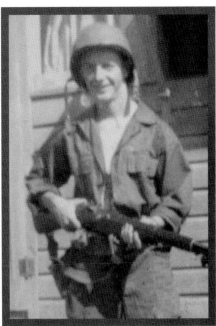

The credo that civilian-cum-US-Army-doctor Raiden Dellinger (TOP LEFT, on RIGHT) practised in 1944–45 overseas included life-saving surgery on comrades just behind the front lines, as well as unexpected first-aid treatment of POWs in the field. On the other hand, US Army infantryman Bill Foley (TOP RIGHT) had different objectives in the Battle of the Bulge—survive front-line combat when it seemed least likely and, as he sketched into his diary (BELOW), cope with military protocol when it seemed least practical.

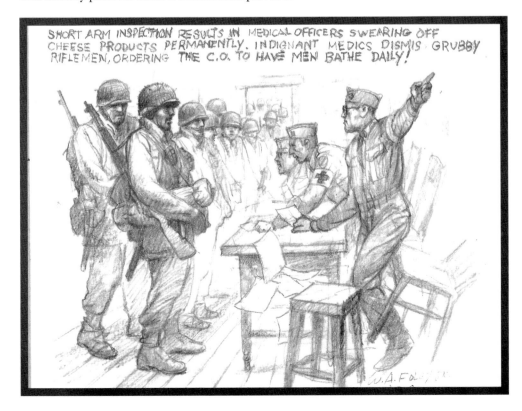

SHORT ARM INSPECTION RESULTS IN MEDICAL OFFICERS SWEARING OFF CHEESE PRODUCTS PERMANENTLY. INDIGNANT MEDICS DISMIS GRUBBY RIFLEMEN, ORDERING THE C.O. TO HAVE MEN BATHE DAILY!

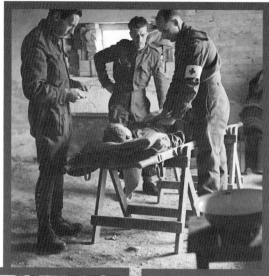

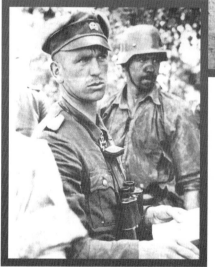

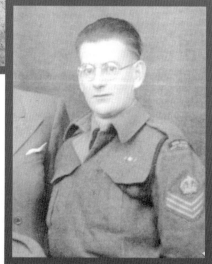

When he landed in Normandy right after D-Day in 1944, Canadian medic Henry Duffield (MIDDLE RIGHT) had to quickly establish a regimental aid post (TOP) to attend to the wounded; his RAP was so close to enemy lines that Duffield faced an unexpected visit from panzer commander Kurt Meyer (MIDDLE LEFT).

Captured in Malaya in January 1942, medical officer Jacob Markowitz (BOTTOM RIGHT) disappeared into a Japanese POW camp where 50,000 Allied prisoners became forced labour on the "Death Railway." Over three years behind the POW wire the doctor performed a thousand amputations, 3,800 transfusions, and 7,000 inoculations, all without actual medical instruments.

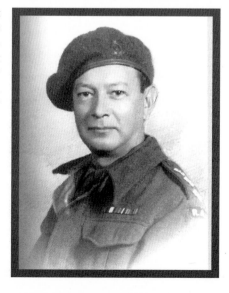

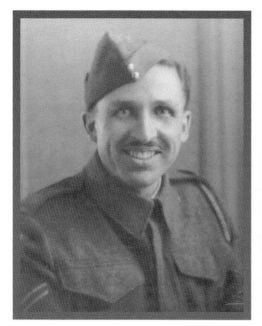

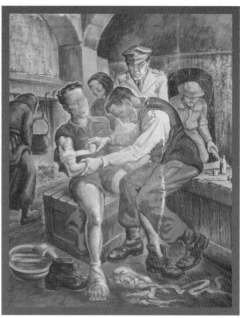

In 1943 medic Arnold Hodgkins (TOP LEFT) tended the wounded in the Italian campaign wherever there was shelter; first as a sketch, then as a painting (TOP RIGHT), Hodgkins captured the experience of attending to a burned tank crewman in a farmhouse near the Moro River.

In 1967, Norm Malayney (MIDDLE LEFT) got his baptism of fire in Vietnam as a medic at the US Air Force hospital in Cam Ranh Bay, near Saigon. Working twelve hours on and twelve hours off through the 1967 US troop surge and the 1968 Tet Offensive, he triaged, packed wounds, and processed the dead in what his comrade called "the worst job in the Air Force."

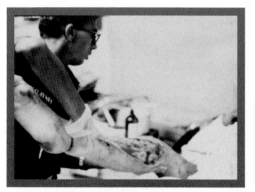

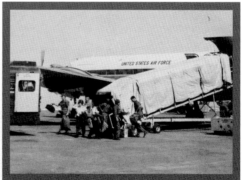

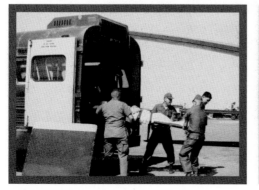

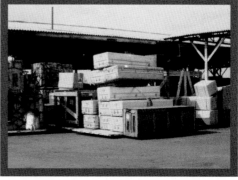

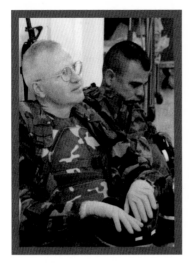

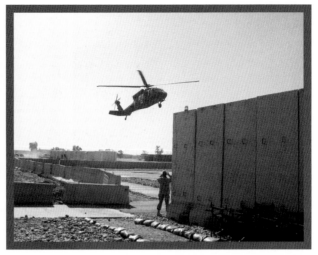

Dane Harden (TOP LEFT, IN FOREGROUND) had already completed overseas deployments for the US Army in Estonia, Bosnia, Kosovo, and Slovenia by 2004, when he began the first of three back-to-back-to-back tours in the Middle East. In Iraq as a flight surgeon, he did much of his service strapped into the midsection of a Black Hawk helicopter (TOP RIGHT), doing emergency medical care on wounded in 110-degree heat as the chopper flew at 140 miles per hour to the nearest base hospital. If a wounded soldier was alive seconds after an injury and a military doctor arrived in that critical time, the patient had a 97 percent chance of survival.

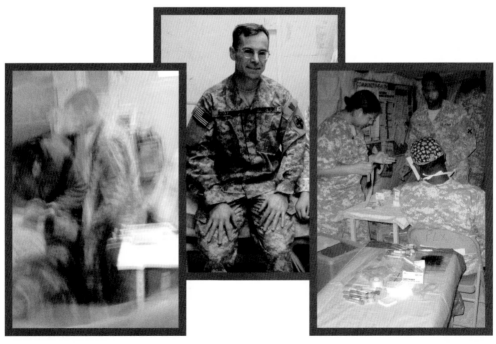

As much as he feared the obvious threats of a war zone—bombs, bullets, and improvised explosive devices—in the Middle East, Herb Ridyard (ABOVE, MIDDLE), surgical chief at a US contingency operating base in Iraq in 2008, worried most about "mass cals" alerts; that's when the massive number of incoming casualties might overwhelm his surgical teams in the operating rooms. The blurred photo (ABOVE LEFT) illustrates the frenzy of such an emergency. In this case, however, Ridyard watched in amazement as personnel from across the base lined up to give blood (ABOVE RIGHT) to compensate for the threat.

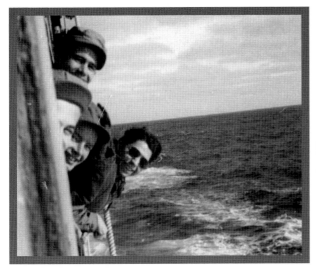

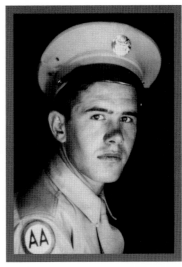

By Christmas 1945, medic Joe Reilly (TOP LEFT IN SUNGLASSES AND TOP RIGHT) was home in Philadelphia. But because of his experiences overseas, he couldn't acclimatize to civilian society until Anne Hubert, a secretary at an elevator company, recognized that all he needed was a chance for a new start. Reilly got a job as a draftsman and his first paycheque and married the secretary.

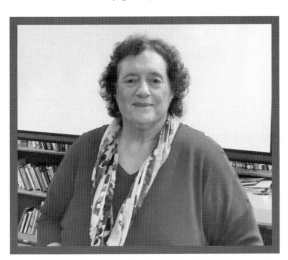

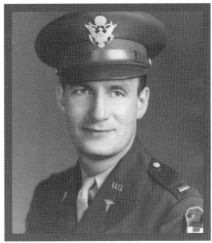

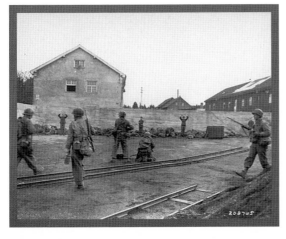

Administering anesthetics during round-the-clock surgeries with the US Army 116th Evacuation Hospital overseas, medical officer David Wilsey (ABOVE RIGHT) faced a final challenge at Dachau concentration camp in May 1945. Writing home, Dr. Wilsey revealed the horrors of treating thousands of prisoners near death while witnessing the execution of Nazi guards by US troops (LEFT). But none of that trauma was known until 2008, when daughter Clarice Wilsey (MIDDLE LEFT) opened a trunk containing her father's wartime citations, letters, and artifacts.

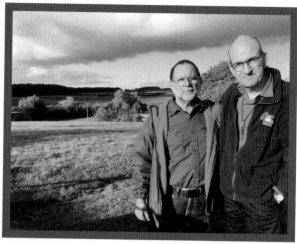

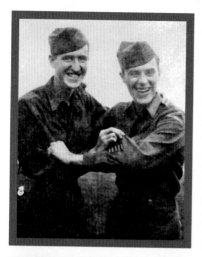

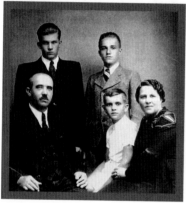

Separated by the war for three years, brothers Alex and Angelo Barris reunited in mid-1945 in Czechoslovakia (TOP LEFT, LEFT TO RIGHT) and kidded each other about their service stripes. Meanwhile, the Czech Krizek family (MIDDLE) billeted Alex, to the delight of their three sons.

During a 2017 tour retracing the 94th Infantry's path in the Battle of the Bulge, German-born American Al Theobald and the author (TOP RIGHT, LEFT TO RIGHT) visited Borg, where in 1945 T/Sgt. Barris established a casualty aid station in Theobald's parents' farmhouse. In Campholz Woods (TOP RIGHT IN BACKGROUND) medic Barris retrieved four wounded US stretcher-bearers and earned a Bronze Star citation (BELOW).

Bronze Star Citation given to Sgt. Alex Barris

Tec 4 Barris is liaison Sgt for this organization whose normal duties are those of maintaining the chain of evacuation from Bn Aid Stations to Coll Co. In this capacity Tec 4 Barris expresses an unselfish devotion to duty. Being without organic transportation, he has managed to maintain perfect liaison by sheer initiative of seeking rides from other units going in his particular direction. Many times when unsuccessful at securing transportation he has walked endless miles, under severe and adverse weather conditions. So intense is his zeal to discharge his duties that on February 15, 16 & 17th, 1945, he refused sleep until all Bn Aid Stations were being properly evacuated. He took to his bed only after being given a direct order to do so. When it became necessary for litter bearers from this company to be placed on special duty with the 302d Regt Battalion Medical Sections due to severe loss in their personnel, Tec 4 Barris personally conducted these squads to their respective duties, sought to their welfare and needs, and was instrumental in their successful discharge of their duties. On 12 February 1945, one litter squad failed to return after an operation by the 1st Bn 302d Regt in Campholz Woods, Germany. Tec 4 Barris personally entered these woods which were heavily sown with mines and booby traps, and located the members of this squad. Two (2) of the members of the squad were wounded and the remaining two were disoriented. He managed to extricate the members of the squad and further their evacuation through medical channels. He has repeatedly expressed initiative and forsight in discharge of his duties as liaison Sgt, and has been greatly instrumental in the success and smooth running of the organization in which he serves. His total disregard for personal safety and his continual service to his organization over and above the call of his particular duties are in keeping with the highest of army traditions.

needed capable corpsmen. Malayney qualified. In April his transport landed in the night at Cam Ranh Bay and he found himself in "the living room war."*

Almost immediately, medic Malayney faced the most horrific of wounds as well as the shortcomings of the treatment system. He dreaded when army wounded arrived with severe burns, because the army did not allow field medics to use Vaseline or other salves on the wounds, only dry gauze packing; when one burn victim arrived and CSU medics removed the field dressing from his back, the man's skin peeled away right down to his muscles, "blue, just like in the textbook." Whenever he found time, Malayney observed experienced nurses packing wounds; by the end of his tour he could handle the toughest dressing assignments as well as any of the nursing staff.

For a while during his tour, Malayney wondered why some of the metal-framed beds had bent bedposts; he discovered that some patients feared the embarrassment of screaming in pain, so they grabbed and pulled on the bedposts instead of shouting out loud. Eventually the CSU got an anesthetist from Khe Sanh who used inhalers with drugs that put a patient into semi-consciousness during painful treatment. Whenever he heard the speaker system announce "Section Eight," Malayney knew it meant a patient had snapped and needed to be put under guard, for his protection and the safety of staff on the base.

---

* On May 31, 1967, American Broadcasting Corporation news anchor Frank Reynolds introduced a report from Vietnam; he suggested to viewers that they were witnessing something unprecedented—a war that TV was delivering to the living rooms of America. President Lyndon Johnson considered the media coverage of the war biased and as undermining popular support for the war. Polls showed that by a margin of 43 to 38 percent (the remainder undecided) Americans disapproved of Johnson's handling of the war.

One patient left a lasting impression on Malayney. The soldier was at Cam Ranh Bay for only about fifteen hours, but during that time Malayney learned the man had been shot not on a battlefield but at an enlisted men's club in South Vietnam where a GI had entered and begun shooting; two died at the scene, but Malayney's patient made it to the 483rd USAF Hospital in time for lifesaving surgery. Norm was assigned to attend the patient until he was shipped out to Japan on a C-141 transport jet the next morning. "I remember this guy. He was semi-conscious, breathing heavily," Malayney said. "I put my hand on the bed and I could feel his heart pounding, each heartbeat through the mattress."

Medical corpsmen were lowest on the totem pole at Cam Ranh Bay, it seemed to Malayney, who was promoted to Airman 1st Class in Vietnam. They were often assigned to night shifts, which meant they had to try to sleep during hot, humid days in huts without any air conditioning. Malayney received his basic service pay of thirty dollars a month, plus hostile-fire pay of sixty dollars a month. Yet they still received equal time off. For every five days of twelve hours on and twelve off, medics got two days off, but they were restricted to base, which meant time off was usually spent trying to catch up on sleep or drinking beer with buddies.

Looking for something different to do when he was off-duty, Malayney took his camera and photographed aircraft, landscapes, and people on the peninsula where the 12th Tactical Fighter Wing was located. He received one out-of-country rest-and-relaxation leave, to Hong Kong in December 1967, and returned to duty just in time for the Tet Offensive on January 31, 1968. That day, some 85,000 North Vietnamese and Viet Cong forces launched simultaneous attacks against five major cities and dozens of military installations in South Vietnam. The offensive left 45,000 casualties on the Communist side and more than 20,000 casualties among US forces. In the first forty-eight hours of the assault, C-141s flew five hundred casualties into Cam Ranh Bay.

"There were no days off during the Tet Offensive; some worked twenty-fours straight," Malayney recalled. "We had one wounded, he was like a mummy. I had just finished dressing his wounds head to foot. [But] they gave him so much antibiotics by IV that it killed the local flora in his gut. He had diarrhea down his legs, through the bedding, to the floor. We had to strip the bed, wash it down, and do his dressings all over again."

Until he landed at Cam Ranh Bay, Malayney had never had to deal with the dead. But in Vietnam, the job of packing the body fell to medical corpsmen, including Malayney. First he had to prepare the body for rigor mortis, tying off the penis and blocking the rectum with cotton to stop either urine or feces from escaping. The corpsman then carefully cleaned the body one last time, finally stringing one identity tag onto a toe and another onto a hand. Then he placed the remains in a body bag. In Vietnam, despite the intense heat most of the year, hospitals the size of the one at Cam Ranh Bay had portable "reefers"—refrigerators—to prevent the bodies from decomposing long enough for air transports to arrive and fly the bodies home to the United States. "Even if it was a hundred degrees outside," Malayney said, "inside where we put the bodies, it was freezing."

Norman Malayney completed his year-long tour of duty, plus an extended tour to overlap with the arrival of new medical corpsmen at Cam Ranh Bay in December 1968. In return for his extension, he earned a thirty-day leave in Europe, visiting England, Holland, Germany, Switzerland, and Italy. By the end of the year the USAF had posted Malayney to MacDill Air Force Base in Tampa, Florida. For six months he tended to injured airmen and some Vietnam veterans at the end of their convalescence, about to be discharged home. One of his patients seemed startlingly familiar. "You were in Vietnam?" Malayney asked.

"Yeah," the man said.

"What happened?"

"I was sitting in an enlisted men's bar, and this guy came in and started shooting people," the vet said.

"Holy smokes, I've heard this story before!"

This, Malayney realized, was the same army soldier he'd attended to in Cam Ranh Bay following the bar shootings, the man whose heavy heartbeat he'd felt through the hospital mattress. For fellow Vietnam veteran Malayney, it was a unique moment; he'd actually witnessed a man he'd tended in an overseas war zone being discharged in good health and heading home.

Before long Malayney was homeward bound too, back to Winnipeg to pursue the other "one of the two greatest experiences of my life"—attending university. Vietnam had given him an excellent education and a sense of self-confidence, but now he wanted the chance to study something of his own choosing, what he'd missed before and during the war. At the University of Winnipeg he gained sufficient training in pharmaceuticals that he was able to build a postwar career in sales around small-town America.

And as for Cal Schuler's claim that Norm had experienced

the worst job in the Air Force? "For the fighter pilots, it was different. They dropped bombs. And the aero-engine mechanics had a tough grind in Vietnam too," Malayney said. "But they didn't have to see the blood and guts and disfigurement that I saw coming through my ward."

2004 TO 2009—IRAQ WAR

COL. DANE HARDEN could definitely relate to Norm Malayney's feeling of satisfaction, years later, at seeing one of his former patients from Vietnam leave the USAF hospital in Tampa fully healed and homeward bound. A veteran flight surgeon of four tours of duty between 2000 and 2005, Harden had triaged, delivered emergency first aid in the field, and kept scores of wounded alive long enough to get them to operating theatres for life-saving medicine, in war zones as challenging as Bosnia, Kosovo, Iraq, and Afghanistan. Nonetheless, by the time American troops were operating in the Middle East, Harden and his medical teams had elevated the science to the point that, if a wounded soldier was alive two seconds after the injury and a military doctor arrived in that critical time, the wounded soldier had a 97 percent chance of survival. Despite the statistics of success, decades after America's involvement in Vietnam, Dane Harden, like his predecessor Norman Malayney, found closure in the simplest of ways.

"Three or four years after I got back from Iraq," Harden said, "I got a letter from a father thanking me for taking care of his son."[21] Flight Surgeon Harden remembered the experience. The man's son had been severely wounded. Fortunately, the system had responded with precision, delivering the soldier through a cascade of care. A combat lifesaver had treated him at the point of injury. Then a combat medic had helped him reach a casualty collection point or a battalion aid station, where a doctor and a physician assistant had likely worked on him. That's where Harden would have flown in to move the wounded man on to the next phase of treatment. Harden felt embarrassed that he'd received all this praise from the father of the wounded man when the whole US Army could be taking credit for it. "The father actually went to the trouble to find out that Doc Harden was the flight surgeon who got his son out of harm's way and got him squared away," he said.

Dane Harden was destined to serve in the US military. During the Second World War, his mother, Anna, had worked at the Glenn L. Martin manufacturing plant building B-29 bombers in Baltimore, while Robert, his father, had served in the Pacific during the liberation of the Philippines and the invasion of Okinawa. Dane's older brothers had both served—Dave with the Marines in Vietnam and later with the 101st Airborne in Kuwait and Iraq, and Darrell in the Army National Guard. The family also had a military lineage going back to the Revolutionary War, the War of 1812–14, the US Civil War, and the Spanish-American War.

Dane's fate was sealed in 1976, when he asked his dad if he could go to college to study engineering; when his father explained that he couldn't afford to send him, the army seemed the next best option for an education. Dane was streamed into combat engineering, "an infantryman with a shovel," building roads, tank traps, and pontoon bridges, conducting demolition, and learning how to map minefields. To add to his credentials, Dane was already a marksman with a National Rifle Association rifle team, had a black belt, and ran cross-country at an elite level.

In eighteen months he'd gone from private to sergeant, and after three years' peacetime training at Fort Knox, Kentucky, he was honourably discharged. He worked part-time as a nursing assistant to help pay for the science courses he was taking at college. And by 1993 he'd also completed his degree as a physician assistant. To add to his resumé, he joined the Maryland Army National Guard, and because of his medical training he automatically became a second lieutenant. Eventually he decided it was time to visit a US Army recruitment office.

"And your credentials?" the recruiter asked.

"Three years as a combat engineer. I kind of miss the military," Harden said. And then he laid out his diplomas, certificates, and other papers, adding, "I'm a physician assistant . . ."

The recruiter nearly leapt over the desk to scoop up the recruit's paperwork. "We're short of medical officers," he said.

So Dane Harden re-entered the US Army as a second lieutenant and was shipped off to Fort Sam Houston, in San Antonio, Texas, for medical officer basic training, where civilian doctors, nurses, and dentists got army familiarization. Later, at Fort Stewart, Georgia, Lt. Harden took his first expert field medical badge test—five days of calling in medevacs, setting up triage casualty collection points, and conducting evacuation procedures; he failed on his first attempt. Undaunted and encouraged by a system desperate to graduate more medical officers, Harden kept training, finally collecting his flight surgeon wings at Fort Rucker, Alabama, in 1998. In the late 1990s and early 2000s, as a member of the Georgia Army National Guard, he received his first overseas deployments, to Estonia, Bosnia, Kosovo, and Slovenia, where he recognized the changing nature of military medicine. Harden learned in those war zones that the enemy was everywhere and had no regard for North Atlantic Treaty Organization guidelines.

"If a doc is in that environment and he pulls his weapon and shoots back, that's actually more valuable and reduces the number of casualties," Harden said. "If I'm in a firefight and I'm trying to save a patient, it's my job to kill the enemy first. And that's an utter shift from the way we normally practise medicine."

In 2004, Maj. Harden was deployed to the Middle East for the first of three back-to-back tours of duty. Much of his service was routine—80 percent doing flight physicals and ground work, but the rest, where the action was, had him airborne in a dual-engine Black Hawk helicopter conducting emergency medical care. In the rear of a chopper en route to and from pick-up points, it was noisy, wide open (the open doors providing the only air conditioning), and, in 110-degree heat, "like basting a turkey." Wearing his fire-resistant Nomex flight suit, helmet, and rubber gloves, Maj. Harden would be belted in. At the point of injury, medics would transfer the wounded soldier from a litter to a carousel aboard the chopper; this would lock the patient into a secured position, allowing Harden to move around him to assess and attend.

In flight, the latest Black Hawks had lights, oxygen, and suction equipment, as well as ventilators with automatic PEEPs—positive end-expiratory pressures—that kept a patient's lungs inflated for better oxygenation. If a soldier went into shock, Harden would request the help of on-board medics working as his assistants to intubate the patient, hook up intravenous fluids, and try to increase blood pressure. All this went on as the Black Hawk crew pushed its aircraft to the limit, at speeds of up to 140 miles per hour, to get Harden's patient to a friendly base and the next level of medical care.

Even though these could be tense situations, Harden went to great lengths to keep his patient calm, by talking his way through the treatment. He would check out airways, breathing, and circulation and make note to both himself and the on-board medic: "I'm listening to your lungs now." He might assure the patient by saying, "I've seen these kinds of wounds before," or "We're going to get you some medication for the pain." Harden called it his mantra—say what you see and see what you say—while completing primary survey, secondary survey, and follow-up. And though it sounded as if Harden were being as personable as possible, in effect he was focusing on what it would take to expedite his patient from the battlefield to the base hospital operating table. Once the delivery was made, his mission was accomplished. Over his career in the military, Dane Harden completed 122 such medevacs.

"I would normally try to find out if the guy lived or died, but after a hundred or so of those cases, you learned that you can't follow them all," Harden said. "I considered that I'd won the battle if they were alive when I got them to the ER."

...

ABOUT EIGHT MILES OUTSIDE the northern Iraq city of Tikrit, US Army Medical Officer Herb Ridyard Jr. worked as the surgical chief of staff at Contingency Operating Base (COB) Speicher* during the second half of the US Army surge in 2008. He wasn't so much concerned about whether he remembered a patient's name or not, just as long as the COB had enough blood on hand whenever the facility experienced a "mass cals"—"massive casualties"—alert. While in the vicinity of the hospital, US forces on the base numbered in the thousands, inside the hospital itself Ridyard led a staff of about a hundred. That meant that if the hospital faced any more than about half a dozen casualties at once, the workload could overwhelm the facility. Despite the fear of that possibility, which was always in the back of his mind, Dr. Ridyard also had to deal with civilian casualties. In fact, on his very first day at the hospital, Christmas Day, Ridyard had to operate on a young Iraqi girl who'd been admitted two days earlier with burns over 60 percent of her body.

"We had suspicions that she was burned because her family had been accused of conspiring with the Americans," Ridyard said.[22] Had the girl gone to a civilian hospital inside the city, it's likely she wouldn't have survived. But at the COB outside Tikrit, the staff pulled out all the stops. The operating room was located in a tent, so contending with blowing sand and the winter temperatures provided several challenges. The staff placed blowers in the tent to keep the air as clean as possible, and they set up heaters to keep the OR at one hundred

---

* Contingency Operating Base Speicher was named after Scott Speicher, the first US Navy pilot shot down in the Gulf War, on January 17, 1991.

degrees Fahrenheit during several weeks of surgeries on the girl. "Everybody had worked above and beyond what was expected," he said. "She was one of our unit's first success stories."

Unlike Dane Harden, who seemed to have armed service in his sights from the time he could shoot a rifle at age nine, Herb Ridyard Jr. came to the US Army as a second or third career, when he was approaching fifty. During the Second World War, his father, Herb Sr., had served as a rifleman in the 301st Infantry Regiment of the 94th Infantry Division; he had helped push back the German *Wacht am Rhein* counteroffensive across the Rhine in the winter of 1945. But the Battle of the Bulge had left its fair share of bad memories, so Herb Sr. had never pushed his son to follow in his army footsteps. Then Herb Jr.'s son John spent two summers at US Marine Corps officer school. The family attended John's graduation, and as Herb Jr. watched his son march smartly across the parade square at Quantico, Virginia, he was struck by the discipline and order he suddenly saw in him.

Herb Jr. listened to the school's officers lament the state of overseas deployment. "We never really have enough surgeons," they said. "They sometimes have gynecologists doing trauma surgery."

"My god," thought Ridyard. "One of these guys is going to get blown up or shot and they're going to have a gynecologist operating on him. Gynecologists don't typically do trauma surgery."

At an American College of Surgeons conference in Boston that same year, the overseas medical shortages emerged again at a military medicine exhibit. The US Army was clearly desperate for general surgeons. "But you can't take somebody who's forty-eight years old," Ridyard told the exhibitor. They said they'd issue him a waiver and take him up to age fifty-two. At home in Windham, Connecticut, where he was assistant chief of staff at a rural hospital, Herb consulted with his wife, Kris; he gave his medical partners his notice, then got an offer for a commission in the medical corps and decided to give it a try.

As a lieutenant colonel he packed up and headed back to school—basic training in San Antonio, at Fort Sam Houston, the training centre for US Army Command and, euphemistically, "the home of the combat medic." At Fort Sam, Ridyard outranked everybody in his class. He had also operated a medical practice longer than most of his classmates had been alive. But he still had to learn how to be a soldier. The culture shock continued right up to the moment he arrived in Iraq in December 2008; that day, he learned that John Pryor, the general surgeon at the Mosul combat support hospital, a man he'd met in training, had been killed in a mortar attack.

Work at the COB seemed surreal for a surgeon who'd led the staff at a rural hospital back in the States. The OR team scrubbed in "third world"–type sinks; blowers helped keep dust from settling on everything; and the surgeons and nurses worked in combat boots and fatigues under their sanitary gowns. Just like in the *M*A*S*H* television series, the COB leapt into action at the sound of helicopters with incoming wounded. Back home, the toughest surgical calls came from multiple-car crashes; in Iraq it was rocket attacks, shell blasts, and IED explosions. On those occasions, the operating theatre would fill with army medical teams attending severe head wounds, carrying out amputations, and conducting surgeries to extract screws, nuts, nails, and other random hardware, the principal projectiles inside IEDs. It wasn't too long into his tour at COB Speicher before the day that Lt. Col. Ridyard most dreaded arrived.

"Six or eight patients came in and they were all pretty bad," he recalled. "We had more patients coming in than we could handle. We made a 'mass cals' call." With the "mass cals" alert, the hospital went into an emergency protocol. There was an immediate call for blood donations. All medical personnel and supplies, not just from inside the base hospital but also from other aid stations around the base, began to converge on the operating theatre. As chief of surgery responsible for organizing the OR, Ridyard soon had a pediatrician on scene, a nurse anesthetist, and a nurse practitioner. At the triage station he posted a gynecologist and other volunteers to process the wounded. Once the casualties were triaged and his two other surgeons had begun their work, Ridyard joined them in the operating theatre and immediately immersed himself in the lifesaving.

But suddenly the operating room had used up its entire blood supply. The COB had hit a wall. "I left the operating room and went out into this other tent," Ridyard said. "To my amazement, there must have been a hundred guys all lined up to give blood. All the techs, soldiers, everybody dropped everything, rolled up their sleeves to donate. It was really something."

At what seemed the darkest moment of his military tour, a base full of Good Samaritans had stepped up and renewed Ridyard's faith in humanity, not to mention replenishing critical units of blood when his patients needed them most.

Herb Ridyard did three four-month tours in Iraq as a hospital surgeon. Dane Harden completed nine deployments overseas as a flight surgeon. As qualified and experienced as they were when they left home, both medical men returned having seen improvements in ways to save lives in traumatic circumstances. Ridyard had his eyes opened by transfusion protocols in Iraq, very different from those followed in civilian blood banks; in Iraq, if they didn't have whole blood, they transfused components (red cells, plasma, and platelets) in a one-to-one-to-one ratio to mimic whole blood. It worked so well that Ridyard used the procedure in his own practice back home. Meanwhile, in northern Kuwait, Harden had worked alongside British medics and surgeons who'd introduced him to polymerized hemoglobin powder; when administered, it acted like a transfusion to expand blood volume and treat shock.

Both Ridyard and Harden received numerous and appropriate service medals for their multiple tours in Iraq. As a flight surgeon, Dane Harden seemed completely at ease assessing the medical state of a patient and dealing with life-threatening needs, all in the open body of a Black Hawk medevac chopper travelling at 140 miles per hour over the Iraqi desert, with temperatures in excess of 110 degrees. Harden considered such a daily routine not advanced trauma life-support skills but more like "what back in Korea might have been called meatball surgery"—trying to stop bleeding, protecting the airway, and preventing shock, all in an attempt to get patients to doctors in an OR. At some levels he considered his profession science, but mostly he thought of it as well-trained reflexes. "I can't imagine doing something more valuable than saving the life of a soldier," Harden said. "It doesn't get any better than that."[23]

Among the lasting impressions Herb Ridyard brought back from Iraq was another civilian case. After much delay and red tape, a young Iraqi boy—carried into the US military facility by his older brother—was rushed into emergency surgery. The patient was unconscious, allegedly hit by a car. Ridyard thought the boy's head wounds looked less like a collision with a car and more like blows from a rifle butt; someone had likely inflicted the wounds because the boy's father was a police officer or in the military. Nevertheless, without missing a beat, he and his ER team put the boy through the works— CT scan, blood transfusion, and surgery for skull fracture and brain injury. "I still remember all the technology and all the people helping when that boy came into the emergency room; fifteen or twenty people all trying to save his life."

Ridyard noted the boy's brother standing off to the side in the ER, watching this scene unfold. "I'm wondering, what does his brother think?" Ridyard concluded. "[Some] think so little of life that they would bash a nine-year-old in the head with a rifle butt, and here we are putting every effort into trying to save him. . . . Those are moments just imprinted on my brain."[24]

CHAPTER TEN

"LIGHT AMONGST THAT EVIL"

F ROM THE TIME I WAS AN ADOLESCENT, I have chased my father's war story. The pursuit has taken me through ancient family suitcases full of photographs and letters; to the National Personnel Records Center in St. Louis to retrieve his military service papers; deep inside a University of Georgia rare books library that housed the wartime diaries and correspondence of my father's regimental comrades; on a personal trek across the German countryside, retracing the path of his medical battalion during the Battle of the Bulge; and eventually to the 94th Infantry Division Historical Society's list of active members, veterans who were still alive. On a summer evening in July 2015, I dialled up Eatontown, New Jersey, and the number of Anthony J. Mellaci. A woman answered and passed the phone.

"I'm looking for Tony Mellaci," I said.[1]

"You've found him," the jovial voice answered.

"Mr. Mellaci, my name is Ted Barris and I'm wondering if you remember my father from the war. He was a medic—"

"Al Barris?" he interrupted.

"Yes . . ."

"The writer? From New York?"

"You knew him?" I asked, my voice shaking.

"Knew him? We served together in the 319th. And I've always wondered whatever happened to him. Is he still alive?"

My father's death in 2004 was the only sad news we shared over the next hour. I was so excited to have found a witness to my dad's other life that I couldn't stop asking Mellaci questions. And Tony, born in 1922, the same year as my father, seemed just as eager to answer them fully. On the phone he led me through story after story of his experiences as a medical corpsman in the war, many of them involving my father. He described their winter of insanity, training at Camp Phillips, Kansas, followed by advanced training, including the live-fire exercises at Camp McCain, Mississippi. He flashed back to the transatlantic trip aboard the troopship *Queen Elizabeth*, landing in France, and then serving as medics all the way to Germany. He touched briefly on his memories of the Bulge, including the night he tried to save the young rifleman whose legs had been horribly smashed during the assault across the River Saar.

But because he knew I wanted something tangible about Dad, Tony also recalled seeing their company captain, Laurence J. Sykora, present the Bronze Star to my father at Krefeld, Germany, just before the 94th pushed its way into Düsseldorf at the end of the war. And he kept coming back to an indelible image of my dad—taking notes, gathering stories, and editing them for publication—almost as if the expenditure of all this creative energy might distract him from the business of war.

"He jotted everything down," Mellaci said. "He talked to everybody, always had jokes to tell. He kept us laughing. He was our battalion journalist."[2]

As I listened to the floodgates of Mellaci's memory open wide with reminiscences, I knew we had to meet face to face. And soon! I sensed that in Mellaci's recollections I might learn a lot about my father's attitude as a medic, about his personality in uniform, and specifically about the events at Campholz Woods in February 1945. I gingerly suggested to Mellaci that, if it were convenient, I could travel there to see him. No pressure. I told him I didn't want to impose. If he could direct me, I'd stay at a nearby motel.

"Come here to New Jersey? Sure. Anytime," he said without hesitation. "And you don't need a motel room. You can stay with us. You're family!"

"You're very kind . . ." I said, and I cried.

"Besides," he concluded, "I have some of your father's paperwork. You know, he wrote about us from training in Kansas all the way to Europe. Like in a battalion newsletter."

The prospect of hearing my father's voice in print grabbed me by the heartstrings. For years I had read and saved some of my father's contemporary writing—from when he was a newspaper columnist in the 1950s; a TV documentary, variety, and sitcom writer in the 1960s and '70s; and as co-author with me on dozens of CBC radio scripts and two non-fiction books in the 1990s and early 2000s. But I had rarely, if ever, heard his writing voice from before I came into his life.

Suddenly one of his affable old war buddies who, like Dad, had left everything about the war behind when he returned to civilian life in the States—in Mellaci's case to take over his father's tavern in Rumson, New Jersey—seemed ready to give me a part of my dad I didn't have, stories of his comrade on or near the front lines of combat in the winter of 1945. It was a part of T/Sgt. Barris I yearned to know. For former S/Sgt. Mellaci, it was a series of mental snapshots of a fellow American, a guy he'd depended on and who'd depended on him, a medical battalion brother, and a man Tony repeatedly referred to as "Al the writer"!

AUGUST 6, 1945—VODŇANY, CZECHOSLOVAKIA

LATE IN THE SPRING OF 1945, during their final days occupying the German city of Düsseldorf, members of my father's umbrella outfit, the 94th Infantry Division, received a special victory edition of its official weekly newspaper. The May 8 edition of *The Attack*, which was typeset and produced in the former printing plant of Nachrichten,[3] the publishing wing of the Communist Party in Germany, had all the latest news of the unconditional German surrender. It also offered words of commendation from the 94th's divisional commander. In an editorial, Maj. Gen. Harry J. Malony congratulated his men, allowing them to bask in the day of victory with a great sense of satisfaction.

In his 250-word statement, titled "We Have Set a Standard," Malony pointed out that the 94th and its various supporting units, including my father's 319th Medical Battalion, had trained and fought for two and a half years and pulled their share of the load. Between February 19 and March 5, 1945, they had breached the Siegfried Switch Line and then mopped up all resistance in the Saar-Moselle Triangle. They had successfully crossed the River Saar against the main Siegfried Line and captured Trier. Between March 13 and 24, the 94th had advanced across the Rhine, liberated two hundred towns and cities, and captured 13,434 prisoners of war. And through seventy-four consecutive days of attack—from September 10, 1944, to March 24, 1945—Malony emphasized, the 94th had virtually never been out of contact with the enemy.

"This Division has never failed in a mission, nor has it ever permanently lost one inch of ground to the enemy," my father's commanding officer wrote in his final congratulatory paragraph. "And whatever may be our next mission, we have set a standard which I ask each one of you to make it his personal business to meet."[4]

For T/ Sgt. Alex Barris, meeting that standard had both obvious and ironic significance. As a medical corps runner on the front lines during most of those seventy-four days of combat, he had processed hundreds of wounded and thousands of wounds to whatever standard could be maintained in such conditions as the Saar-Moselle Triangle posed that winter. If that standard had meant following orders, he'd done so. If that standard had included living up to his responsibilities as a medical corps section leader, the events of February 12, 1945, in Campholz Woods showed that he'd met and exceeded it. However, if that standard were the one Gen. Patton repeatedly told members of the 94th they could never reach because he considered them all "slackers," then it's unlikely that either Maj. Gen. Malony or T/Sgt. Barris could ever have convinced him otherwise.

Still, in his continuing service following the publication of the VE-Day edition of *The Attack*, it must have occurred to my father and others in his unit that one standard worth practising and upholding in the European victory was the principle of free speech, especially inside the most powerful military force on the planet at that moment. Thus, in the summer of their Czech occupation my father and his medical corps buddies launched a new internal periodical, the *B Company Bull Farm*, in whose opening pages were printed the publication's principles and guidelines. They read much like the First Amendment to the US Constitution, enshrining the rights of its contributors and editors.

"With this first issue, we start a monthly magazine given over entirely to the expression of the opinions of, and to stories and other items by the members of Company B," read the *Bull Farm*'s mission statement. "If you disagree with an opinion set forth in an article, we would like you to write a reply. . . . The only limitations will be those of space and good taste."[5]

The inaugural edition featured a short history of their Czech cohabitants during the occupation and their centuries-long fight for liberty, written by co-editor Cornelius Clifford. Contributing editor William Griswold offered a practical photography primer for Company B corpsmen who had suddenly found themselves in the possession of "new and strange cameras."[6] The third of four editors, Walter Clark, offered his thoughts about Chief Justice Oliver Wendell Holmes, "a man of ideals and deep-seated convictions, ever willing to uphold justice against all odds, even to the extent that he became known as 'the great dissenter' on the Supreme Court."[7] But in this first issue of the *Bull Farm*, fourth editor Al Barris chose to reflect on the publication date of the magazine, in an editorial titled "A Year Ago Today." It was a veteran's commentary on the challenges and outcomes, the idiosyncrasies and conformities, the commanders and the enlisted men of a medical unit that had come through a year of war together, all summarized with the benefit of 20/20 hindsight.

A year to the day before, the 319th Medical Battalion had been stationed at Camp Shanks, New York, the largest army port of embarkation in the United States, the place GIs nicknamed "Camp Last Stop USA." Recalling the battalion's priorities then, *Bull Farm* editor Al Barris wrote that "the Battle of the Duffle Bags wasn't over yet. . . . In France, Carlyles [wound dressing packets] were being saturated with blood faster than they could be supplied, but here we were grumbling, 'Why in Hell do we have to carry these aid kits?' . . . Then the 'march of death' with full field packs and duffle bags. You could have launched a battleship with the sweat that rolled down our weary faces. . . . And then the gangplank. The sharpest bookie in the world could have stood there and offered fantastic odds that we'd never again be as miserable as this, and he wouldn't have drawn a bet.

"But how naïve we were!" he continued. "If anyone had told Mike Sciortino that in about eight months he'd be riding a horse through an artillery barrage in Taben, Germany, the Bandit would have laughed. Or, if anyone had tried to describe the horror of a place called the Campholz Woods, we would have shaken our heads sadly and then returned to the business of feeling sorry for ourselves, because we had to climb a gangplank with a full field pack and a duffle bag."[8]

That first issue of the *B Company Bull Farm* was dated

August 6, 1945. On that same day—unknown to the corpsmen of my father's company in faraway Czechoslovakia, but
of immediate impact on both sides in the Pacific War—a US
Army Air Force bomber had dropped the world's first atomic
weapon on the Japanese city of Hiroshima. Three days later,
a similar bomb landed on its target: Nagasaki, Japan. And on
August 15 the capitulation of Imperial Japan officially brought
the Second World War to an end. But when my father wrote
his editorial "A Year Ago Today," he finished it by summing
up the "three hundred and sixty-five tightly packed, unique
days. Days of doing things we had never done before, and,
pray God, we will never have to do again!"[9]

Between the lines, his commentary shared a common sentiment among members of his medical company and, for that
matter, among all military personnel returning home after
warfare: the war had changed everything—in particular, everything about *them*.

AUGUST 23, 1944—NORMANDY, FRANCE

THE WAR MOST CERTAINLY CHANGED orderly Tony Burns.
In fact, he could pinpoint the moment; he described it as "the
night I died."[10] It happened in the same hospital—Basingstoke,
the neurological and plastic surgery hospital in Hampshire,
England—where in 1942 he had trained to become an operating room assistant in the Royal Canadian Army Medical
Corps. Expecting that he'd one day get the call to cross the

Channel and join the invasion force, Pte. Burns familiarized himself with the instruments of his wartime trade: aneurysm needles, forceps, drills, scissors, retractors, saws, scalp clips, traction tongs, suction tubing, and anesthetic gases. Fully qualified, Pte. Burns landed on Juno Beach, the Canadian sector of the Normandy invasion force, as an orderly with No. 1 Canadian Mobile Neurosurgical Unit (CMNSU), shortly after D-Day. The CMNSU's specialty was administering first aid to soldiers with head wounds.

In its first month ashore in Normandy the CMNSU handled more than two hundred cases. Then, on August 23, 1944, Burns became the unit's first casualty. About noon, the trailer in which the surgeons and operating room assistants worked came under attack. An explosion outside the operating tent capsized an instrument sterilizer full of hot water on Pte. Burns, scalding him across his back and arms. His medical colleagues immediately anesthetized him to treat his burns. They feared infection might set in, so they transferred him back to Basingstoke.

"I fell into a deep coma," he said. "I remember my eyes were closed. I wasn't able to move a muscle. But I could hear every word being said. I could feel the chaplain near me giving me the last rites."[11]

When he finally woke up, Burns found himself back in England, in a room full of wounded, each bandaged from head to toe. He was in the burns ward, where every day the nursing staff wheeled patients to bathe in a tub of warm saline water. Though his scalded skin began to heal, the daily rhythm of soaking and bandaging proved excruciating. He felt guilty about complaining in a ward with men more severely wounded than he was, but the pain still nearly drove him mad. "One day, after several months of pain, I couldn't take it anymore," he said. "So, I took the rosary my father gave me, covered my head with a blanket and died."

Apparently it wasn't his time. Burns awoke fifty hours later surrounded by many of the doctors and nurses who had trained him, including his commanding officer. Maj. William Keith of the CMNSU gave Tony Burns a reason to live: Keith told him the unit would one day need him back on duty. Indeed, when Burns recovered sufficiently to re-cross the Channel—where he caught up with his comrades in Ghent, Belgium—Dr. Keith was there to greet him; not only did Burns get his old job back, but there was also an added surprise.

"Dr. Keith threw a greatcoat over my shoulders to keep me warm," Burns said. "The coat had two pips [lieutenant stripes] on it. I started to take it off, but Dr. Keith smiled and said they were my pips as long as I was with the unit. A battlefield promotion, I guess."[12]

On June 6, 2003, Tony Burns returned to Normandy to join D-Day observances as well as the opening of the Juno Beach Centre, a veteran-sponsored museum commemorating Canadians' service during the Second World War. In particular, he felt compelled to pay homage to his brother, Lt. Dan Burns, who'd served with the Royal Canadian Regiment and died in action on January 1, 1945, during the Italian campaign. He said he felt guilty that he'd once wished he were dead in that burns ward at Basingstoke. Unlike his brother Dan, Tony Burns had been able to serve out the rest of the war with a vital unit in the medical corps; after VE-Day he'd enjoyed a triumphant repatriation to Halifax, a return to peacetime pursuits, a wife and family, and a full life to old age.

"Peace—so many millions never experienced it," he said. "What a pity."

SEPTEMBER 1946—PHILADELPHIA, PENNSYLVANIA

JOE REILLY HAD SOME UNDERSTANDING of the impact the war had on its veterans. He'd heard the terms "shell shock" and "battle fatigue" before, but he didn't consider himself a victim. At least not right away. Drafted into the US Army in April 1943, shortly after his twentieth birthday, and assigned to the medical detachment of the headquarters battery of the 489th AAA Automatic Weapons Battalion, S/Sgt. Reilly had served for twenty-five months with the 4th Armored Division of the US Army in northwestern Europe.

From the moment he'd landed in Normandy in July 1944, Reilly and the 4th Armored had spearheaded Gen. Patton's Third Army breakout across France. Next, through the winter of 1945, they'd turned their attention to Patton's counteroffensive against the German Bulge. And finally, in May 1945, they'd worked to establish a bridgehead across the River Otava in Strakonice, Czechoslovakia. Following several months of occupation duty—with his volunteer medals and meritorious Bronze Star award in his hands and sufficient service points as a veteran to get him home quickly—Joe Reilly shipped out of Le Havre, France, aboard US Army Transport *Edmund B. Alexander*, arriving in New York Harbor just before Christmas 1945.*

Intent on getting home, all Reilly remembered about the westbound transatlantic trip was that it took just days for the *Alexander* to get to North America, whereas the convoy to Europe, two years before, had taken two weeks. The only other memory of the trip home was that the ship was filled beyond capacity; there were 6,000 GIs all jammed aboard this modest transport vessel, he said. And the ship's company was nearly her undoing on the last leg of the passage into New York. As the *Alexander* approached Liberty Island, everybody rushed to the side of the transport closest to the Statue of Liberty. "The ship tilted. There was nobody on the side opposite the Statue of Liberty," Reilly said. "I swear to God, I thought the damned thing was going to tip over!"[13]

The *Alexander* did eventually dock safely at Camp Kilmer, New Jersey, where S/Sgt. Reilly disembarked and received his mustering-out pay, about $300, and five dollars for transport home to Philadelphia. He remembered a military debriefing that was more brief than it was substantive. US Army demobilization officials told him that his job was to rehabilitate himself back into civilian life. They told the Battle of the Bulge veteran to "suck it up and get on with life," and that he could join the

---

* Not obvious in the ship's name, US Army Transport *Edmund B. Alexander* began life in 1905 as a German-built passenger liner, *Amerika*. During the latter stages of the First World War, she became USS *America* and was then redesignated USAT *America*. Modernized during the Second World War as *E.B. Alexander*, she made transport runs between the United States, North Africa, and Europe, including the repatriation of US troops overseas.

"52-20 Club." That meant the federal government would pay him twenty dollars a week for the first year of his repatriation, provided that each Friday, when he arrived to claim his stipend, he had proof he'd applied for civilian work sometime during the previous seven days. For half of 1946, Reilly recalled whiling away the time between the 52-20 cheques. "I joined the literary guild so I could get all kinds of novels to read," Reilly said. "At night I'd join [friends] and we'd have a couple of beers. That was my life. . . . I was turning into a bum."

It never occurred to him, or anybody else—least of all the military authorities who told him to work his own way back into civilian society—that someone should perhaps assess Joe Reilly's state of mind after ten months of service on the front lines in Europe. It wasn't part of US Army protocol, post–Second World War, to debrief a man whose military unit had endured more than a dozen critical military engagements in France, Belgium, Luxembourg, Germany, and Czechoslovakia. There appeared to be neither the expertise nor the desire among anybody processing him back to civvy street to invite him to explain what he had seen, heard, or felt during his tour of duty as a medic overseas from July 1944 to May 1945. Not that he ever complained; in fact, quite the opposite. Joe Reilly's personality and ethical compass often pushed him to step up and volunteer for more than his share.

During medic training at Fort Bliss, in El Paso, Texas, Pfc. Reilly repeatedly offered to assist the battalion doctor; he said it accelerated his on-the-job learning, including how to deal with people's gripes, real and imagined. He learned to anticipate what might be needed (bandages, adhesive, morphine) and earned the nickname "Little Beaver" for his agility and attitude. During his unit's first days on the Continent in July 1944, the 489th AAA Automatic Weapons Battalion had joined the Third Army breakout in Normandy.

Under normal circumstances, anti-aircraft batteries directed their fire—from 37 mm cannons and .50-calibre machine guns mounted on half-track vehicles—skyward at incoming enemy aircraft. During the Battle of the Hedgerows through Saint-Lô, however, the 489th resorted to firing the same weapons with a level trajectory (horizontally) at enemy troops and armoured vehicles. Jimmy Wyant, a medic with Battery A, reported to Reilly that the firefight he'd experienced was so intense he'd been thrown into the rear of the half-track truck with bullets ricocheting all around him inside the vehicle.

"I'm not going back," Wyant told Reilly during a pause in the fighting. The Battery A medical corpsman was shaking, in a state of shock. "I can't go through that again."

Reilly tried to calm his fellow medic, but the man was inconsolable; Wyant was chain-smoking, Reilly recalled, butting out the cigarettes in the palm of his hand. "Okay, Jimmy, we'll find a replacement . . ."

No doubt playing on Reilly's mind so early in the campaign to liberate France was his experience at Fort Livingston, Virginia, just weeks before—the last stop before the 489th embarked for the posting overseas. Reilly remembered stern-faced indoctrination officers screening a 1943 training film, *Kill or Be Killed*, and lecturing the American troops about what they would face in combat with the enemy in Europe. "You're going to war," the officers had drilled into them. "You're going to be fired on and put in a situation to cause you to run away. But you cannot go to war to fight for your country and then run away." For three days in a row, four times each day, Reilly remembered, the officers—none from his regiment—lectured him and his comrades in no uncertain terms: "You have to know that if you try to run away, you will be shot!" Clearly the dilemma of sending shell-shocked medic Jimmy Wyant back into the front line at Saint-Lô wasn't something the indoctrination officers at Fort Livingston had considered. Reilly was forced to improvise. He asked for a volunteer from among his subordinates to replace Jimmy Wyant. Nobody stepped up. "I'm not going to force anybody," Reilly said, and so he took Wyant's place himself. "Little Beaver" Reilly remained Battery A's medical sergeant for the rest of the war.

Later, in January 1945, when the 489th had raced to the assistance of Allied troops in the Battle of the Bulge in western Belgium, Reilly's battery came under intense enemy fire again. German mortars and artillery shells seemed to arrive from every direction. Reilly leapt into a foxhole with one of the 489th battery gunners. The two hunkered down to wait out the barrage, but before long they could hear calls for a medic out in the battlefield. With his now seasoned reflexes in play, Reilly gathered his medic's kit and began crawling out of the foxhole. The gunner grabbed Reilly to keep him from leaving the safety of the foxhole, but Reilly shook himself loose and—driven by his training and moral compass—dashed to a nearby Jeep, where a GI lay conscious but with a severe head wound. Shrapnel had struck the right side of the man's skull. Reilly was doing a quick check of the man's vital signs just as an army warrant officer (WO) arrived to help remove the wounded soldier.

"Don't you think you should put some sulphonamide powder

on it?" the WO asked Reilly, thinking that such a deep gash needed the disinfectant to prevent infection.

Reilly had never dealt with a head wound like this one before. He could see the inner surface of the man's head because the hair and skin were gone. But, oddly, there was no bleeding. The cut was clear, but there was no visible hemorrhaging.

"If I put the powder on it, they're going to have to clean it off at the aid station," Reilly told the WO; instead he took out a Carlyle bandage, covered the wound and bound it to the man's head. "Since it's not bleeding, all I want to do is protect it, so that they can treat it as soon as he gets there."

The warrant officer seemed to accept Reilly's assessment and made note of both the medic's rapid reflexes, dashing from the foxhole without regard for his own safety, and his cool-headed treatment of the severely wounded GI under fire. He subsequently recommended the medic for a Bronze Star.[14] Reilly never did see the citation acknowledging his actions; what mattered to him was that the soldier with the head wound remained conscious all the way to the aid station. He probably survived.

That spring of 1945, during the final days of the Third Reich, S/Sgt. Reilly's 489th AAA Automatic Weapons Battalion awaited orders in a field near the city of Worms, Germany. Finally they were told to advance toward a German army headquarters building. They found it abandoned. Inside, documents and maps lay strewn across office desks and walls. The captured papers would no doubt be useful acquisitions for American intelligence, but what Reilly considered the most valuable prize of the day was a two-by-five-foot crimson flag with a German swastika at its centre.

As senior NCO he claimed it as his personal souvenir, only later recognizing its dark significance. "When I got home, I realized it was a symbol of hatred and brutality," Reilly said, "and it bothered me."[15]

It's little wonder that Joe Reilly felt out of step with the civilian life he returned to on Catharine Street in Philadelphia in 1946. No surprise either that he retreated into the novels his literary guild supplied him as a kind of sanctuary, or that he relied on the mindless routine of waiting for each Friday to pick up his 52-20 Club instalment. None of the jobs Joe Reilly had secured before the war was held for him: not the one making screen doors and windows, not the one on a drill press at a machine shop, not even his job as a dispatch runner for the Pennsylvania Railroad. He'd been so effective at deliveries that the railroad had issued him a card guaranteeing him free passage anywhere the company operated between Philadelphia and St. Louis. But that was all before the war. In 1946, work wasn't as plentiful and guarantees were out of date.

Nevertheless, that summer he answered five ads in the *Philadelphia Record* newspaper. He finally got a response. A secretary at the Energy Elevator and Dumb Waiter Company phoned and invited him to an interview for a drafting position. He was so nervous he said he didn't know how to get there. She gave him exact instructions, right down to the last trolley transfer, and he arrived punctually for an interview with the owner.

"We had 125 applications for this job," co-owner James Currie told Reilly. "I picked five and you're one of the five."

"I'm primarily interested in improving my mechanical drawing," Reilly said, and then put all his cards on the table, "which means I'd be depending on your instruction."

Currie must have appreciated the veteran's honesty. He called Reilly back in early August.

"Are you going to hire me?" Reilly asked.

"Yes, but I take my family on a two-week vacation the last two weeks in August, so I don't want to see you until the first week in September," Currie said.

Reilly was over the moon. After a week on the job—the pay for which had been advertised as twenty-nine dollars a week— Reilly got a cheque for thirty-five dollars. He asked about the confusion, but his next paycheque was even higher. "After two weeks at Energy, I was making forty dollars," Reilly said. "But the other surprise was, the girl who'd called me and directed me to the job that first day, the secretary, was Anne Hubert."

Anne and Joe were married in 1949, and while she then had to leave the company (according to its no-married-couples policy), his income helped them buy a house and raise a family of six children. He later came to understand the reason why he was so out of step with civilian life when he returned from overseas in 1945: he was suffering from post-traumatic stress syndrome. "Little Beaver" Joe Reilly died in 2016 at age ninety-three.

MAY 1945—DACHAU, GERMANY

WHILE SOME FORMER MEDICS struggled to find a career path stateside, David Wilsey, who had served in the US Seventh Army as an anesthesiologist, quite logically chose to pick up his medical career right where he'd left it before the war. After receiving an honourable discharge, Dr. Wilsey and his family settled in Spokane, Washington, where he established a medical practice as a physician. There in the South Hill residential area of the city, Dr. Wilsey was also reunited with his wife, Emily, and their toddler son, Terry. Throughout his overseas service in 1944 and 1945, Dr. Wilsey had written letters home often, daydreaming about the son he affectionately knew as "Thump," a nickname he'd gained because he kicked so much inside his mother's womb.

"Whenever I see ol' Thump in a snapshot just a-workin' away fixin' or investigatin' something," he wrote to Emily on May 25, 1945, "I just purr all over at his intelligent, cute, lovely, facial expressions. They are so nice."[16]

Capt. Wilsey's light-hearted descriptions of a son he'd not seen in a year, and the easygoing cursive writing on his letter paper home to Emily, masked the man's true state of mind. As with so many who'd seen what he'd seen, the scars were deep. Wilsey had crossed the Atlantic for Europe in 1944 with the 116th Evacuation Hospital. When the United States entered the war in 1941, its medical treatment planners had organized a system of general hospitals, station hospitals, surgical hospitals, and evacuation hospitals, the latter to deliver medical assistance to soldiers and civilians liberated from prison camps. But by March 1943, the US War Department had re-evaluated its medical needs and increased its capacity to 140 station hospitals, twenty-seven general hospitals, fourteen field hospitals, two convalescent hospitals, three surgical hospitals, and twenty-three evacuation hospitals in all theatres of war.

In May 1945, when wartime hospital facilities reached their peak of operation, US military hospitals had 335,000 fixed beds and about 87,000 mobile beds attending to wounded in all theatres; in the European theatre alone, seven hundred hospitals were functioning at that time. In the last two years of the war, US military medical staff tended more sick and wounded personnel—more than five million patients—than at any time previously in the history of the US Army.[17] Capt. Wilsey's 116th Evacuation Hospital was one of twenty-three such facilities following the US infantry in its trek eastward to liberate Europe. The work proved to be nothing at all like the treatment Wilsey had delivered in peacetime America. "My father was an internist before the war," his daughter Clarice Wilsey explained. "He'd never dealt with severed limbs or bellies ripped open by shrapnel."[18]

Evacuation hospitals were located some distance behind the division clearing stations. Typically they housed between 400 and 750 beds, and they kept their patients longer than did the field hospitals. Capt. Wilsey and his medical staff never stayed in one place, however, keeping up with an offensive, moving into a new area, erecting tents, and receiving first casualties all within a few hours. During such large operations as the Battle of the Bulge, for example, when casualties accumulated to their highest levels in Europe, the 116th could have ten to twelve operating tables in use twenty-four hours a day; in a year on the Continent an average evac hospital performed more than 10,000 operations.[19]

"My father delivered thousands of anesthesias," Clarice Wilsey continued. "There might be seven operating tables working at once, and he would just continue going round and round, continuously administering anesthetics."[20]

In the citation that accompanied the Bronze Star awarded

to Capt. David Wilsey, the narrative recognized that "approximately five thousand procedures were performed by the Anesthesia Section. Due to his efforts, no time was lost . . . His superior professional skill, keen judgement . . . and tireless devotion to duty contributed inestimably to the success of each operation."[21] The document was signed by his superior officer and covered the period of Wilsey's service from November 30, 1944, to May 1, 1945. That very day, just a week before VE-Day, Wilsey sat down to write his wife, Emily, back in Elko, Nevada, that the end of the war and their long-anticipated reunion were near.

"The war could end any hour, yet we keep moving, racing, working just as if it weren't over," he lamented, and pointed out that his unit was en route to a new location. He signed off his letter as he often did, with "I love you."[22] However, this time he'd written the phrase nine times, in four long rows at the bottom of the letter.

Almost as he mailed this latest missive to Emily, Capt. Wilsey and other American troops, including members of the 157th Infantry Regiment, had been liberating Dachau, the Nazi concentration camp just outside Munich, in southern Germany. Though the capture of the camp involved some combat with enemy forces, the Americans suffered few if any losses and quickly overran the area. What the liberators of Dachau quickly discovered was a huge complex of ramshackle huts, mortuaries overflowing with bodies, a crematorium, and literally thousands of prisoners suffering from malnutrition, typhus, and a complete absence of hygienic conditions. Capt. Wilsey and members of the 116th Evacuation staff seem to have arrived right after the GIs seized the camp.

"We roared through the gates of Dachau figuratively minutes after its liberation," Wilsey wrote Emily a week later, "while 40,000 wrecks-of-humanity milled, tore, looted, screamed, cried as/like depraved beasts which the Nazi SS has made them."[23]

What Capt. Wilsey experienced in the next hours and days of May 1945 took another sixty-three years to come to light. On December 1, 1945, Capt. Wilsey arrived home in the United States. In 1946 he received his honourable discharge and returned to his medical practice in Nevada. He taught for a few years at the University of Minnesota Medical School and then moved to Spokane, Washington, to establish his Physicians Anesthesia practice. He and Emily raised three children—Terry, Sharon, and Clarice—and were married for fifty-two years. One day, when Clarice was six, she opened a dining room drawer and pulled out several black-and-white images of corpses, left over from the war.

"You're not supposed to look at these," Dr. Wilsey scolded his daughter. "This is something a little girl shouldn't know about."[24] Clarice's father immediately stowed the photos in a trunk in the attic. Anytime the notion of exploring the trunk came up, it was met with a terse "No. Never." from her father.

Once, when Clarice was an adult, conversation with some neighbours revealed that Dr. Wilsey had been among the first to arrive at Dachau. "The prisoners had their arms wide open, needing to be hugged," Dr. Wilsey said, and Clarice recalled her dad explaining that "[I] embraced them even though they were covered in lice and smelled." He went so far as to recount that "when the American physicians went in there, [we] couldn't eat, and were constantly vomiting because of what [we] saw."[25]

"That really touched me," Clarice remembered.

Dr. Wilsey died in 1996, before his daughter could ask him questions about such things. But everything suddenly gelled one day in 2006, when Clarice visited the United States Holocaust Memorial Museum in Washington, DC. Stepping from an elevator, she looked up at a screen showing archival film footage of US troops at a Second World War concentration camp. "And there was my father," she said. "I started shaking." An archivist told her the film was shot at Dachau.

The last piece of the puzzle fell into place after Clarice's mother died in 2008, when the three Wilsey children finally opened the forbidden trunk. In it they found Wilsey's wartime memorabilia—the Bronze Star and citation, a Red Cross arm band, cameras, guns, broken microscope slides, a Nazi swastika flag, and letters he'd sent to their mother, Emily. When Clarice found those letters—written about the time of the liberation of Dachau—the significance of her father's responsibility inside the camp struck her. He was likely the only American in the liberating group who spoke German. "He had to talk to [the prisoners] and convince them they were good doctors . . . there to help them," she said.[26]

The letters revealed how conflicted he was about treating wounded and sick German soldiers, doling out fragments of penicillin pills to them, knowing that American prisoners of war weren't likely getting nearly the same care at German POW camps in Germany and Poland. Then Clarice discovered the darkest secret of the trunk in the attic. In one of his letters addressed to her mom, whom Dr. Wilsey called "My Most Precious Being," she learned what also had happened when American troops and medics entered Dachau.

"In those early minutes, I saw captured SS tortured against the wall and then shot in . . . cold blood," he wrote. "But Emily! God forgive me if I say I saw it done without a single disturbed emotion BECAUSE THEY SO HAD-IT-COMING after what I had just seen and what every minute more I have been seeing of the SS beasts' actions."[27]

The images, the passages, the anger, the distress, the pain cascaded from one letter to the next to the next. Clarice said that while reading the letters, looking at the photographs, and realizing how much her father's service had wounded him, she had never cried so hard in her life.

"For over 8 days, I've seen-lived-smelled-existed it as one of 28 doctors to try to correct the medical-horror component of THE-Hell-On-Earth," Wilsey wrote. Clarice read through these passages that amplified the black-and-white photos she'd stumbled upon in the family dining room drawer years before. He described bodies piled like cordwood, shower rooms used as a ruse to disguise the gas chambers, and the ovens used to dispose of the evidence. After the winter that Wilsey and his medics had endured patching up wounded in the Battle of the Bulge, the prospect of facing this miserable place as well seemed insurmountable. "Stepping high as you walk to work over dead bodies in the street—Storm troopers (the SS), not prisoners, and man-eating Doberman pinscher dogs—all rotting!" Wilsey wrote.[28]

And the deeper Clarice dug into the letters from her father's time at Dachau, the more she recognized that the experience had damaged him permanently. She reflected on the short movie clip at the Holocaust Museum and the intense look on her father's face that the wartime camera had captured on film. "I'd seen that look in my dad before," she said. But there was more intensity, more hurt in subsequent letters to Emily.

"Did I confess how PASSIVELY my canteen cup was used to pour ice river water down SSers' half-naked backs as they stood for hours with a two-arm-up-Heil-Hitler . . . ?" he wrote on May 22, 1945.[29] A combat engineer from California had asked Wilsey if he could borrow the cup. Another staff member with the 116th Evacuation Hospital witnessed the torture as three SS soldiers, stripped to the waist, were forced to stand with their arms outstretched in the Nazi salute. Medic Al Bacchetta said the combat engineer had lost his brother to the SS during the war and "poured water on them from the neck down and it was a cold day in May, and if they moved . . . but it didn't last long, because the GI took all three into a concrete guard house and shot 'em all."[30]

In the weeks following the liberation of Dachau, reports of US troops killing up to fifty SS soldiers who'd either surrendered or been captured were disclosed. Within a month, by June 1945, the US military had gathered evidence and issued a report, "Investigation of Alleged Mistreatment of German Guards at Dachau," which concluded that several GIs accused of the abuses should be court-martialled. Stories abounded, apparently apocryphal, that Gen. George Patton had been so incensed by the recommendations that he'd personally ordered the reports to be burned.[31] Despite the rumour, however, the US Seventh Army eventually acquired all the documentation. But not until the Wilsey children decided to donate their father's memorabilia and letters to the Holocaust Museum was the shroud lifted on this personal horror story.

By the middle of July 1945, Capt. Wilsey had come out the other side of his concentration camp assignment, in the place he called "Damn, Dastardly, Dirty, Dismal, Den Dachau." He and his 116th Evacuation Hospital staff had converted the dormitories where SS officers had housed their mistresses into mass treatment wards. The doctors and medics had attended to hundreds and hundreds of Holocaust survivors for tuberculosis, typhus, lice infestations, and malnutrition. At the end of it all, he'd sent back pictures to Emily of the piles of bodies of the victims they couldn't save. "This, Madam, AND ALL THE WORLD, is just a sample of what we saw and lived days after we hit Dachau," he wrote, and should anyone not believe his story, he signed off, "P.S. YOU BET! I WAS THERE!"[32]

Clarice Wilsey and her siblings have spent much of their time since 2008 sharing the contents of their father's wartime trunk with museums, libraries, and education centres in the United States and abroad. She considers the work her calling in life and that she is her father's voice today. It remains for Clarice a painful exercise to revisit and review this extraordinary collection from a medical officer who endured too much. Indeed, she still searches for answers to questions she wishes she could have asked her father.

"There's a sort of emptiness, not being able to talk to him about it," she said. "But . . . I'm so glad [he was] such a loving healing person for these people. He was a light amongst that evil."[33]

...

MARCH 28, 2011—ORLEANS, ONTARIO

FROM THE MOMENT SHE BEGAN her deployment training for Afghanistan, in 2006, medic Alannah Gilmore learned to keep her ears and eyes open to activity five or ten feet in front of her, off to the side, and even behind her. Quite literally, that distance might be all that would separate her from a remotely activated improvised explosive device, with even less distance and time to react and avoid its consequences. Lay people might call it knowing one's environment; Gilmore called it "situational awareness."[34] Throughout her tour in the Panjwaii district during Operation Medusa, and in Kandahar City, M/Cpl. Gilmore paid serious attention to any and all intelligence available to her in the Canadian Army. As the crew commander of a Bison ambulance, she'd listen to other crew commanders, fellow medics, and engineers about the latest on firefights with the enemy. Then she'd run scenarios through her head, expecting the worst. What weapons might she be facing if called upon to defend her ambulance? Were insurgents suddenly packing IEDs inside soapboxes? If there was one suicide bombing, could a secondary bomber be lurking nearby?

"We wake up one morning, around 7:15, with a big explosion outside our gate," she said. "A guy detonated a bomb in his vest, full of ball bearings. But I had nightmares. What if they sent two suicide bombers together?"

This was no figment of her imagination, no *Call of Duty* shooter fantasy. During her first tour, in the Panjwaii district, M/Cpl. Gilmore and her crew responded to an incident involving a Canadian convoy of Bison armoured vehicles. Canadian soldiers Robert Girouard and Albert Storm were shuttling Christmas presents to a forward operating base; en route, a suicide bomber drove into their vehicle, killing both Canadians. The carnage at the scene illustrated the randomness of Taliban attacks; the suicide bomber had set off the explosive near a market and an orphanage. It occurred to Gilmore that she and her crew could be racing right into the centre of a bombing with a second bomber lurking. In a Canadian deployment following Gilmore's tour in Afghanistan, two medics—Kristal Giesebrecht and Andrew Miller—responded to a report of a mine found in the doorway of a building outside Kandahar City. When they arrived on the scene, their vehicle triggered an IED. Both died in the secondary explosion. "Even though you're responding to one bomber, there was always the potential of another," Gilmore said.

As much as Gilmore would have preferred to leave what she'd experienced in Afghanistan behind her, she couldn't. Upon her return home in 2007, she reconnected with the Canadian sniper she'd attended to in January of that year, at Masum Ghar. Jody Mitic had begun rehabilitation in the aftermath of the land-mine explosion that had forced the amputation of both feet. Alannah helped Jody adjust to life after Afghanistan; they had much in common in that regard and settled down together, having a child soon after. And though she had worked for a while helping to train the next contingent of Canadians—3rd Battalion RCR—deploying to Afghanistan, she never really fully removed herself from her own deployment. The attention to detail and preparedness she'd developed in training and active service over there were impossible to shake. Try as she might, she could never completely shut down that reflex back home. She even tried medication to calm that part of her brain. In spite of those efforts, and even without the daily demands of active service in a theatre of war, her muscle memory remained intact.

Then it happened. On a Sunday in late March 2011, Alannah and Jody were travelling on a main thoroughfare in Ottawa when they approached a five-car collision in which one vehicle had T-boned a van. A police officer was on the scene, but he had just arrived and had his hands full. Jody said to Alannah, "It's go time."

Gilmore's reflexes responded to the crisis almost involuntarily. First she did a run-around, telling one driver to turn off his ignition. Then she found a woman, a nurse, leaning into the van; the side door had buckled, pinning a small girl. The mother was crying hysterically. Alannah shut everything else out and got inside the van, crawling as close to the girl as she could, manually trying to maintain a clear airway. When firefighters arrived, she began calling to them for life-saving equipment and oxygen. "I was like, 'Thank God! Just hand it to me! I need this! I need that!'" she recalled, attending to the girl as quickly as first responders could get her the gear.

When the paramedics arrived, Gilmore remained next to the little girl and completed the handover to them. Despite every effort, however, the child later died. Small consolation, perhaps, but Gilmore had responded with the same authority and skill as she had on deployment in Afghanistan. Her muscle memory had not failed her. Nor would it on another occasion, when she came across a vehicle with a woman slumped over the steering wheel. The woman's daughter had pulled the car off the road, but the mother had passed out while suffering a heart attack. Alannah and another bystander pulled the woman from the car. "She came out like a rag doll, like she was dead. No pulse," Alannah said. "We did CPR and then the paramedics arrived."

Thanks to the quick response by Alannah and the bystander, the woman recovered completely. Gilmore was later awarded a Chief of Defence Staff Commendation and a Chief of Military Personnel Commendation.*

"Medics on the whole—we're not a very familiar trade," she said. "I'm basically a glorified first-aider. I have knowledge and I will use whatever I need to. I'll MacGyver whatever I have to, to make it happen."

NOVEMBER 11, 2014—PORT PERRY, ONTARIO

BACK ON CIVVY STREET IN 2011, Alannah Gilmore recognized that while she could take the medic out of the war zone, taking the war zone out of the medic was a tougher proposition. When army medic Arnold Hodgkins was demobilized back to Canada after the Second World War, he faced a similar predicament. His experience with the No. 2 Canadian Light Field Ambulance overseas—more than three years attached to the Ontario Tank Corps, fighting from Sicily and Italy to France, Belgium, Holland, and Germany—had trained his body to respond to medical trauma in the battlefield, but it

---

* Gilmore had already received two commendations for her military service—in 2004, the CO's Commendation for Service in Alert, and the Commander in Chief Commendation for her deployment to Afghanistan, 2006–7. In all, she put in twenty-three years of service in the Canadian Forces.

had also created muscle memory of a different sort: an urge to sketch and paint what he saw.

Growing up in rural southwestern Ontario, Arnold had delved into many vocations—junior banker, bookkeeper, truck driver, and construction worker—but his mother, Frances, encouraged avocations such as piano playing, sketching, and painting. In 1928, on her deathbed, Frances entreated him to continue his pursuit of art; he composed his first song, "Lonely," and then "Muskoka Moon," made famous by orchestra leader Luigi Romanelli. During the Depression he wrote, directed, and performed in musical plays while helping to feed the family by assisting the local undertaker, embalming and digging graves. He married Iola Houser in 1934 and they took over a funeral business and started a sign shop in Campden, Ontario. All the while, Arnold continued teaching himself to paint. In the first year of the war, the Hodgkins had a son, Gary, and then Arnold enlisted in the Royal Canadian Army Medical Corps.

His light ambulance unit embarked for Britain in June 1941, and while his medic's kit and manual occupied most of his attention, his daily journal of personal observations, travel commentary, and sketches was always within reach. Training and preparing for an invasion occupied his next year, in the United Kingdom. He experienced his first contact with casualties at Newhaven on the south coast, where the first wounded from Dieppe arrived late in the day on August 19, 1942; in his journal he called it "a thunder in the channel . . . And the breath of death was blowing. Down the shore where heroes crept."[35] Then, with broken bones set, wounds packed, and drugs administered to the wounded, Sgt. Hodgkins and his ambulance comrades found comfort in their peacetime hobbies—stamp collecting, antique buying, and jewellery making.

"It had been my good fortune to build up rather a widely representative art portfolio," he wrote, "sketches of Loch Lomond . . . Edith Cavell's monument . . . the grey, time-smoothed multi pillars of Westminster."[36] One sketch was a pastel of a young British pilot looking brave, determined, and braced for the unknown. "He was killed in action twelve hours after the sketch," Hodgkins said.[37]

By December 1943, Sgt. Hodgkins and his No. 2 Canadian Light Field Ambulance unit had moved with their armoured regiment, the Ontario Tanks, from Sicily onto the boot of Italy. They had smashed through the Germans' fallbacks—the Hitler Line and the Gustav Line—and were advancing toward the German stronghold at Ortona. Members of the Canadian medical corps had handled more than 2,300 casualties during the fighting in Sicily, and another 650 in the approaches to Ortona. With a medical officer (Laurence Alexander, the captain decorated for his service at Dieppe), a corporal, four combat orderlies, three combat drivers, two ambulance drivers, a truck driver, a Jeep driver, a batman, a dispatch rider, and medic Hodgkins, also on a motorcycle, the No. 2 Field had travelled and treated their armoured comrades every step of the way.

A week into December, the Ontario Tanks had dug in north of San Vito while combat engineers prepared a Canadian assault across the Moro River toward Ortona. That gave Hodgkins time to repair a flat on his motorcycle, nicknamed "Gariola." "It is disappointing to realize that ugly destruction lurks at every hairpin bend of the mountain roads. . . . Too much depends upon getting men, guns and tanks across [the

Moro] to work on [Field-Marshal Albert] Kesselring's famous line," he wrote.[38]

As the tankers and ambulance corps awaited completion of the engineers' handiwork at the river, Hodgkins and the rest of his field ambulance crew settled in and around a *casa*, a farmhouse (with the farm family going about its daily chores); for several days a large front room with a fireplace in the farmhouse became the No. 2's regimental aid post. Very quickly, wounded arrived from just ahead of them.

A badly burned tank driver was rushed in. One orderly retrieved fresh water for Doc Alexander to clean the driver's wounds, while Hodgkins pulled gauze from his medic's kit. They learned the wounded man's Sherman tank had been hit by a German 88 shell, which blew the hatches off the tank and set the vehicle on fire, killing or wounding the rest of his crew. In minutes Alexander had sulpha powder covering the man's wounds, and Hodgkins prepared the last step in the treatment.

"A long strip of gauze, Sergeant," Alexander told Hodgkins.[39]

Working from the man's shoulder downward to the wrist and hand, Alexander wound the dressing firmly over the burned flesh.

"Want me to take over?" Hodgkins asked.

The doctor nodded and began to work on the driver's other arm.

"Water?" Hodgkins asked the driver, and the tanker smiled yes.

Following the first aid, Hodgkins caught his breath and allowed himself to think about the lives of the men about him in the room. Instinctively the field medic's thoughts turned to his refuge. "The old itchiness to sketch something of the fleeting scene assails me. Anything," Hodgkins wrote later. "And so I sketch it. It is of no value as a picture, but will serve to remind me one day (should Lady Fortune ever break down and dish out) that I have not always slept in expensive hotels."[40]

Lady Fortune appeared to abandon Arnold Hodgkins completely just twenty-four hours later. On December 10, 1943, as the sergeant medic drove Gariola through the Moro River crossing with the No. 2 Field Ambulance crew, his bike ran over a Teller mine that exploded and badly tore the muscles in both his lower legs and additionally wounded his right arm and head. He was evacuated to the coastal town of Vasto, where surgeons determined they needed to amputate both legs; Hodgkins protested, and instead his legs were salvaged. In Malta for three months to recuperate, the wounded medic craved his favourite pastime; a nursing sister travelled miles to obtain art supplies so her patient could return to his sketching.[41]

Evacuated to England in the spring of 1944, Hodgkins went through a difficult rehab. One afternoon he passed a closet mirror and caught sight of himself. "I am startled to behold the reflection of a stranger," he wrote in his journal. "His face is ghastly white beneath the tan. There gleams an expression of cold flint from narrowed eye-lids. No love, no patience, no peace can be found written on that grim countenance. Only dull, frozen fury . . . My God! Is that me?"[42]

Despite the lingering after-effects of his wounds—shrapnel in his legs, a resulting limp, and periodic blackouts—Hodgkins was eager to rejoin the active medical corps during the invasion of France. He took a demotion to private so that he could serve with No. 6 Field Dressing Station under Laurence Alexander, the medical officer with whom he'd served in Sicily and Italy. Ashore in France in the summer of 1944, with the Canadians liberating the country, the then thirty-three-year-old medic happened on a jail in Livarot where the Maquis (French Resistance) were evening the score with Nazi collaborators. He sketched the dingy prison, the young Maquis guard, the rabid mob eager for revenge, and the shamed collaborators, their heads shorn clean. He showed his sketch to a comrade. "He does not criticize me for drawing the ugly thing," Hodgkins wrote. "He knows it is the logical means of removing something off a man's mind."[43]

With this sketch and hundreds more in his medic's satchel, Pte. Hodgkins completed his overseas service with the Royal Canadian Army Medical Corps, returned to the United Kingdom in time for VJ-Day in Piccadilly Circus in London, and was repatriated to Canada in September 1945. His son Gary was five when Arnold Hodgkins came home from the war. Family noted that Arnold was not the same man, that time and war had scarred him. "Now he walked with a limp and carried a new portfolio of memories,"[44] a friend wrote. The very next month he enrolled in courses at the Ontario College of Art in Toronto (completing the four-year course in three) and launched his career as a professional artist. Upon graduation, Hodgkins operated art studios, gave art instruction, and took commissions in portraiture in Toronto; then the veteran and artist developed the Deerfoot Art Settlement and Gallery near Leaskdale, Ontario.

It took years, his daughter Carol Hodgkins-Smith said, but Arnold's war sketches eventually took shape as paintings. Like the sketching he did after Dieppe, at the *casa* near the

Moro River, while recuperating in Malta, and at the prison in Livarot, once home, Hodgkins faced his demons by putting the "portfolio of memories" to paint on canvas.

In time, Carol Hodgkins-Smith began displaying her father's war art privately on the walls of her home in Port Perry, Ontario. In 2014, in time for Remembrance Day observances on November 11, she opened her home for the public to see the art of his wartime journey—soldiers in crisis, a nurse, civilians in flight, villages in ruin, medics attending wounded. Once, while still overseas, Arnold Hodgkins was so desperate to respond to this urge to record what he'd seen that one evening he pleaded with a French civilian for a table and a small light to allow him to sketch.

"I would gladly pay," Hodgkins explained.

"*Non, non, Monsieur*," she replied. "We have no oil, no candles. The Boche, he took everything when he passed through."

Eventually a fellow medic found Hodgkins a lighted compartment in an ambulance.

"I try it," Hodgkins wrote later. "But it is futile. There is far too much to divert from the cool strong flow of reasoning. . . . Maybe tomorrow."[45]

OCTOBER 2017—CAMPHOLZ WOODS, GERMANY

LIKE BOTH CLARICE WILSEY and Carol Hodgkins-Smith, I needed to grow into adulthood before I could seek out my father's wartime hell. And I found it on an October afternoon in 2017. To me the place looked pretty tranquil. In the distance, tri-bladed turbines turned lazily in the breeze. Off to one side, a white-fenced paddock and an affluent-looking complex of horse barns and riding stables seemed to give order to the landscape. The only ones taking notice of me—a couple of horses, their bodies blanketed, their cannons wrapped—lifted their heads in unison but, recognizing no apparent threat, returned to their grazing. Where I stood, at the edge of a freshly cultivated farm field, I could see the shadows the sun cast along perfectly furrowed rows. And just beyond the rolling earth, a bluff of trees at the end of their season's growth showed off amber and golden leaves. On my map that forest was called Campholz Woods. To me, in October of 2017, the place seemed bucolic.

But not to my father when he first saw it. Not tranquil. Not orderly. Not peaceful. Definitely threatening.

The first time he learned about these woods, T/Sgt. Alex Barris saw them as an amoeba-like grey blob on a topographical map at an improvised first-aid station in Borg, Germany. And at that time—the first week of February 1945—Campholz Woods, just west of the River Moselle, wasn't considered pastoral. It was a military objective, a place to be seized, overrun, if necessary destroyed, and its enemy occupants killed or captured.

My father, barely twenty-two, served as a platoon leader in the medical battalion and was responsible for about a dozen medics. On February 12, 1945, he had dispatched a group of stretcher-bearers and junior medics to retrieve American wounded from a battle raging somewhere out there in that same Campholz Woods. When they failed to return, my father quickly recognized that it was up to him to find them—in the dark, in the snow—and if possible lead them out of the woods and back to that first-aid station, a vacated farmhouse on the reverse side of a hill in Borg, about a mile south of the woods.

When I walked part of that mile in October 2017, it was

in broad daylight and the air was warm. I had joined a tour, principally members of an American historical society commemorating the anniversary of the 94th Infantry Division's liberation of this part of Germany in 1945. I had asked for time to myself—away from the thirty or so other travellers—to retrace my father's steps alone. Thirteen years after his death in 2004, I had come all the way from North America to be at this spot, to imagine what my father had experienced during the Second World War. Until that day I had never walked on the war-torn ground he had known as a military medic. I'd never come this close to my father's hell. I began striding out over the farm field, heading north toward Campholz Woods alone, the way he had. For me it was nothing to cross that ground, stepping over the furrows at a leisurely pace. I started my cellphone recorder—as if verifying aloud with my dad what he had experienced there—and was overcome by emotion.

"You walked here, Dad," I said into the recorder. "Crossed this very ground, not in fall but in winter, through knee-deep snow. Not across a plowed farm field but across a battlefield sown with *Schü* mines. Not in daylight, but in darkness!"[46]

My walk at a steady pace toward the woods took ten minutes. I was a tourist in Germany, walking freely. His repeated crossings of that ground must have taken hours. His was a life-and-death mission. Campholz was deceptive. From across the field the forest looked accessible, easy to penetrate. But the closer I drew to the woods, the fewer seemed my options for entry. The view ahead darkened as the crowns of the trees overhead obscured the light, and the dense brush nearer the ground blocked my path at every turn. Eventually, when I discovered a way in, I had to crouch, protect my face with my arms and force my way through the brush. I'm sure the config-uration of the woods would have been different the night my father slogged through snow here, over seventy years ago. But somehow Campholz's present impenetrable exterior sharp-ened the sensations I felt.

"You had sent your medics out here to bring back the wounded from the woods. Now you had to find them and guide them back," I said through tears into my cellphone. "You were responsible for them. You had to bring as many back alive as possible. How? How the hell did you do this?"

DECEMBER 1945—MANHATTAN, NEW YORK

IT WAS THE ODDEST WELCOME HOME he could ever have imagined. Just a week before Christmas in 1945, a few days after his honourable discharge from the US Army, my father, the now former wartime medic, hopped on the New York City subway and travelled from the family home in Jackson Heights, in Queens, to 59th Street and 10th Avenue. There in midtown Manhattan, Alex Barris returned to his alma mater, Haaren High School, from which he'd graduated—the only member of his family ever to finish high school—in 1939. It wasn't a nostalgia trip: my dad wanted to retrieve his senior matriculation records in case he needed them when upgrading his skills or searching for work.

In its prime, Haaren had been the largest high-school build-ing in America, offering vocational programs that ranged from basic art classes to the building of internal combustion engines.

Among its distinguished alumni were Herman Badillo, the first Puerto Rican elected to the US House of Representatives; John Worth, iconic designer of model aeronautics; Paul Rand, ADC Hall-of-Fame illustrator and creator of, among other things, the corporate logos for IBM, Westinghouse, and ABC; photojournalist Ed Feingersh, whose subjects were as diverse as Marilyn Monroe and the Korean War's Battle of Pork Chop Hill; Irish poet Padraic Fiacc; Soviet spy David Greenglass; and actors Albert Salmi and Robert Mitchum.

But my father, the ex–US Army tech sergeant returning to the school this December day in 1945, was not among those illustrious alumni. The war was over. He'd completed his voluntary service. At twenty-three, and like hundreds of thousands of other ex-GIs, seeking celebrity status didn't figure into his future plans. Dad just needed to find his way back to civvy street, land a job, maybe reconnect with his friend Koula Kontozoglou, and get his life back on track.

As he waited to meet with the school registrar about collecting his high-school records—just in case he ever decided to go to college under provisions of the Servicemen's Readjustment Act, or GI Bill—my father paused in front of a recently renovated wall in the school's main foyer. As with many American high schools, where pride in armed service ranked highest among those attributes recognized and commemorated on the school premises, Haaren had updated its honour roll to include the names of former students killed in the recently ended war. Having graduated from Haaren some six years before, my father did not expect to find anyone he knew among the columns of names etched alphabetically on the plaque. He couldn't think of anybody from the 94th killed in action who might be commemorated on the Haaren High School honour roll.

"Alumni Who Gave Their Lives in World War II," it said across the top of the commemorative wall. Beneath the heading the list was lengthy. My father recounted how he'd been startled at the number of names filling the columns on the wall— dozens and dozens, arranged alphabetically. After a time, Alex found himself counting the names rather than reading them. By the time he'd reached the bottom of the last column, he'd counted fifty-six. Then the most incredible thing happened. He called it "a frozen second." He saw his own name etched there in the bronze. Dead. Honoured. But it was a mistake.

"That's crazy," Alex said.[47] And he turned for the office where the school registrar was retrieving his records.

"Your transcript is ready," she said, meeting him at the office door. "Here you are, and good luck to you, young man."

My father took the paper, but he was still shaken by what he'd just read at the honour roll. "Thank you," he said, and then added, "but there's another thing. That scroll out there in the hallway has a mistake on it. It says I'm dead. But I'm not."

Rather than responding with some empathy for the mix-up, the woman's face grew disapprovingly into a frown. "That isn't a thing to joke about, soldier. I just don't know what it is that the war has done to some of you boys."

"Ma'am," he said as calmly as he could. "I'm not joking. I'll mail you a photostatic copy of my army discharge, so someone can correct that error out there."

My father remembered the woman blushing with embarrassment. She blurted out an "Oh my. Someone will be in trouble over this . . ." and she returned to her office.

Alex saw no point in lingering. He mumbled a final thank-you and walked back down the hallway toward the exit. He remembered that he couldn't help but pause to read his name one more time on that scroll of honoured dead. And there was yet an additional irony to the inscription. The bronzed honour roll displayed the name *Alex Barbaritis*. That was my father's name when he'd attended Haaren in the 1930s, all right. But, in a way, the war had even changed that. My father's older brother, Angelo, who had joined the US Army a year before Alex, got sick and tired of people completely mis-pronouncing the family surname, making it sound like a scalp disease. Even worse, my uncle couldn't stand his army buddies using the pejorative oversimplification of Angelo Barbaritis to "Angelo the Greek." And since their mother had separated from their father years earlier, the contraction of Barbaritis to Barris seemed to solve a lot of problems. It did not, however, resolve the mistaken conclusion by Haaren High School that my father had been killed in action.

"The correction," my father later wrote, "was never made. The old Haaren building was torn down sometime in the 1980s, so I guess my premature demise was eventually rescinded, or else demolished along with the building."[48]

For whatever reason—perhaps because he was too polite to demand that the honour roll be corrected, its content reviewed, and its deadly inscription removed—my father chose not to pursue the matter. After all, he certainly didn't consider himself among the school's illustrious grads with bur-geoning high-profile careers. He was just another GI with just another honourable record of service in the war just won. He had enlisted on December 12, 1942, not as a patriot intent on winning the Congressional Medal of Honor but because he knew that, eventually, the war consuming Europe and (after December 1941) the Pacific would come looking for him.

In fact, my father never let any inflated sense of his three years of service—which ended with an honourable discharge on December 18, 1945—get the better of his ego. Except for one of his active service awards, his discharge papers—which I tracked down at the National Personnel Records Center in St. Louis, Missouri—appeared pretty standard; he'd been awarded the requisite World War II Victory Medal, the American Service Medal, the European–African–Middle Eastern Campaign Medal, and the Good Conduct Medal. His Bronze Star had been one of 2,538 awarded to members of the US Army 94th Infantry Division.

It could be that the most persuasive of my father's reasons not to fuss over the error on the Haaren honour roll came from a memory of one of his high-school teachers and the warning she'd offered in the late 1930s. In a memoir my father composed in the 1980s, *Growing Up Greek*, he recalled the wisdom of a history instructor, a Mrs. Aaronson. He admired her because she was outspoken, fearless, and controversial in front of her students. When Adolf Hitler defied the League of Nations in 1936 and began to remilitarize the Rhineland, that buffer between Germany and France, his beloved history teacher told her pupils they should be alarmed. How many Depression-era teenagers had even a glimmering of what the Rhineland was or what its importance might be to world affairs? Still, my father recalled her dire prediction: "It is quite possible, even probable," Mrs. Aaronson had warned the class, "that Hitler's aggressive moves will lead to war. And believe me if it becomes a large war, it will change your lives forever . . . forever!"[49]

Had my father only known. Not only was Mrs. Aaronson's premonition accurate in its scale and impact, but also, in the case of my father's war service specifically, in its reference to the location where she said the greatest threat lay. It was in that so-called buffer between France and Germany, the Rhineland, where the toughest and most indelible part of my father's war would take place. Alex's haphazard streaming by his military superiors into becoming a medical corpsman, the timing of his arrival in Europe and the coincidental circumstances surrounding the Battle of the Bulge, and his own instinctive sense of looking out for others—perhaps ingrained during those moments of candour in Mrs. Aaronson's history class—would determine my father's military fate and the fates of those who depended on him in the bloody winter of 1944–45.

But while Mrs. Aaronson got it right, Haaren High's record-keepers did not. They determined that Alex Barbaritis, who was really Alex Barris, had died overseas. "You cannot begin to imagine what a chilling experience it is to see yourself listed as killed in action," Dad wrote later.[50]

More than that, at least symbolically, they had erased the story of a citizen who recognized the perceived threat of the time, responded to his country's call to arms, accepted the military's assignment to train and serve in the medical corps, and learned to survive and improve the chance of others' survival to the best of his ability. He learned that he would be sworn to do all of this while armed only with a medic's bag slung around his neck, a Red Cross emblem displayed on his helmet, and little more than the wits in his head and the devotion in his heart to meet that commitment until that war was won.

Finally, I think, my father came to understand the most hazardous aspect of his job description as a member of a medical battalion deployed to a killing zone. While others in the heat of combat on the front line might ultimately choose to flee from the perceived or real danger, it was his duty and moral obligation to rush toward it. His story—and the stories of those men and women who choose to meet that lethal challenge—deserve to be remembered.

SOURCES

Unpublished Sources

AUTHOR INTERVIEWS

Marion Andros, New York, NY, November 29, 2014
Alex Barris, Agincourt, ON, June 1964
Angelo Barris, New York, NY, November 28, 2014
Stephen Bell, Uxbridge, ON, May 21, 1993
Keith Besley, Toronto, ON, July 17, 1997
Jim Brittain, Oshawa, ON, October 22, 2014
Tony Burns, Halifax, NS, May 24, 2004
Frank Cullen, Toronto, ON, July 17, 1997
Dennis Daniel, Colorado Springs, CO, August 30, 2014
Bill Davis, Portland, ON, November 6, 1977
Jim and Ray Duffield, Toronto, ON, August 15, 2015
Jerome Fatora, Luxembourg City, Luxembourg, October 5, 2017
Don Flieger, Kitchener, ON, April 15, 1998
Bill Foley, Dallas, TX, September 8, 2015
Mary Gaudet, Charlottetown, PEI, March 11, 2019
Alannah Gilmore, Ottawa, ON, October 13, 2017
Dane Harden, Windsor, ON, August 13, 2016
George Hodgkinson, Pembroke, ON, July 29, 2016
Reg Hodgson, St. Albert, AB, February 14, 2018
Harry Helms, West Brandywine, PA, July 12, 2015
John Meirion Jones, Tholthorpe, UK, July 26, 2018
Greg Leperides, Parsippany, NJ, November 22, 2015
Dave Lewis, Uxbridge, ON, April 9, 2016
Norman Malayney, Winnipeg, MB, June 1, 2016
Frank Matthews, Triangle, VA, July 2014
Sharon and Tony Mellaci, Eatontown, NJ, August 18 and 19, 2015
David Mitchell, Atlanta, GA, June 2015

Jody Mitic, Ottawa, ON, May 17, 2016

Anne and Joe Reilly, Warminster, PA, August 20, 2015

Herb Ridyard Jr., Trier, Germany, October 10, 2017

Herb Ridyard Sr., Luxembourg City, Luxembourg, October 5, 2017

Marketa Schusterova, Toronto, ON, October 2016

Al Theobald, Borg, Germany, October 6, 2017

Clarice Wilsey, Spokane, WA, September 12, 2016

Bill Wilson, Borden, ON, November 23, 2004

OTHER INTERVIEWS

Bob Donaldson, interview with Al Bachetta, November 14, 2011

Vladimir Krizek, interview with Marketa Schusterova, Vodňany, Czech Republic, October 2016

Herbert Thistle, interview with Alex Barris, St. John's, NL, August 24, 1993

Grace MacPherson, interview with CBC Radio, March 9, 1963, Part 1, Library and Archives Canada, RG41, vol. 22

Unpublished Works

Barris, Alex. *Growing Up Greek*, unpublished manuscript, author's collection.

———. *Moonshine Glory*, unpublished manuscript, author's collection.

Drake, Harriet, *World War I Letters and Newspaper Clippings of Nursing Sister Harriet Drake*, Martha E. McKenna, ed., Osler Library, McGill University Archives, 2007.

Elliott, O.A. *Personal Diary O.A. Elliott, No. 5 Canadian Field Ambulance.*

Gurd, Fraser B. Unpublished diaries, diagrams, and case studies, George Metcalf Archival Collection, Canadian War Museum, accession 201550239.

Hodgkins, Arnold. Unpublished diaries, War Journey Series, Book No. 3, 1942; Book No. 5, 1943; Book No. 16, 1943; Book No. 17, 1943; Book No. 18, 1944; Book No. 19A, 1944, courtesy of Carol Hodgkins-Smith.

Kennedy, John Jack Campbell. Unpublished diary and letters, courtesy of Lisa Boyce.

Macpherson, Cluny. "An Episode at the War Office, 1915," *Reflections of a Newfoundlander*, Notebook #2, Faculty of Medicine Founders' Archive, Health Sciences Library, Memorial University, St. John's, NL.

MacPherson, Grace. Personal diaries, 1916–18, courtesy of Diana Filer.

Van Nest, Paul. "Remembering Richard," speech, Fredericksburg Civil War Roundtable, Jepson Alumni Center, Mary Washington University, Fredericksburg, VA, May 28, 2008.

319th Medical Battalion, Regimental Aid Station Log, 94th Infantry Division Collection, Hargrett Rare Book and Manuscript Library, University of Georgia, Athens.

PUBLISHED SOURCES

BOOKS

Alexander, Larry. *Biggest Brother: The Life of Major Dick Winters, the Man Who Led the Band of Brothers*. New York: Penguin, 2005.

Ambrose, Stephen E. *Band of Brothers: E Company, 506th, 101st Airborne from Normandy to Hitler's Eagle's Nest*. New York: Simon & Shuster, 1992.

———. *Citizen Soldiers: The U.S. Army from the Normandy Beaches to the Bulge to the Surrender of Germany, June 7, 1944–May 7, 1945*. New York: Simon & Shuster, 1997.

———. *D-Day June 6, 1944: The Climactic Battle of World War II*. New York: Simon & Shuster, 1995.

Auer, George Scott. *Soldiers of the Soil: Grey County Goes to War, 1914–1918*. Owen Sound, ON: Ginger Press, 2016.

Barrett, Harry B. *Port Dover's Nursing Sisters of World War I: Memories of Minnie and Laurel Misner*. Simcoe, ON: Who-Did-It Club, 2013.

Barris, Alex, and Ted Barris. *Days of Victory: Canadians Remember, 1939–1945*, Toronto: Macmillan, 1995.

Barris, Ted. *Days of Victory: Canadians Remember 1995–1945*, sixtieth anniversary edition, Toronto: Thomas Allen, 2005.

———. *Deadlock in Korea: Canadians at War, 1950–1953*. Toronto: Macmillan, 1999.

———. *Juno: Canadians at D-Day, June 6, 1944*. Toronto: Thomas Allen, 2003.

———. *Victory at Vimy: Canada Comes of Age, April 9–12, 1917*, Toronto: Thomas Allen, 2007.

Benz, Wolfgang and Barbara Distel, eds. *Dachau and the Nazi Terror, Vol. II Studies and Reports*. Brussels: Comite International de Dachau, 2002.

Bessner, Ellin. *Double Threat: Canadian Jews, the Military, and World War II*. Toronto: New Jewish Press, 2018.

Betts, Amanda, ed. *In Flanders Fields: 100 Years*. Toronto: Alfred A. Knopf Canada, 2015.

Booton, Herndon. *The Unlikeliest Hero: The Story of Desmond T. Doss, Conscientious Objector Who Won His Nation's Highest Military Honor*. Boise, ID: Pacific Press Publishing, 1967.

Boyko, John. *Blood and Daring: How Canada Fought the American Civil War and Forged a Nation*. Toronto: Alfred A. Knopf Canada, 2013.

Bruce, Jean. *Back the Attack: Canadian Women During the Second World War—At Home and Abroad*. Toronto: Macmillan, 1985.

Byrnes, Laurence G., ed. *History of the 94th Infantry Division in World War II*. Washington, DC: Infantry Journal Press, 1948.

Cambon, Kenneth. *Guest of Hirohito*, Vancouver: PW Press, 1990.

Campbell, Ian J. *Murder at the Abbaye: The Story of Twenty Canadian Soldiers Murdered at the Abbaye d'Ardenne*. Ottawa: Golden Dog Press, 1996.

Canadian Jews in World War II, Part I, Decorations. Montreal: Canadian Jewish Congress, 1947.

Cassel, Robert, ed. *94th Infantry Division Association Commemorative History*. Dallas: Taylor Publishing Co., 1989.

Catton, Bruce. *The Civil War*. New York: American Heritage Press, 1960.

Churchill, Winston S. *The Second World War: The Hinge of Fate*. Boston: Houghton Mifflin Company, 1950.

Clarkson, Adrienne. *Norman Bethune*. Toronto: Penguin, 2009.

Coco, Gregory A. *A Vast Sea of Misery: A History and Guide to the Union and Confederate Field Hospital at Gettysburg, July 1–November 20, 1863*. Gettysburg, PA: Thomas Publications, 1988.

Cook, Tim. *At the Sharp End: Canadians Fighting the Great War, 1914–1916*, Volume One. Toronto: Viking, 2007.

———. *No Place to Run: The Canadian Corps and Gas Warfare in the First World War*. Vancouver: University of British Columbia Press, 1999.

———. *Shock Troops: Canadians Fighting the Great War, 1917–1918*, Volume Two. Toronto: Viking, 2008.

———. *The Secret History of Soldiers: How Canadians Survived the Great War*. Toronto: Penguin, 2018.

Copp, Terry and Bill McAndrew. *Battle Exhaustion: Soldiers and Psychiatrists in the Canadian Army, 1939–1945*. Montreal and Kingston: McGill-Queen's University Press, 1990.

Cowdrey, Albert E. *Fighting for Life: American Military Medicine in World War II*. New York: Simon & Shuster, 1994.

———. *The Medic's War: United States Army in the Korean War*. Washington, DC: Center of Military History, US Army, 1987.

Cross, Robin. *The Battle of the Bulge: Hitler's Last Hope, December 1944*. London, UK: Amber Books, 2014.

Dancocks, Daniel J. *Welcome to Flanders Fields: The First Battle of the Great War, Ypres 1915*. Toronto: McClelland & Stewart, 1988.

Dauphin, Marc. *Combat Doctor: Life and Death Stories from Kandahar's Military Hospital*. Toronto: Dundurn Press, 2013.

Desai, Ashwin and Goolam Vahed. *The South African Gandhi: Stretcher-Bearer of Empire*. Stanford, CA: Stanford University Press, 2016.

Eberhart, Carolyn J. *The Shifting Sands of Cam Ranh Bay: RVN 1965–1972: A True Story of the U.S. Air Force Combat Nurses*. Shifting Sands, 2012.

Edmonds, Sarah Emma. *Nurse and Spy in the Union Army: The Adventures and Experiences of a Woman in Hospitals, Camps, and Battle-Fields*. Hartford, CT: W.S. Williams & Co., 1865.

Egger, Bruce E., and Lee McMillan Otts. *G Company's War: Two Personal Accounts of the Campaigns in Europe, 1944–1945*. Tuscaloosa: University of Alabama Press, 1998.

Entin, Martin A. *Edward Archibald: Surgeon of the Royal Vic*. Montreal: McGill University Libraries, 2004.

Farquharson, Robert H. *For Your Tomorrow: Canadians and the Burma Campaign 1941–1945*, Victoria, BC: Trafford Publishing, 2004.

Feinstein, Anthony. *Battle Scarred: Hidden Costs of the Border War*. Cape Town, SA: Tafelberg, 2011.

Fencl, Florian. *Soumrak A Svitani Es Vodnan, 1939–1945*. Spolek Ve Vodnanech, 1948.

Fetherstonhaugh, R.C., ed. *No. 3 Canadian General Hospital (McGill) 1914–1919*. Montreal: Gazette Printing, 1928.

Foley Jr., William A. *Visions from a Foxhole: A Rifleman in Patton's Ghost Corps*. New York: Ballantine Books, 2003.

Gaudet, Mary F., ed. *From a Stretcher Handle: The World War I Journal and Poems of Pte. Frank Walker*. Charlottetown, PEI: Institute of Island Studies, 2000.

Gelbart, Larry. *Laughing Matters: On Writing M*A*S*H, Tootsie, Oh, God!, and a Few Other Funny Things*. New York: Random House, 1998.

Ginn, Richard V.N. *The History of the U.S. Army Medical Service Corps*. Washington, DC: United States Army, 2008.

Gordon, David A. *The Stretcher Bearers*. Stroud, ON: Pacesetter Press, 1995.

Graham, Ian. *The Ultimate Book of Imposters*. Naperville, IL: Source Books, 2013.

Granatstein, J.L., and Desmond Morton. *Canada and the Two World Wars*. Toronto: Key Porter, 2003.

Graves, Dianne. *A Crown of Life: The World of John McCrae*. St. Catharines, ON: Vanwell Publishing, 1997.

Grescoe, Audrey, and Paul Grescoe. *The Book of War Letters*. Toronto: McClelland & Stewart, 2003.

Gurd, Fraser N. *The Gurds, The Montreal General and McGill: A Family Saga.* Burnstown, ON: General Store Publishing House, 1996.

Gwyn, Sandra. *Tapestry of War: A Private View of Canadians in the Great War.* Toronto: HarperCollins Publishing, 1992.

Harless, Nancy Leigh, ed. *Nurses Beyond Borders: True Stories of Heroism and Healing Around the World.* New York: Kaplan, 2010.

Harris, Robert, and Jeremy Paxman. *A Higher Form of Killing*, London, UK: Chatto and Windus, 1982.

Horton, Charles H., and Dale le Vack, ed. *Stretcher Bearer! Fighting for Life in the Trenches.* Oxford, UK: Lion Hudson, 2013.

Hyatt, A.M. Jack, and Nancy Geddes Poole. *Battle for Life: The History of No. 10 Canadian Stationary Hospital and No. 10 Canadian General Hospital in Two World Wars.* Waterloo, ON: Laurier Centre for Military Strategic and Disarmament Studies, 2004.

Kessel, Lipmann. *Surgeon at Arms.* London, UK: William Heinemann, 1958.

King, Martin. *Searching for Augusta: The Forgotten Angel of Bastogne.* Guilford, CT: LP Globe Pequot, 2017.

Kingsmill, Suzanne. *Francis Scrimger: Beyond the Call of Duty.* Toronto: Dundurn Press, 1991.

Klinck, Carl F. *Robert Service: A Biography.* Toronto: McGraw-Hill Ryerson, 1976.

———, ed. *William 'Tiger' Dunlop.* Toronto: Ryerson Press, 1958.

Le Tissier, Tony. *Patton's Pawns: The 94th US Infantry Division at the Siegfried Line.* Tuscaloosa: University of Alabama Press, 2007.

Letterman, Jonathan. *Medical Recollections of the Army of the Potomac.* New York: D. Appleton and Company, 1866.

Leddy, Mary Jo. *Memories of War: Promises of Peace.* Toronto: Lester & Orpen Dennys, 1989.

Litwak, Leo. *The Medic: Life and Death in the Last Days of World War II.* Chapel Hill, NC: Algonquin Books, 2001.

MacDermot, H.E. *Sir Thomas Roddick, His Work in Medicine and Public Life.* Toronto: MacMillan Company, 1938.

MacDonnell, George S. *One Soldier's Story, 1939–1945: From the Fall of Hong Kong to the Defeat of Japan.* Nepean, ON: Baird, O'Keefe Publishing, 2000.

Macphail, Sir Andrew. *Official History of the Canadian Forces in the Great War: The Medical Services, 1914–1919.* Ottawa: F.A. Acland, 1925.

Martin Day, Frances, Phyllis Spence, and Barbara Ladouceur, eds. *Women Overseas: Memoirs of the Canadian Red Cross Corps.* Vancouver: Ronsdale Press, 1998.

Mauldin, Bill. *Back Home.* New York: William Sloane Associates, 1947.

———. *Up Front.* New York: W.W. Norton & Company, 1945.

McMullen, Michael K., and Michael J. Morris. *The Chapleau Boys Go To War*. North Charleston, SC: Createspace, 2015.

Messenger, Charles. *World War Two Chronological Atlas*. London, UK: Bloomsbury, 1989.

Meyer, Kurt. *Grenadiers*. Translated by Michael Mendé. Winnipeg: J.J. Fedorowicz Publishing, 1994.

Mitic, Jody. *Unflinching: The Making of a Canadian Sniper*. Toronto: Simon & Shuster, 2015.

Morrison, J. Clinton. *Hell Upon Earth: A Personal Account of Prince Edward Island Soldiers in the Great War, 1914–1918*. Summerside, PEI: privately printed, 1995.

Nasmith, George Gaillie. *On the Fringe of the Great Fight*. Toronto: McClelland, Goodchild and Stewart, 1917.

Nichol, John, and Tony Rennell. *Medic: Saving Lives—from Dunkirk to Afghanistan*. London, UK: Penguin, 2010.

Nicholson, Lt.-Col. G.W.L. *Official History of the Canadian Army in the Second World War, Volume II, The Canadians in Italy, 1943–1945*. Ottawa: Queen's Printer, 1957.

——. *Seventy Years of Service: History of the Royal Canadian Army Medical Corps*. Ottawa: Borealis Press, 1977.

Norris, Marjorie Barron. *Medicine and Duty: The World War I Memoir of Captain Harold W. McGill, Medical Officer, 31st Battalion C.E.F.* Calgary: University of Calgary Press, 2007.

——. *Sister Heroines: The Roseate Glow of Wartime Nursing*. Calgary: Bunker To Bunker, 2002.

O'Keefe, David. *One Day in August: The Untold Story Behind Canada's Tragedy at Dieppe*. Toronto: Alfred A. Knopf Canada, 2013.

Patton George. *War As I Knew It*. Edited by Beatrice Banning Ayer Patton. Boston: Houghton Mifflin, 1947.

Prefer, Nathan N. *Cracking the Siegfried Line: Patton's Ghost Corps*. Novato, GA: Presidio, 1998.

Primono, John W. *The Appomattox Generals: The Parallel Lives of Joshua L. Chamberlain*. Jefferson, NC: McFarland & Co., 2013.

Quinn, Shawna M. *Agnes Warner and the Nursing Sisters of the Great War*. Fredericton, NB: Goose Lane Editions, 2010.

Rasky, Frank. *Gay Canadian Rogues: Swindlers, Gold-diggers and Spies*. Toronto: Thomas Nelson and Sons, 1958.

Rawling, Bill. *Death Their Enemy: Canadian Medical Practitioners and War*. Ottawa: self-published, 2001.

Robertson, Ian Bruce. *While Bullets Fly: The Story of a Canadian Field Surgical Unit in the Second World War*. Victoria, BC: Trafford Publishing, 2007.

Robertson, Terrence. *The Shame and the Glory: Dieppe*. Toronto: McClelland & Stewart, 1962.

Rogers, Major R.L. *History of the Lincoln and Welland Regiment*. Montreal: Industrial Shops for the Deaf, 1954.

Ross, Josephine, ed. *The Vogue Bedside Book*. London, UK: Hutchinson, 1984.

Service, Robert. *Ballads of a Bohemian*. Toronto: Barse & Hopkins, 1921.

Scott, Eric, ed. *Nobody Ever Wins a War: The World War I Diaries of Ella Mae Bongard, R.N*. Ottawa: Janeric Enterprises, 1998.

Schurz, Carl. *The Reminiscences of Carl Schurz, Volume 2, 1852–1863*. New York: D. Appleton and Company, 1866.

Skaarup, Harold. *New Brunswick Hussar: Corporal Harold Jorgen Skaarup, G753, 5th Armoured Regiment–8th Princess Louise New Brunswick Hussars*. Lincoln, NE: Iuniverse, 2001.

Souhami, Diana. *Edith Cavell: Nurse, Martyr, Heroine*. London, UK: Quercus, 2010.

Stacey, Col. C.P. *Official History of the Canadian Army in the Second World War, Volume III, The Victory Campaign, The Operations in North-West Europe, 1944–1945*. Ottawa: Queen's Printer, 1960.

Stewart, Roderick, and Sharon Stewart. *Phoenix: The Life of Norman Bethune*. Montreal and Kingston: McGill-Queen's University Press, 2011.

Swettenham, John. *McNaughton, Volume 1: 1887–1939*. Toronto: Ryerson Press, 1968.

Tait, Carrie. "Dieppe Remembered, 70 Years Later through a Grandfather's Red Leather Journal." *Globe and Mail*, August 19, 2012.

Time-Life. *Time Capsule/1945*. New York: Time-Life Books, 1968.

Wafer, Francis M. *A Surgeon in the Army of the Potomac*. Edited by Cheryl A. Wells. Kingston: McGill-Queen's University Press, 2009.

Webster, David Kenyon. *Parachute Infantry: An American Paratrooper's Memoir of D-Day and the Fall of the Third Reich*. Baton Rouge: Louisiana State University Press, 1994.

Wells, Cheryl A. *Civil War Time: Temporality and Identity in America, 1861–1865*. Athens: University of Georgia Press, 2005.

Whitaker, Denis, and Shelagh Whitaker. *Dieppe: Tragedy and Triumph*. Toronto: McGraw-Hill Ryerson, 1992.

Whitman, Walt. *Memoranda During the War*. Boston: Applewood Books, 1990.

Willes, John A. *Out of the Clouds: The History of the 1st Canadian Parachute Battalion*. Port Perry, ON: Port Perry Printing, 1981.

OTHER PUBLISHED SOURCES

The Attack, newsletter of the 94th Infantry Division (later its association and historical society). Issues contained in the 94th Infantry Division Collection, Hargrett Rare Book and Manuscript Library, University of Georgia, Athens.

Canada Department of Militia and Defence. "Report Upon the Suppression of the Rebellion in the North-West Territories, and Matters in Connection Therewith in 1885." Ottawa, 1886.

———. "Report of Operations Performed on the field at Battle of Batoche, May 9th to 13th, 1885."

The Company B Bull Farm, newsletter editions 1945. Published by 319th Medical Battalion, 94th Infantry Division, U.S. Army. Courtesy of Tony Mellaci.

The McGilliken (formerly *The McGill Daily*), published by students of McGill University, 1915–16, Osler Library, McGill University Archives, Montreal.

Roddick, Thomas. "Report of Deputy Surgeon-General to D. Bergin, Surgeon-General, Militia, Montreal, May 10, 1886. Roddick, Thomas. "Report of Deputy Surgeon-General to D. Bergin, Surgeon-General, Militia, Montreal, May 10, 1886.

U.S. War Department. "Record of Proceedings (revised) of the Trial by Canadian Military Court of S.S. Brigadeführer (Major-General) Kurt Meyer."

The Weekly Dose, newsletter editions 1943–1945. Published by 319th Medical Battalion, 94th Infantry Division, U.S. Army. Courtesy of Tony Mellaci and 94th Infantry Division Collection, Hargrett Rare Book and Manuscript Library, University of Georgia, Athens.

PERIODICALS, NEWS FEATURES, BROADCASTS, JOURNALS, PAMPHLETS, VIDEOS, AND WEBLOGS

Alexander, Laurence. "Doc Alexander: The Second World War journals of Dr. L.G. Alexander." https://docalexander.wordpress.com.

Archibald, Edward. "Colonel F.A.C. Scrimger, V.C." Obituary. Osler Library, McGill University Archives, c. 1937.

Avery, Marjorie. "Bastogne Desolate After Liberation: Survivors Tell of Blood and Fire of Hospital Bombed Christmas Eve." *Detroit Free Press*, December 30, 1944.

Bell, William. "Arnold Hodgkins: The Man and His Art." n.d.

Blair, Eric Arthur (a.k.a. George Orwell). "You and the Atomic Bomb." *Tribune* (London), October 19, 1945.

Boule Margie. "One Northwest Doctor's Legacy: A Light amid the Evil at Dachau." *The Oregonian*, January 24, 2010.

Burton, Sarah. "Edith Cavell." *The Independent*, November 11, 2010.

Clare, David Wesley. "Doctor at Dieppe." *Canadian Medical Association Journal* (November 1992).

Collard, Edward Andrew. "Of Many Things . . . McCrae of 'Flanders Fields.'" *Montreal Gazette*, November 4, 1978.

———. "Of Many Things . . . A Voice for the dead." *Montreal Gazette*, November 11, 1978.

Cooke, Britton B. "McGill Hospital Is a Marvel of Efficiency." *Toronto Star*, reprinted in *McGill Daily*, November 6, 1915.

Cosgrave, Lawrence. "McCrae Wrote Classic In Twenty Minutes." *Toronto Star*, May 14, 1919.

"Eavesdrop with Eva." *Morning Albertan*, August 11, 1962.

"Edith Cavell," https://firstworldwarhiddenhistory.wordpress.com/2015/09/23/edith-cavell-1-the-constant-patriot.

Firstbrook, J.B. "Thomas Roddick: 1846–1923." *Annals of the Royal College of Physicians and Surgeons* 13, no. 3 (July 1980).

Gallagher, C.A.W. "Extraordinary Privates Extraordinarily Happy." *The McGilliken*, November 26, 1915.

Gelbart, Larry and Gene Reynolds (developed by). *M*A*S*H*, Los Angeles: 20th Century Fox Television, 1972–83.

Goellnitz, Jenny. "Civil War Medicine: An Overview of Medicine." Ohio State University. https://ehistory.osu.edu/exhibitions/cwsurgeon/cwsurgeon/cwsurgeon/introduction.

Hawkley, Maj. Gen. Paul R. "That Men Might Live: The Story of the Medical Service—ETO." Pamphlet published by the Orientation Branch, Information and Education Division, ETOUSA, 1945.

Hersey, Linda. "A Royal Filly," *Legion*, September 1, 2003.

Howell, W.B. "Letter Diary." *Canadian Medical Association Journal* (March 1938).

Jones, Donald. "In praise of Toronto's most valorous heroes." *Toronto Star*, June 4, 1994.

Keirstead, David. "Hampton History: The Royal Lady Arrived 70 Years Ago." *Hampton Herald*, March 7, 2016.

SOURCES

Kershaw, J.B. "Richard Kirkland, the Humane Hero of Fredericksburg." *Charleston News & Courier*, 1880.

Kings County Record, April 4, 1946.

McKenzie, F.A. "Nurses Disdain Death to Help Wounded Men" *Toronto Star*, May 25, 1918.

Mulligan, Robert, dir. *The Great Imposter*. Los Angeles: Universal Pictures, 1961.

Nessel, Leandra. "Behind the Front Lines: The M.H. Mitchell, Inc./94th Division Collection." *Attack*, 2009.

Padawer, Ruth. "Going Silent: Augusta Chiwy, She Saw So Much and Could Say So Little about It." *New York Times Magazine*, December 23, 2015.

Peate, Les. "The Case of the Spurious Sawbones." *Esprit de Corps Magazine*, April 1996.

Penfield, Wilder. "Edward Archibald, 1872–1945." *Canadian Journal of Surgery* 1, no. 2 (January 1958).

"Princess Louise: Canada's Equine War Hero." *Horse Canada*, December 9, 2013.

Prior, Jack. "The Night Before Christmas—Bastogne, 1944." *Bulletin of the Onondaga County Medical Society*, December 1972.

Scher, Len. "Nurse, Soldier, Spy." *National Post*, November 9, 2002.

———. "Emma's Battles: North America's First Female Soldier." Independent film documentary, 2002.

Scrimger Wootton, John C. "Francis Alexander Carron Scrimger: Surgeon, Soldier and Teacher, 1881–1937," May 30, 1978. Osler Library, McGill University Archives.

"Silver Star Citation: Captain Irving L. Naftulin." *Syracuse Post Standard*, November 25, 2007.

Swettenham, John. "The Final Drive to Victory." *Legion*, May 1970.

Swinton, W.E., "Physicians in Literature. Part I: John McCrae, Physician, Soldier, Poet." *Canadian Medical Association Journal*, November 8, 1975.

Van Nest, Paul. "The 2nd Battle of Ypres and John McCrae." Kingston Historical Society, Kingston, ON, November 2014.

War Diary of No. 1 Canadian General Hospital, May 19, 1918. https://camc.files.wordpress.com/2010/01/1cgh-may-1918.

Warshofsky, Fred. "Saga of the 94th Infantry Division." *SAGA: The Magazine for Men*, February 1961.

Wells, Leonard "Scotty." "Tales from the Sea: Memories of Adventure, Danger and Intrigue Serving Aboard the HMCS *Cayuga* during the Korean War." *Our Canada*, October/November 2014.

Wilcox, Herbert, dir. *Nurse Edith Cavell*. New York: Imperadio Pictures, 1939.

"Youthful Courage, Not Weapons, Won Epic Battle of Belgium Bulge." *Asbury Park Press*, January 14, 1945.

NOTES

CHAPTER ONE

1. Alex Barris, interview with the author, Agincourt, ON, June 1964.
2. Alex Barris, *Growing Up Greek* (unpublished manuscript, author's collection), 231.
3. Alex Barris, *Moonshine Glory* (unpublished manuscript, author's collection), 130–31.
4. John R. Koellhopper, quoted in Laurence G. Byrnes, ed., *History of the 94th Infantry Division in World War II* (Washington, DC: Infantry Journal Inc., 1948), 245.
5. 319th Medical Battalion, Regimental Aid Station Log, 0915–2136 hours, February 10, 1945, 94th Infantry Division Association, M.H. Mitchell, Inc. 94th Infantry Division Collection (Hargrett Rare Book and Manuscript Library, University of Georgia, Athens).
6. Bronze Star citation, issued by Headquarters, Co. "B" 319th Medical Battalion, APO 94, US Army, March 4, 1945 (National Personnel Records Center, St. Louis, MO).
7. Time-Life, eds., *Time Capsule/1945* (New York: Time-Life Books, 1968), 222–23.
8. John A. Willes, *Out of the Clouds: The History of the 1st Canadian Parachute Battalion* (Port Perry, ON: Port Perry Printing, 1981), 144.

CHAPTER TWO

1. National Personnel Records Center (St. Louis, MO) to author, June 30, 2015.
2. Clinical Record Brief no. 1566, Station Hospital, Camp Phillips, Kansas (National Personnel Records Center, St. Louis, MO), 1.
3. Clinical Record Brief no. 1566, 5.
4. Angelo Barris, interview with the author, New York, NY, November 27, 2014.
5. Tony Mellaci, interview with the author, Eatontown, NJ, August 19, 2015.
6. Mellaci, interview.
7. Tony Mellaci, interview with the author, Eatontown, NJ, August 18, 2015.
8. Barris, *Growing Up Greek*, 219.
9. Mellaci, interview, August 19, 2015.
10. Barris, *Moonshine Glory*, 47–50.
11. Jody Mitic, *Unflinching: The Making of a Canadian Sniper* (Toronto: Simon & Shuster, 2015), 18.

12. Jody Mitic, interview with the author, Uxbridge, ON, May 17, 2016.

13. Mitic, interview.

14. Mitic, *Unflinching*, 146.

15. Mitic, *Unflinching*, 195.

16. Mitic, interview.

17. Mitic, *Unflinching*, 197.

18. Alannah Gilmore, interview with the author, Ottawa, ON, October 13, 2017.

19. John W. Primono, *The Appomattox Generals: The Parallel Lives of Joshua L. Chamberlain* (Jefferson, NC: McFarland, 2013), 53.

20. Primono, *Appomattox Generals*, 52.

21. Walt Whitman, *Memoranda During the War* (Boston, MA: Applewood Books, 1990), 8–9.

22. Paul Van Nest, "Remembering Richard," speech, Fredericksburg Civil War Roundtable, Jepson Alumni Center, Mary Washington University, VA, May 28, 2008.

23. Quoted in J.B. Kershaw, "Richard Kirkland, the Humane Hero of Fredericksburg" (Charleston, SC: Charleston News & Courier, 1880).

24. Van Nest, "Remembering Richard."

25. Jenny Goellnitz, "Civil War Medicine: An Overview of Medicine," Ohio State University, https://ehistory.osu.edu/exhibitions/cwsurgeon/cwsurgeon/introduction.

26. Carl Shurz, *The Reminiscences of Carl Schurz, Vol. 2, 1852–1863* (New York: McClure, 1907), chapter 7.

27. Jonathan Letterman, *Medical Recollections of the Army of the Potomac* (New York: D. Appleton, 1866), 51.

28. Richard V.N. Ginn, *The History of the U.S. Army Medical Service Corps* (Washington, DC: United States Army, 2008), 14.

29. Ginn, *History of the U.S. Army Medical Service Corps*, 46.

30. Ginn, *History of the U.S. Army Medical Service Corps*, 70

31. Ginn, *History of the U.S. Army Medical Service Corps*, 73.

32. John Boyko, *Blood and Daring: How Canada Fought the American Civil War and Forged a Nation* (Toronto: Alfred A. Knopf Canada, 2013), 129.

33. Whitman, *Memoranda*, 21.

34. Bruce Catton, *The Civil War* (New York: American Heritage Press, 1960), 164.

35. Letterman, *Medical Recollections*, 154.

36. Jonathan Letterman, Gettysburg Report, Headquarters Army of the Potomac, Medical Director's Office, near Culpeper Court House, Virginia, October 3, 1863.

37. Letterman, *Medical Recollections*, 186.

38. Ginn, *History of the U.S. Army Medical Service Corps*, 73.

CHAPTER THREE

1. Harry Helms, interview with the author, West Brandywine, PA, July 12, 2015.

2. David Mitchell, interview with the author, Atlanta, GA, June 2015.

3. Quoted in Leandra Nessel, "Behind the Front Lines: The M.H. Mitchell, Inc./94th Division Collection," *Attack*, 2009.

4. Byrnes, *History of the 94th*, 23.

5. Byrnes, *History of the 94th*, 49.

6. Barris, *Growing Up Greek*, 230.

7. Byrnes, *History of the 94th*, 69.

8. Fred Warshofsky, "Saga of the 94th Infantry Division," *SAGA: True Adventures for Men* 23 (February 1962): 52.

9. Barris, *Moonshine Glory*, 129–30.

10. Byrnes, *History of the 94th*, 80.

11. Byrnes, *History of the 94th*, 84.

12. Tony Le Tissier, *Patton's Pawns* (Tuscaloosa: University of Alabama Press, 2007), 35.

13. Guy Fisher, "A Front-Line Infantryman's View (When He Dared to Look)," quoted in *94th Infantry Division Association Commemorative History*, ed. Robert Cassel (Dallas, TX: Taylor, 1989), 152.

14. Richard Bertz to Robert Cassel, February 1955, courtesy 94th Infantry Division Association.

15. Bertz to Cassel.

16. Byrnes, *History of the 94th*, 184.

17. Byrnes, *History of the 94th*, 184.

18. R.C. Fetherstonhaugh, ed., No. 3 *Canadian General Hospital (McGill), 1914–1919* (Montreal: Gazette Printing, 1928), 5.

19. Edward William Archibald Fonds, P88, Osler Library Archives Collection, McGill University.

20. Quoted in Martin A. Entin, *Edward Archibald, Surgeon of the Royal Vic* (Montreal: McGill University Libraries, 2004), 2–3.

21. Wilder Penfield, "Edward Archibald, 1872–1945," *Canadian Journal of Surgery* 1, no. 2 (January 1958): 167–74.

22. Fetherstonhaugh, No. 3 *Canadian General Hospital*, 10.

23. Quoted in Fetherstonhaugh, No. 3 *Canadian General Hospital*, 10.

24. Letter dated May 6, 1915, quoted in Martha E. McKenna, ed., *World War I Letters and Newspaper Clippings of Nursing Sister Harriet Drake* (Montreal: McGill University Libraries, 2007).

25. McKenna, *World War I Letters*.

26. Letter dated May 16, 1915, quoted in McKenna, *World War I Letters*.

27. John McCrae to Tom McCrae, March 30, 1915, Guelph Museum Papers.
28. Edgar Andrew Collard, "Of Many Things . . . McCrae of 'Flanders Fields,'" *Montreal Gazette*, November 4, 1978.
29. John McCrae to Tom McCrae, March 30, 1915.
30. Tim Cook, *At the Sharp End: Canadians Fighting in the Great War, 1914–1916*, vol. 1 (Toronto: Viking, 2007), 199.
31. Sir Andrew Macphail, *Official History of the Canadian Forces in the Great War: The Medical Services* (Ottawa: F.A. Acland, 1925), 106.
32. George Gaillie Nasmith, *On the Fringe of the Great Fight* (Toronto: McClelland, Goodchild and Stewart, 1917), 93.
33. Quoted in Daniel J. Dancocks, *Welcome to Flanders Fields: The First Battle of the Great War, Ypres, 1915* (Toronto: McClelland and Stewart, 1988), 115.
34. Tim Cook, *No Place to Hide: The Canadian Corps and Gas Warfare in the First World War* (Vancouver: UBC Press, 1999), 25.
35. Paul Van Nest, "The 2nd Battle of Ypres and John McCrae," Kingston Historical Society, Kingston, ON, November 2014.
36. Quoted in John Swettenham, *McNaughton, Vol. 1, 1887–1939* (Toronto: Ryerson Press, 1968), 44–45.
37. J. Clinton Morrison, *Hell upon Earth: A Personal Account of Prince Edward Island Soldiers in the Great War, 1914–1918* (Summerside, PEI: privately printed, 1995), 71.
38. Robert Harris and Jeremy Paxman, *A Higher Form of Killing* (London: Chatto and Windus, 1982), 3.
39. John McCrae to Janet McCrae, April 20, 1915, Guelph Museum Papers.
40. Dianne Graves, *A Crown of Life: The World of John McCrae* (St. Catharines, ON: Vanwell, 1997), 194.
41. J. George Adami, *The War Story of the C.A.M.C., 1914–1915, Vol. 1, The First Contingent* (London: Musson, 1918), 118–19.
42. Lawrence Cosgrave, "M'Crae Wrote Classic in Twenty Minutes," *Toronto Star*, May 14, 1919.
43. Graves, *Crown of Life*, 203.
44. Archibald Fonds.
45. Entin, *Edward Archibald*, 48.
46. Archibald Fonds.
47. Fetherstonhaugh, No. 3 *Canadian General Hospital*, 19.
48. Archibald Fonds.
49. Archibald Fonds.
50. Quoted in Fetherstonhaugh, No. 3 *Canadian General Hospital*, 22.
51. Britton B. Cooke, "McGill Hospital Is a Marvel of Efficiency," *Toronto Star*, reprinted in *McGill Daily*, November 6, 1915.

52. Archibald Fonds.

53. Fetherstonhaugh, No. 3 *Canadian General Hospital*, 27.

54. Archibald, letter to his mother, begun September 1, 1915, Archibald Fonds.

55. Archibald Fonds.

56. Archibald Fonds.

57. Archibald Fonds.

58. C.A.W. Gallagher, "Extraordinary Privates Extraordinarily Happy," *The McGilliken* (newspaper started by former students who worked on the *McGill Daily*), November 26, 1915.

59. Harriet Drake, "World War I Letters and Newspaper Clippings of Nursing Sister Harriet Drake," letter dated May 31, 1915.

60. Archibald Fonds.

61. Archibald Fonds.

62. Archibald Fonds.

63. Madame Manoel of the Scottish Women's Hospital, quoted in Fetherstonhaugh, *No. 3 Canadian General Hospital*, 32.

64. Elder, quoted in Fetherstonhaugh, *No. 3 Canadian General Hospital*, 32.

65. McKenna, *World War I Letters*, December 5, 1915.

66. McKenna, *World War I Letters*.

67. Archibald Fonds.

Chapter Four

1. Barris, *Moonshine Glory*, 159–61.

2. Barris, *Moonshine Glory*, 159–61.

3. Barris, *Moonshine Glory*, 159–61.

4. Le Tissier, *Patton's Pawns*, 84.

5. Nathan N. Prefer, *Patton's Ghost Corps: Cracking the Siegfried Line* (Novato, CA: Presidio Press, 1998), 81.

6. Sarah Emma E. Edmonds, *Nurse and Spy in the Union Army: The Adventures and Experiences of a Woman in Hospitals, Camps, and Battle-Fields* (Hartford, CT: W.S. Williams, 1865), 38.

7. Edmonds, Nurse and Spy, 39.

8. Edmonds, Nurse and Spy, 43.

9. Edmonds, Nurse and Spy, 47.

10. Boyko, Blood and Daring, 108.

11. Edmonds, Nurse and Spy, 371.

12. Len Scher, "Nurse, Soldier, Spy," National Post, November 9, 2002.

13. Scher, "Nurse, Soldier, Spy."

14. John C. Scrimger Wootton, "Francis Alexander Carron Scrimger: Surgeon, Soldier and Teacher, 1881–1937," May 30, 1978, Osler Library, McGill University, 14.

15. Francis Scrimger diary, April 24, 1915, McGill University Archives.

16. Edward Archibald, "Colonel F.A.C. Scrimger, V.C.," obituary, Osler Library, McGill University, c. 1937, 2.

17. Suzanne Kingsmill, *Francis Scrimger: Beyond the Call of Duty* (Toronto: Dundurn Press, 1991), 17.

18. E.F. McDonald, quoted in *Selected Articles, Canadian Journal of Medicine and Surgery*, January 1920, Osler Library, McGill University, vol. 47, 32.

19. Quoted in W.B. Howell, "Letter Diary," *Canadian Medical Association Journal* (March 1938): 280.

20. Archibald, "Colonel F.A.C. Scrimger, V.C.," 4.

21. Kingsmill, *Francis Scrimger*, 49.

22. Cluny Macpherson to Gordon-Taylor, October 6, 1958, courtesy Faculty of Medicine Founders' Archive, Health Sciences Library, Memorial University, St. John's, Newfoundland.

23. Macpherson to Taylor, October 6, 1958.

24. Cluny Macpherson, "An Episode at the War Office, 1915," *Reflections of a Newfoundlander*, Notebook #2, 128–32, courtesy Faculty of Medicine Founders' Archive, Health Sciences Library, Memorial University, St. John's, Newfoundland.

25. Macpherson to Taylor, October 6, 1958.

26. Macpherson, "An Episode at the War Office, 1915."

27. Macpherson to Taylor, October 6, 1958.

28. Macpherson to Taylor, October 6, 1958.

29. Macpherson to Taylor, October 6, 1958.

30. Macpherson, "An Episode at the War Office, 1915."

31. Macpherson, "An Episode at the War Office, 1915."

32. Macpherson, "An Episode at the War Office, 1915."

33. Cluny Macpherson to Paddy Grace, July 13, 1940, courtesy Faculty of Medicine Founders' Archive, Health Sciences Library, Memorial University, St. John's, Newfoundland.

34. Macpherson to Taylor, October 6, 1958.

35. Macpherson, "An Episode at the War Office, 1915."

36. Jim Brittain, interview with the author, Oshawa, ON, October 22, 2014.

37. Brittain, interview.

38. Maj. R.L. Rogers, *History of the Lincoln and Welland Regiment* (Montreal: Industrial Shops for the Deaf, 1954), 141.

39. Brittain, interview.

40. D. Wesley Clare, "Doctor at Dieppe," *Canadian Medical Association Journal* (November 1992): 1351.

41. Clare, "Doctor at Dieppe."

42. Clare, "Doctor at Dieppe."

43. Stan A. Kanik, quoted in Denis Whitaker and Shelagh Whitaker, *Dieppe: Tragedy and Triumph* (Toronto: McGraw-Hill Ryerson, 1992), 151.

44. Laurence Alexander, "Doc Alexander: The Second World War Journals of Dr. L.G. Alexander," courtesy of Rob Alexander, https://docalexander.wordpress.com.

45. Alexander, "Doc Alexander."

46. Alexander, "Doc Alexander."

47. Alexander, "Doc Alexander."

48. Stephen Bell, interview with the author, Uxbridge, ON, May 21, 1993.

49. Clare, "Doctor at Dieppe."

50. Alexander, "Doc Alexander."

51. Terence Robertson, *The Shame and the Glory: Dieppe* (Toronto: McClelland & Stewart, 1962), 387.

52. Quoted in Carrie Tait, "Dieppe Remembered, 70 Years Later Through a Grandfather's Red Leather Journal," *Globe and Mail*, August 19, 2012.

CHAPTER FIVE

1. Byrnes, *History of the 94th Infantry Division*, 280.

2. Jerome Fatora, interview with the author, Luxembourg City, Luxembourg, October 5, 2017.

3. Le Tissier, *Patton's Pawns*, 157.

4. Le Tissier, *Patton's Pawns*, 157.

5. Byrnes, *History of the 94th*, 289.

6. Barris, *Growing Up Greek*, 233.

7. Barris, *Growing Up Greek*, 234.

8. Mellaci, interview, August 18, 2015.

9. Mellaci, interview, August 18, 2015.

10. Dr. Darby Bergin, quoted in Canada Department of Militia and Defence, "Report Upon the Suppression of the Rebellion in the North-West Territories, and Matters in Connection Therewith in 1885" (Ottawa, 1886), 50.

11. Quoted in H.E. MacDermot, *Sir Thomas Roddick: His Work in Medicine and Public Life* (Toronto: MacMillan, 1938), 51.

12. F.J. Shepherd, quoted in J.B. Firstbrook, "Thomas Roddick: 1846–1923," *Annals of the Royal College of Physicians and Surgeons* 13, no. 3 (July 1980): 241.

13. Quoted in Firstbrook, "Thomas Roddick," 241.

14. Thomas Roddick, "Report of Deputy Surgeon-General to D. Bergin, Surgeon-General, Militia," Montreal, May 10, 1886.

15. "Report of Operations Performed on the Field at Battle of Batoche, May 9th to 13th, 1885," in Department of Militia and Defence, *Medical and Surgical History of the Canadian North-West Rebellion of 1885, as told by Members of the Hospital Staff Corps* (Montreal: John Lovell & Son, 1886), 33.

16. H.H. Chown, quoted in MacDermot, *Sir Thomas Roddick*, 83.

17. "Report of the Surgeon General to the Minister of Militia and Defence, May 13, 1886," in Department of Militia and Defence, *Medical and Surgical History of the Canadian North-West Rebellion of 1885*, 5.

18. Bill Rawling, *Death Their Enemy: Canadian Medical Practitioners and War* (Ottawa: Self-published, 2001), 76.

19. Quoted in Charles Horton and Dale le Vack, eds., *Stretcher Bearer! Fighting for Life in the Trenches* (Oxford: Lion Hudson, 2013), 56.

20. Boyde Beck, "You Have No Idea: Stretcher Bearers in the Great War," in *From a Stretcher Handle: The World War I Journal and Poems of Pte. Frank Walker*, ed. Mary F. Gaudet (Charlottetown, PEI: Institute of Island Studies, 2000), xiv.

21. Horton and le Vack, *Stretcher Bearer!*, 58.

22. Horton and le Vack, *Stretcher Bearer!*, 58.

23. Journal entry, September 30, 1916, in Gaudet, *From a Stretcher Handle*, 105.

24. Gaudet, *From a Stretcher Handle*, 105.

25. Journal entry, October 6, 1916, in Gaudet, *From a Stretcher Handle*, 107.

26. Gaudet, *From a Stretcher Handle,* 107.

27. Gaudet, *From a Stretcher Handle*, 108.

28. Beck, "You Have No Idea," xiv–xv.

29. Gaudet, *From a Stretcher Handle*, 122.

30. John "Jack" Campbell Kennedy, letter to granddaughter Lisa Boyce, Montreal, February 3, 1967, with permission.

31. Fryniwyd Tennyson Jesse, quoted in *The Vogue Bedside Book*, ed. Josephine Ross (London: Hutchinson, 1984).

32. Grace MacPherson interview, March 9, 1963, Part 1, Library and Archives Canada, RG41, vol. 22, 7.

33. Quoted in Sandra Gwyn, *Tapestry of War: A Private View of Canadians in the Great War* (Toronto: HarperCollins, 1992), 446.

34. MacPherson interview, 1.

35. Gwyn, *Tapestry of War*, 447.

36. Grace MacPherson, diary entry, August 21, 1916, courtesy Diana Filer.

37. MacPherson interview, 2.

38. MacPherson interview, 15.

39. MacPherson interview, 5.

40. Ted Barris, *Victory at Vimy: Canada Comes of Age, April 9–12, 1917* (Toronto: Thomas Allen, 2007), 180.

41. MacPherson interview, 12.

42. MacPherson interview, 5.

43. Katherine Macdonald, letter to mother, c. April 6, 1917, Canadian War Museum, accession 19950037-58A 1 114.9.

44. Macdonald, letter to mother and sister, November. 7, 1917.

45. Macdonald, letter to mother and sister, March 24, 1918.

46. Macdonald, letter to mother and sister, May 18, 1918.

47. F.A. McKenzie, "Nurses Disdain Death to Help Wounded Men," *Toronto Star*, May 25, 1918.

48. *War Diary of No. 1 Canadian General Hospital*, May 19, 1918, https://camc.files .wordpress.com/2010/01/1cgh-may-1918.

49. Maj. S.J.M. Comoton (Canadian Chaplain Service) to Capt. Ballantyne (Macdonald's fiancé), June 2, 1918, Canadian War Museum, accession 19950037-013.

50. Quoted in "Canadian Nurses Tell of Hun Attack," *Morning Albertan*, June 7, 1918.

51. "Canadian Nurses Tell of Hun Attack."

52. Capt. Donald Martyn, quoted in Gwyn, *Tapestry of War*, 457–58.

CHAPTER SIX

1. Alex Barris to Koula Kontozoglou, April 3, 1945, author's collection.

2. Barris to Kontozoglou, April 3, 1945. All quotations from Barris's letters to Kontozoglou in this section are taken from this source.

3. Harold McGill–Emma Griffis Fonds, Glenbow Alberta Institute Archives (hereafter referred to as GAI-MG), letter dated December 5, 1915.

4. GAI-MG, letter dated June 16, 1916.

5. Marjorie Barron Norris, *Sister Heroines* (Calgary: Bunker to Bunker, 2002), 99.

6. "Eavesdrop with Eva," *Morning Albertan*, August 11, 1962.

7. Marjorie Barron Norris, ed., *Medicine and Duty: The World War I Memoir of Captain Harold W. McGill, Medical Officer, 31st Battalion CEF* (Calgary: University of Calgary Press, 2007), 205.

8. Norris, *Medicine and Duty*, 205

9. Teddy Barnes, quoted in Norris, *Medicine and Duty*, 220.

10. GAI-MG, letter dated October 1, 1916.

11. GAI-MG, letter dated October 1, 1916.

12. GAI-MG, letter dated February 5, 1917.

13. Norris, *Medicine and Duty*, 109.

14. GAI-MG, letter dated July 12, 1917.

15. GAI-MG, letter dated August 2, 1917.

16. Author correspondence with Donna Henderson, granddaughter of Fred Lailey, Toronto, ON, December 8, 2018. All quotations from Fred Lailey in this section are taken from this source.

17. Bill Murphy, quoted in J.L. Granatstein and Desmond Morton, *Canada and the Two World Wars* (Toronto: Key Porter, 2003), 266.

18. Granatstein and Morton, *Canada and the Two World Wars*, 267.

19. Quoted in Linda Hersey, "A Royal Filly," *Legion*, September 1, 2003. Gerald Kelly's recollections of the event in this section are all taken from this source.

20. Quoted in David Keirstead, "Hampton History: The Royal Lady Arrived 70 Years Ago," *Hampton Herald*, March 7, 2016.

21. Quoted in Hersey, "Royal Filly."

22. *Kings County Record*, April 4, 1946.

23. Magistrate Arthur J. Kelly, quoted in "Hampton History."

24. Quoted in "Princess Louise: Canada's Equine War Hero," *Horse Canada*, December 9, 2013.

25. Jack Prior, "The Night Before Christmas—Bastogne, 1944," *Bulletin of the Onondaga County Medical Society*, December 1972.

26. Augusta Chiwy, interview with Martin King, September 28, 2009, in *Searching for Augusta* (Guilford, CT: Lyons Press, 2017), 191, with permission.

27. Prior, "Night Before Christmas."

28. Marjorie Avery, "Bastogne Desolate after Liberation: Survivors Tell of Blood and Fire of Hospital Bombed Christmas Eve," *Detroit Free Press*, December 30, 1945.

29. Avery, "Bastogne Desolate."

30. Prior, "Night Before Christmas."

31. The first meeting between Capt. Jack Prior and Registered Nurse Augusta Chiwy is recounted in King, *Searching for Augusta*, 66–67.

32. Chiwy interview with King, October 2, 2009, with permission.

33. Prior, "Night Before Christmas."

34. Jack Prior, quoted in King, *Searching for Augusta*, 71, with permission.

35. Ruth Padawer, "Going Silent: Augusta Chiwy, She Saw So Much and Could Say So Little about It," *New York Times Magazine*, December 23, 2015.

36. Prior, "Night Before Christmas."

37. "Silver Star Citation: Captain Irving L. Naftulin," *Syracuse Post Standard*, November 25, 2007.

38. King, *Searching for Augusta*, 216.

39. Prior, "Night Before Christmas."

40. Chiwy interview with King, October 8, 2009, with permission.

41. Chiwy interview with King, October 8, 2009, with permission.

42. Quoted in King, *Searching for Augusta*, 138.

43. King, *Searching for Augusta*, 150.

44. Quoted in King, *Searching for Augusta*, 195.

45. Jeffrey Prior, correspondence with Martin King, in *Searching for Augusta*, endnotes.

46. Prior, "Night Before Christmas."
47. Barris to Kontozoglou, April 3, 1945 (author's collection).
48. "Youthful Courage, Not Weapons, Won Epic Battle of Belgium Bulge," *Asbury Park Press*, January 14, 1945.
49. Winston Churchill, British House of Commons, January 18, 1945.
50. George Patton, *War As I Knew It*, ed. Beatrice Banning Ayer Patton (Boston: Houghton Mifflin, 1947), 40.

CHAPTER SEVEN

1. Mellaci, interview, August 18, 2015.
2. Barris, *Moonshine Glory*, 44.
3. William A. Foley Jr., *Visions from a Foxhole: A Rifleman in Patton's Ghost Corps* (New York: Ballantine, 2003), 43.
4. Foley, *Visions from a Foxhole*, 145–46.
5. Foley, *Visions from a Foxhole*, 145–46.
6. George P. Whitman, "Memoirs of a Rifle Company Commander in Patton's Third U.S. Army," in Le Tissier, *Patton's Pawns*, 35.
7. Byrnes, *History of the 94th Infantry Division*, 146.
8. Byrnes, *History of the 94th Infantry Division*, 224–25.
9. Raiden Dellinger, letter to parents (from New York), September 25, 1939, courtesy of David Mitchell.
10. Dellinger, letter to parents (from France), December 7, 1944, courtesy of David Mitchell.
11. Dellinger, letter to wife (from France), February 1945, courtesy of David Mitchell.
12. Byrnes, *History of the 94th*, 477.
13. Dellinger, letter to parents (from Germany), March 27, 1945, courtesy of David Mitchell.
14. Bruce E. Egger and Lee McMillan Otts, *G Company's War: Two Personal Accounts of the Campaigns in Europe, 1944–1945* (Tuscaloosa: University of Alabama Press, 1998), 110.
15. David Kenyon Webster, *Parachute Infantry: An American Paratrooper's Memoir of D-Day and the Fall of the Third Reich* (Baton Rouge: Louisiana State University Press, 1994), 41.
16. Stephen E. Ambrose, *Citizen Soldiers: The US Army from the Normandy Beaches to the Bulge to the Surrender of Germany, June 7, 1944, to May 7, 1945* (New York: Simon & Schuster, 1997), 325.
17. EBR, quoted in Canadian War Museum document, 1937 (no other identifying information available).
18. EBR.

19. EBR.

20. Albert E. Cowdrey, *Fighting for Life: American Military Medicine in World War II* (New York: Simon & Schuster, 1994), 251–52.

21. Quoted in Kenneth Cambon, *Guest of Hirohito* (Vancouver: PW Press, 1990), 180–81.

22. Cambon, *Guest of Hirohito*, 182.

23. Winston Churchill, *The Second World War: The Hinge of Fate* (Boston: Houghton Mifflin, 1950), 92.

24. Jacob Markowitz, speech delivered to Dominion Network, April 11, 1946, Markowitz Papers, University of Toronto Archives.

25. Jacob Markowitz, quoted in *Canadian Jews in World War II*, Part I, *Decorations* (Montreal: Canadian Jewish Congress, 1947), 15–16.

26. Robert H. Farquharson, *For Your Tomorrow: Canadians and the Burma Campaign, 1941–1945* (Victoria, BC: Trafford, 2004), 126.

27. John Nichol and Tony Rennell, *Medic: Saving Lives from Dunkirk to Afghanistan* (London: Penguin, 2009), 76.

28. Markowitz, speech, April 11, 1946.

29. Ellin Bessner, *Double Threat: Canadian Jews, the Military and World War II* (Toronto: New Jewish Press, 2017), 13.

30. Jacob Markowitz, curriculum vitae, University of Toronto Archives.

31. Nichol and Rennell, *Medic*, 76.

32. Markowitz, in *Canadian Jews in World War II*, 15.

33. *Order of Battle of the German Army, March 1945*, War Department, Washington, DC, 343; *Record of Proceedings (revised) of the Trial by Canadian Military Court of S.S. Brigadeführer (Major-General) Kurt Meyer*, especially 617–19 (testimony of Meyer).

34. Herbert Thistle, interview with Alex Barris, August 24, 1993, St. John's, NL.

35. Thistle, interview.

36. Ray Duffield, interview with the author, August 15, 2015, Toronto, ON.

37. Kurt Meyer, *Grenadiers: Memoir by SS Brigadeführer Kurt Meyer*, trans. Michael Mendé (Winnipeg, MB: J.J. Fedorowicz, 1994), 124.

38. Jim Duffield, interview with the author, August 15, 2015, Toronto, ON.

CHAPTER EIGHT

1. Larry Gelbart, AZ Quotes, https://www.azquotes.com/quote/957703.

2. Barris, *The Weekly Dose*, March 6, 1943, courtesy of Tony Mellaci.

3. Larry Gelbart, *Laughing Matters: On Writing M*A*S*H, Tootsie, Oh, God! and a Few Other Funny Things* (New York: Random House, 1998), 48.

4. Barris, *Growing Up Greek*, 234.
5. George S. Patton to Gen. Harry J. Malony, March 29, 1945, quoted in Brynes, *History of the 94th*, 450.
6. Mellaci, interview, August 18, 2015.
7. Bronze Star citation, issued by Headquarters, Co. "B" 319 Medical Battalion, APO 94, US Army, March 4, 1945, National Personnel Records Center, St. Louis, MO.
8. Diana Souhami, Edith Cavell: Nurse, Martyr, Heroine (London: Quercus, 2010), 351.
9. "Edith Cavell: Patriot Nurse, Underground Agent," https://firstworldwarhidden history.wordpress.com/2015/09/23/edith-cavell-1-the-constant-patriot.
10. "Edith Cavell," firstworldwarhiddenhistory.
11. Souhami, *Edith Cavell*.
12. Hugh S. Gibson, quoted in Wikipedia, https://en.wikipedia.org/wiki/Edith_Cavell.
13. Gibson, Wikipedia.
14. Quoted in Sarah Burton, "Edith Cavell," *The Independent*, November 11, 2010.
15. Shawna M. Quinn, *Agnes Warner and the Nursing Sisters of the Great War* (Fredericton, NB: Goose Lane Editions, 2010), 130.
16. Burton, "Edith Cavell."
17. *Nurse Edith Cavell*, dir. Herbert Wilcox (New York: Imperadio Pictures, 1939).
18. Bill Davis, interview with the author, Portland, ON, November 6, 1997.
19. Davis, interview.
20. Ian Graham, *The Ultimate Book of Imposters* (Naperville, IL: Source Books, 2013), 230.
21. Don Flieger, interview with the author, Kitchener, ON, April 15, 1998. All of Flieger's recollections in this section are taken from this source.

CHAPTER NINE
1. Barris, *Growing Up Greek*, 236.
2. Barris, *Growing Up Greek*, 236.
3. Barris, *Moonshine Glory*, 237.
4. Barris, *Moonshine Glory*, 237.
5. Barris, *Growing Up Greek*, 237.
6. Vladimir Krizek, interview with Marketa Schusterova, October 2016, Vodňany, Czech Republic.
7. Jaroslava Svatkova, quoted in Florian Fencl, *Soumrak a Svitani es Vodňany, 1939–1945; Twilight and Dawn: National Chronicle of Vodňany, 1939–1945* (Pamatnikovy spolek Vodňany, 1948) (published by the Remembrance Society of Vodňany, 1948).

8. Krizek, interview.

9. Byrnes, *History of the 94th*, 490.

10. Krizek, interview.

11. Angelo Barris, interview. All Angelo Barris quotations in this section are taken from this source.

12. Barris, *Growing Up Greek*, 239.

13. George Orwell [Eric Arthur Blair], "You and the Atomic Bomb," *Tribune* (London), October 19, 1945.

14. Frank Cullen, interview with the author, July 17, 1997, Toronto, ON.

15. Cullen, interview.

16. Keith Besley, interview with the author, July 17, 1997, Toronto, ON.

17. Besley, interview.

18. Norman Malayney, interview with the author, June 1, 2016, Winnipeg, MB.

19. Carolyn J. Eberhart, *The Shifting Sands of Cam Ranh Bay; RVN 1965–1972: A True Story of the U.S. Air Force Combat Nurses* (Shifting Sands, 2012), 8.

20. Malayney, interview. All of Malayney's recollections in this section are taken from this source.

21. Dane Harden, interview with the author, August 13, 2016, Windsor, ON. All of Harden's recollections in this section are taken from this interview.

22. Herb Ridyard Jr., interview with the author, October 10, 2017, Tier, Germany. All of Ridyard's recollections in this section are taken from this interview.

23. Harden, interview.

24. Ridyard Jr., interview.

CHAPTER TEN

1. Tony Mellaci, interview with the author, July 23, 2015, Eatontown, NJ.

2. Mellaci, interview, July 23, 2015.

3. Byrnes, *History of the 94th*, 477.

4. Quoted in Byrnes, *History of the 94th*, 279.

5. Cornelius Clifford, Walter Clark, William Griswold, and Al Barris, eds., *B Company Bull Farm*, August 6, 1945, 3.

6. William Griswold, "Practical Photography," *B Company Bull Farm*, 15.

7. Walter Clark, "The Readers' Corner," *B Company Bull Farm*, 16.

8. Al Barris, "A Year Ago Today," *B Company Bull Farm*, 4–5.

9. Barris, "A Year Ago Today," 6.

10. Tony Burns, correspondence with author, February 3, 2003.

11. Burns, correspondence.

12. Tony Burns, interview with the author, Halifax, NS, May 24, 2004.

13. Joe Reilly, interview with the author, Warminster, PA, August 20, 2015. All of Reilly's recollections in this section are taken from this source.

14. Headquarters 4th Armored Division, A.P.O. 254, General Orders Number 124, Section II: "To Technician Third Grade Joseph F. Reilly 33598288 MD, 1944–1945, France, Belgium, Luxembourg and Germany. Entered military service from Pennsylvania." Courtesy of Joe Reilly.

15. Reilly, interview.

16. David Wilsey to Emily Wilsey, May 25, 1945, courtesy of Clarice Wilsey.

17. WW2 U.S. Medical Research Centre, www.med-dept.com.

18. Clarice Wilsey, interview with the author, Spokane, WA, September 12, 2016.

19. Maj. Gen. Paul R. Hawkley, Chief Surgeon, Medical Service, European Theater of Operations, "That Men Might Live: The Story of the Medical Service—ETO," pamphlet published by Orientation Branch, Information and Education Division, ETOUSA, c. 1945, 20.

20. Clarice Wilsey, interview.

21. Citation for Award of Bronze Star Medal, courtesy of Clarice Wilsey.

22. David to Emily, May 1, 1945 (from Germany), courtesy of Clarice Wilsey.

23. David to Emily, May 8, 1945, courtesy of Clarice Wilsey.

24. Clarice Wilsey, quoted in Margie Boule, "One Northwest Doctor's Legacy: A Light amid the Evil at Dachau," *The Oregonian*, January 24, 2010.

25. Quoted in Boule, "One Northwest Doctor's Legacy."

26. Quoted in Boule, "One Northwest Doctor's Legacy."

27. David to Emily, May 8, 1945.

28. David to Emily, May 8, 1945.

29. David to Emily, May 22, 1945 (from Germany), courtesy of Clarice Wilsey.

30. Bob Donaldson, interview with Al Bachetta, November 14, 2011, https://furtherglory.wordpress.com/tag/116th-evacuation-hospital/.

31. Wolfgang Benz and Barbara Distel, eds., *Dachau and the Nazi Terror, Vol. II, Studies and Reports* (Brussels: Comité International de Dachau, 2002), 159.

32. David to Emily, July 1945 (from Dachau, Germany), courtesy of Clarice Wilsey.

33. Quoted in Boule, "One Northwest Doctor's Legacy."

34. Gilmore, interview. All of Gilmore's recollections in this section are taken from this source.

35. Arnold Hodgkins, War Journey Series, book 3, 1942, courtesy of Carol Hodgkins-Smith.

36. Hodgkins, War Journey Series, book 5, 1943, courtesy Carol Hodgkins-Smith.

37. William Bell, "Arnold Hodgkins: The Man and His Art," n.d., 10.

38. Hodgkins, War Journey Series, book 16, December 7, 1943, courtesy of Carol Hodgkins-Smith.

39. Hodgkins, War Journey Series, book 17, December 8, 1943, courtesy of Carol Hodgkins-Smith.

40. Hodgkins, War Journey Series, book 17, December 9, 1943.

41. Bell, "Arnold Hodgkins," 11.

42. Hodgkins, War Journey Series, book 18, May 18, 1944, courtesy of Carol Hodgkins-Smith.

43. Hodgkins, War Journey Series, book 19A, August 28, 1944, courtesy of Carol Hodgkins-Smith.

44. Bell, "Arnold Hodgkins," 12.

45. Hodgkins, War Journey Series, book 19A, August 28, 1944.

46. Author's notes, October 6, 2017.

47. In the 1960s, Alex Barris decided to capture many of his wartime recollections in a novel about a medic serving in the Battle of the Bulge. The unpublished manuscript was titled *Mooshine Glory*. As much of the novel is based on his actual experiences—including his return to Haaren High School in 1945—I have borrowed the re-creation of his encounter with the school registrar.

48. Barris, *Growing Up Greek*, 246.

49. Barris, *Growing Up Greek*, 134.

50. Barris, *Growing Up Greek*, 245.

PHOTO CREDITS

First Insert

Page 1: Winter fighting background, dragon's teeth, and Alex Barris in Red Cross helmet: author's collection; Tony Mellaci at Nantes: courtesy of Tony Mellaci.

Page 2: Jonathan Letterman at US Civil War military camp and field ambulance: Library of Congress, National Archives Still Picture Unit.

Page 3: Canadian General Hospital in tents in France: courtesy of Florence Watkinson and the Port Dover Harbour Museum; Edward Archibald, No. 3 Canadian General Hospital x-ray unit, operating theatre, and Queen Mary's visit: Osler Library of the History of Medicine, McGill University.

Page 4: First World War stretcher-bearers: courtesy of Glenn Warner and Glenn Kerr (Central Ontario Branch of the Western Front Association) and Library and Archives Canada, William Rider-Rider Collection, O-2202; Francis Scrimger: Osler Library of the History of Medicine, McGill University; April 22, 1915, German gas attack: courtesy of Glenn Warner and Glenn Kerr (Central Ontario Branch of the Western Front Association) and Canadian War Museum, George Metcalf Collection, 19700140-077; Cluny Macpherson and soldiers in gas masks: Faculty of Medicine Founders' Archive, Health Sciences Library, Memorial University.

Page 5: Wesley Clare: courtesy of Scott Clare; Laurence Alexander and Dieppe battle scene: courtesy of Rob Alexander; Members of the Regimental Aid Party of the Cameron Highlanders of Ottawa: Library and Archives Canada, MIKAN no. 3206448; Jim Brittain: courtesy of Ron Brittain.

Page 6: Thomas Roddick and Batoche medical scene: courtesy of Osler Library of the History of Medicine, McGill University; Alannah Gilmore in Bison ambulance: courtesy of Alannah Gilmore.

Page 7: John Kennedy and fellow medic of No. 9 Field Ambulance: courtesy of Lisa Boyce; Frank Walker and fellow medics of No. 1 Field Ambulance: courtesy of Mary Gaudet; Grace MacPherson and her VAD ambulance: Canadian War Museum AN-19920085-357.

Page 8: Katherine Maud Macdonald and John McCrae with Bonfire and Bonneau: Osler Library of the History of Medicine, McGill University; No. 7 Canadian General Hospital after May 19, 1918, bombing: courtesy of Florence Watkinson and the Port Dover Harbour Museum.

SECOND INSERT

Page 1: Envelope and letter background and Alex Barris photo: author's collection; Harold McGill at dressing station (NA-4938-17), Emma Griffis outside Calgary Hospital (NA-4938-10), Harold W. McGill portrait (NA4938-16): all Glenbow Alberta Institute Archives.

Page 2: Louise Ann Spry: courtesy of Donna Henderson and City of Toronto Archives, Fonds 234, Series 1200, Subseries 3, File 1; Frederick Charles Lailey: courtesy of Donna Henderson and City of Toronto Archives, Fonds 556, File 13; Princess Louise horse mascot: courtesy of Harold Skaarup, Tom McLaughlan, and Library and Archives Canada, MIKAN no. 3240626; Jack Prior and Augusta Chiwy: courtesy of Martin King.

Page 3: Raiden Dellinger and comrade in France: courtesy of David Mitchell; Bill Foley at training camp and medics sketch: courtesy of Bill Foley.

Page 4: Personnel of Royal Canadian Army Medical Corps with wounded Canadian soldier: Library and Archives Canada, MIKAN no. 3587617; Kurt Meyer: J.J. Fedorowicz Publishing; Henry Duffield: courtesy of the Duffield family; Jacob Markowitz: University of Toronto Archives, John P. Robarts Research Library.

PHOTO CREDITS

Page 5: Arnold Hodgkins portrait and painting: courtesy of Carol Hodgkins-Smith; Norm Malayney in Vietnam (four photos): courtesy of Norm Malayney.

Page 6: Dane Harden in theatre: courtesy of Dane Harden; Black Hawk helicopter landing, "mass cals" image, Herb Ridyard Jr. in theatre, and blood donation line: courtesy of Herb Ridyard Jr.

Page 7: Joe Reilly and comrades coming home, and Joe Reilly in uniform: courtesy of the Reilly family; Clarice Wilsey presenting talk, David Wilsey in uniform: courtesy of Clarice Wilsey; Dachau concentration camp: Arland B. Musser photo, no. 208705, US Seventh Army.

Page 8: Alex and Angelo Barris in Czechoslovakia, 1945, Al Theobald and Ted Barris in front of Campholz Woods, Germany, and Sgt. Alex Barris Bronze Star citation: author's collection; Krizek family portrait: courtesy of the Krizek family.

INDEX

Page numbers in italic followed by *n* refer to footnotes.

INDEX

nurse, 10, 12, 43, 64–66, 69, 70, 84, 85, 90,
92, 93, 99–103, 105, 113, 114, 146,
151, 152, 168–172, *172n*, 179–181,
184–188, 190–192, 199, 202, 206,
208–210, 212–215, 217, 222, 231,
232, 252, 256, 257, *258n*, 260–263,
292, 295, 301, 306, 307, 319, 320,
339, 344, 346
Nurse and Spy in the Union Army (book), 102
Nurse Cavell (movie), 216
Nurse Edith Cavell (movie), 262
nursing sister, 12, 84, 90, 92, 93, 170–172,
172n

"O Canada," 69
occupation, 3, 51, 54, 73, 120, 126, 181, 186,
242, 256, 257, 275, 280–285, *280n*,
314, 316, 321
O'Keefe, David, *126n*
"olive drab," 61, 137, 238
Olympic, RMS, 187
One Day in August (book), *126n*
Ontario College of Art, 345
operating room/theatre (OR), 12, 33, 34, 39,
40, 85, 191
Operation Basher, 123
Operation Jubilee, 125–133
Operation Medusa, 27, 32, 337
Operation Plunder, 253
Operation Rocket Man, 27
Operation Totalize, 122
Operation Watch on the Rhine, 55, 56, 200,
201, 203, 207, 305
orderly (medical attendant), 8, 11, 12, 18,
84, 85, 88, 89, 144, 148, 149, 152,
153, 158, 168, 178, 215, 222, 235,
237, 244, 247, 252, 292, 318, 319,
342, 343
Order of St. George, 119
Order of St. Michael, 119
Order of the British Empire (OBE), 241
Orscholz (Germany), 59–62
Orwell, George, 284, 285
Osler, Revere, 71
Osler, William, 68, 71
Oxford University (UK), 68

Packing Out (poem), 158
pacifist, 11
Pah-Ute, 41
Panjwaii (Afghanistan), 27, 28, 32, 337
parade ground, 23
Paris (France), 55, 56, 109, 116, 132, 176
Passchendaele (Belgium), 73
Pathé, 116, 117

pathology, 79, 91, *94n*, 217
Patrol Base Wilson (Afghanistan), 32
Patton, George S., 56, 57, 59, 95–98, *96n*, 141,
143n, 176, 203, 214, 215, 219, 223,
253–255, 315, 321, 335
addressing 94th, 96–98
at Bastogne, 214
burns records, 335
campaign in France, 56, 176, 321
campaign vs. Bulge, 57, 59, 141, 203, 253
crossing Rhine, 254
praise for 94th, 254
Patton's Ghost Corps (book), *143n*
Pearl Harbor (Hawaii), 20, 228, 233
pediatrician, 307
Peninsula campaign (US Civil War), 41, 101
Pennsylvania Railroad, 327
Peru (Indiana), 277
pharyngitis catarrhal acute, 16, *16n*
Philadelphia (Pennsylvania), 321, 322, 327
Philadelphia Record (newspaper), 327
photo reconnaissance, 54
Pierce, Hawkeye (Alan Alda), 267, 268
Pilckem Ridge (Belgium), 77
pillbox, 7, 54, 59, 61, 62, 126
Pilsen (Czechoslovakia), 277, 282
plasma, 21, 145, 205, 308
Plomer, James, 264
pneumonia, 16, *16n*, 44, 70, 98, 104, 149, 251
poison gas, 74–79, 104, 111
effect on troops, 76–79
German gas attacks, 74–79, 111, 112, 118,
127
Porter, Cole, 278
Port Perry (Ontario), 340, 346
positive end-expiratory pressures (PEEPs), 303
Post Mason, Charles, 262
post-mortem, 78, 86, 88
Potter, Sherman T. (Harry Morgan), 267, 268
Potts, Louis, 230
Pozières Wood (France), 153, 155, 181
Prague (Czechoslovakia), 3
Prefer, Nathan N., *143n*
Pridham, Dave, 32
Prince (horse), 198
Prince Albert (Saskatchewan), 244
Princess Louise (horse), 196–198
Princess Louise II (horse), 198
Prior, Jack, 200, 203–206, 208–218
air raid, 210, 211
at Noville, 203–205
makeshift hospital, 205–209
praises nurses, 212, 213
response to racism, 213, 214
reunion with Chiwy, 217, 218